Singing in the Rain

Weathering the Storm of Dementia with Humor, Love, & Patience

by Vicky Ruppert
and Ann Henderberg

Singing in the Rain:
Weathering the Storm of Dementia with Humor, Love, & Patience
by Vicky Ruppert & Ann Henderberg
Copyright © 2013

This book contains anecdotes, opinions, and suggestions pertaining to the authors' personal experiences with dementia caregiving. The information herein is not a substitute for the reader's own medical, financial, or other professional advice.

Some names have been changed to protect the privacy of the individual/or family.

Permission to use "There is always tomorrow to do it better" was given by Angela Dentz.

Permission to use "Courage doesn't always roar. Sometimes courage is the quiet voice at the end of the day, saying, 'I will try again tomorrow'" was given by Mary Anne Radmacher.

Cover design by Barb Anderson
Photos of authors by Kelly Elizabeth Portrait Studio

The Rain Group Press
PO Box 1152
Pittsford, NY 14534-9152
www.survivingdementiacaregiving.com
theraingrouppress@gmail.com

ISBN: 978-1489598592

Foreword

In 2006, I met Vicky and Jim Ruppert. They had generously agreed to participate in a report on Alzheimer's disease for the NBC Nightly News. In a long career, I have met many families where one is afflicted with a terrible disorder. I quickly realized that Vicky and Jim were among the warmest, kindest, and most intelligent. I was especially struck by their obvious affection for one another despite circumstances that would try the most compassionate.

By then Jim, age 58, was four years past his Alzheimer's diagnosis and many years beyond when he first noticed memory problems. Jim, whose family carried a strong history of late onset Alzheimer's, was aware of his condition and quite articulate even though the problems were obvious.

At one point I asked if he was glad to know his diagnosis. He responded, "You really have no choice with this disease, you know. It's there every second of the day. Forgetting 50 times a day what you're doing sometimes gets really frustrating, and I forgot your question. I didn't get around to answering it."

This book begins three years after my first meeting with the Rupperts when Jim's disease had progressed significantly. It is the story of the friendship, affection, and support of Vicky Ruppert and the co-author Ann Henderberg. Ann's husband, Ralph, suffered a different form of progressive dementia, but ultimately diagnosis matters far less than the enormous burden on those who care for loved ones with damaged brains.

Vicky and Ann met in a support group arranged by the Alzheimer's Association, a terrific organization that is allowing millions to know they are not alone as caregivers for someone with dementia. The two women kept their frequent correspondence and their own diaries. Through their experiences Vicky and Ann illustrate some key points. No one person with dementia is the same as another. A person with dementia can change day to day, even from minute to minute. And most importantly, nothing is more valuable than the support by someone else who is experiencing the same ongoing 24 hour a day tragedy.

Their experiences and insights in dealing with their husbands at home, with their families, in the community, and with their health care system can be heartbreaking. But they are also enormously compelling and instructional for all the others who are or will be taking the same terrible journey.

The book ends with a long list of specific, practical advice on caring for a loved one with dementia and on coping with matters including legal papers, dealing with the health care system, and arranging for nursing home care.

I always hoped I would have the opportunity to report on a cure for Alzheimer's. It does not appear that will happen anytime soon. This book is a compelling portrait of and a guidebook for caregivers, those who bear the burden until there is a cure.

Robert Bazell, Yale University
Formerly Chief Science & Health
Correspondent, NBC News

Acknowledgements

The idea of writing a book would not have been possible were it not for our families who encouraged us to begin, and gave their blessings having no idea what we would write or how specific we would be. ~I thank the memory of James Sr. & Marion Ruppert for showing us how to live with this disease, and to Nancy (Ruppert) & Marty Salzbach for enduring the disease twice, caring for both parents, one after the other. Thank you to my sister Carol Crompton for her continuing loving support........Vicky. ~My grateful thanks for the love and support of my family. I couldn't have done it all without you: daughter Nancy and Lou Bellina, son Brian and Shino Henderberg, grandson Alan and Christine Henderberg, grandkids Amanda and Robert Schank, Hassan and Aisha Henderberg, and great granddaughters Brittany VandeMar and Marissa Henderberg, my sister Norma Ogley........Ann.

Heartfelt thanks to my coworkers who endured my tales of woe, cheered me up, and laughed with me at the comical descriptions that this disease sometimes presents. "It's going in the book" became a reality! (Karen Salmon, Sheila Noble, Debra Jesien, David Kelsey, Maria Humphrey, Gail Sheridan, Lori Lincourt, Pat Carson, & Jean Foley. I would also like to express my gratitude to my bosses for allowing me time off for doctor appointments and emergencies that cropped up when I least expected them: Debra Jesien, Susan Raub, Sharon Petry, Dr. Dwight Hardy) A very special 'Thank You' goes to Jim's boss and coworkers for helping him make retirement with special accommodations for his handicaps. This allowed him to retire with his self-worth and to see that he left as a skilled family therapist: John Campolieto, Marty Mowers, Patricia Denhoff, Becka Heurtley, Joan Riesenberger, and Ellen Rusling. You were doing what is right for your staff way before anyone else ....Vicky.

Although many who are diagnosed with dementia find that their circle of friends becomes very small, ours did not change. ~Kudos to you all, with special thanks to Jim & Judy Shafer, Barry Fry, Bonnie Seitz, Ken Harris, Howard & Carole Camp, Geri Meloni, Karen Duffy, and Laurene & Manville Jennings as well as our Scuba friends. Thanks to Brian McCarty who began as a companion for Jim, and turned into a very special friend to Ann and me........Vicky ~Thanks also for the help and understanding of special friends: Will and Launa Bellucci, Bob and Rose Reid, Dorothy Young, Anne Gunn, Anne Chapman, Betty Worden, Wayne Lee, Dave Griffin, Laurene and Manville Jennings, Lou and Marilyn Baskin, and my Oasis Tappers dance troupe........Ann.

Cheers to our neighbors who always kept their eyes out for our men, and were very instrumental in helping them find their way home when they needed it.

We would also like to thank the staff of the Alzheimer's Association for all their programs and assistance through our journey. ~Jim and I became active members in the Alzheimer's Association years ago. Thanks to Teresa Galbier, Sharon Boyd, Debbie Houck, and Paula Casselman for giving Jim a second career as a facilitator, speaker, and advocate.......Vicky. ~We are both so grateful to Fern Speer

Acknowledgements (cont.)

and Cindy Krutell for the years of support and friendship as our support group facilitators...we couldn't have done it without you, nor could we have done it without our support group friends who shared their lives to help make ours better.

To Mary K. Dougherty of Bootstrap Publishing and Barb Anderson of DM BookPro for showing us how to get our book from mere paper to printed book form.

Our appreciation to Dr. Robert Bazell of Yale University, formerly Chief Science and Health Correspondent, NBC Universal for writing our foreword.

Thanks to Dr. Christine Borghi-Cavallaro and Dr. Louis J. Papa for your continuing support and special thanks to our neurologists: Dr. Pierre Tariot, Dr. Anton Porsteinsson, Dr. Charles J. Duffy, and his social worker Susan Ruhlin.

Our gratitude to St. John's Meadows and St. John's Home for all their help.

To Kip Ruppert who inherited the people skills of his dad, and lived with his dad's Alzheimer's for half his life, "Thank You" for being here every time I needed you, for being my sounding board at all hours, giving me reassurance, and for being my unwavering friend through the rest of my life........Vicky.

To Ann ~ Thank you for your broad shoulders, your wit and skill in knowing how to break my mood and make me laugh. You made it bearable........your forever friend, Vicky.

To Vicky ~ My soul sister, I'm forever grateful to you for being my rock and companion on this sad journey.

To Jim and Ralph most of all, no greater courage have we seen than in these two gentle souls.

~Jim ~ I'd marry you again in a minute if I had a 'Do Over.'........ Vicky

~My sweet husband, Ralph~ The night before you entered St. John's Home, you told me you felt you had more to accomplish. You were remarkably clear and fluent when you said you wished you could do something to help folks with problems like yours. Well, honey, as this book goes into print, it seems you got your wish.........Ann

To Ralph, To Jim...

My weary travelers, lay down your heads, it is time to sleep.

You have made your long journey uphill and down,

You have offered your thoughts to those who would listen,

You have fought your way through the fog and the storms.

You have wrestled this disease every step of the way,

Now your mind and body are spent, you are tired.

You must go and feel your peace at last . . .

You lived the best of lives because you dared.

Forever Yours,

Ann and Vicky

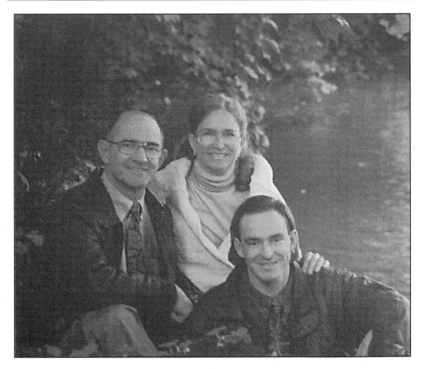

Jim, Vicky, & Kip Ruppert about 1994

Jim High School Grad '66

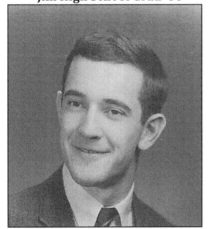

Vicky & Jim 2002, Alberta CA

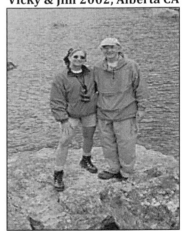

Ann & Ralph at the wedding of their daughter, 2005.

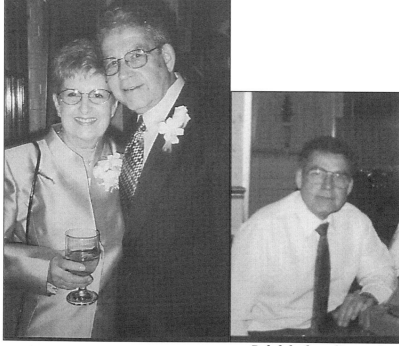

Ralph before diagnosis

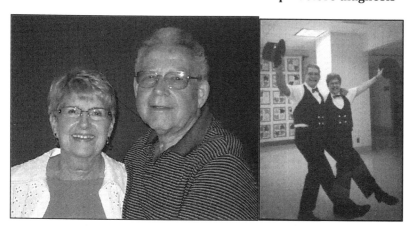

Ann's 75th birthday, 2009   Ann & Ralph - Oasis Tappers

Table of Contents

Table of Contents cont.

~Introducing Ann ~

By today's standards I was a child bride. However in 1953, while not the norm, marriage at 18 (me) and 22 (Ralph) was hardly unusual. Ralph was a friend of my brother, and having an older brother was a great source of potential boyfriends. We dated for 2½ years and then began the typical 50's lifestyle: Dad being the breadwinner and Mom fulfilling the role of homemaker. This was before the 'liberation' movement so we were content in our assigned roles.

We raised four children; three born two years apart and the fourth coming along eight years later. At one time we had a kindergartner and a senior in high school. In time we became grandparents and great-grandparents. We were busy and happy, and the years flew by.

Ralph was a model maker at Eastman Kodak Company, making authentic prototypes of cameras, projectors, etc. from designers' drawings. His inner creative urge kept nudging him, though, and in the late sixties, he enrolled in and graduated from the School for American Craftsmen at RIT.

After retiring in '89, Ralph was able to follow his passion and joined a number of art groups. He created beautiful sculptures, jewelry, and furniture from both common and exotic woods. He branched out into photography and was in a number of 'photography as art' gallery shows.

The first signs of dementia appeared in mid-2004 after shoulder surgery. The jury is still out as to whether anesthesia contributes to or exacerbates dementia, especially in older folks. Ralph was 74 at the time. He was tested and diagnosed with dementia at the Memory Disorders Clinic in the summer of 2005. The most common cause of dementia is Alzheimer's disease (AD). It is clear, however, that there are many other causes of dementia.

Ralph remained a puzzle throughout the course of his disease. At various times, he was diagnosed with progressive aphasia, fronto-temporal dementia, Lewy body disease, and MSA (multiple system atrophy). At this point in time a definitive diagnosis can only be made post-mortem. His neurologist said from the beginning that it was not AD, but most probably one of the other above dementias.

I can't say enough good things about both Ralph's neurologist and the Alzheimer's Assoc. here in Rochester. The Assoc. provides help and support for all the dementias and it was here, at the monthly support group, that we met Vicky and Jim Ruppert. Our particular group catered to both the caregiver and patient, patients in one room and caregivers in another, each with their own facilitator. While Vicky and I were bonding and becoming friends, Jim and Ralph were fast becoming good friends in their own group. The four of us began meeting for lunch every month and began melding our families and social events. I think dementia-grounded friendships are especially sweet because no matter how much love and support one receives from family and friends, it takes another caregiver to relate in a deeper, mutual understanding. Vicky and I began e-mailing as a way of pouring out our frustrations, woes, and general day to day anecdotes about life and marriage in this tango of constant challenge. We don't know exactly when, but at some point one of us suggested turning these e-mails into a book for fellow caregivers. The following is the result.

~ Introducing Vicky~

I have known my husband for most of my life. We lived in the same town, and although my family moved around the country, we always came home to Whippany, New Jersey where it began. We dated seriously our senior year in high school after meeting again in Advanced Biology class, and have been together ever since. The draw to Jim was his sweet and gentle nature and his shoulders...he was a gymnast, wrestler, and pole vaulter. He had beautiful muscles! We married the summer of our junior year in college, finished our studies at separate schools, and then began our life together.

Jim was first a school psychologist. After further training in social work, he became a family therapist for B.O.C.E.S 1 in Rochester, New York. I became a clinical microbiologist for the University of Rochester Medical Center. We settled down in the outskirts of Rochester, and began ticking away the years while raising our son, Kip. About the time that Kip was in high school and college, both of us began shouldering increased amounts of stress. My father died in 1989 of post-polio syndrome and heart disease. One month after the funeral my mom called from Florida to divulge that she had an abnormal contour of her left breast, something she had noticed months before, but had ignored. She just couldn't deal with it while taking care of Dad, too. So we moved her up to Rochester where the cancer care was top notch, and she moved in with us for the operation and initial recovery. She then moved to a place of her own nearby. She eventually died from the metastases of the cancer in 1995.

In the early 90's Jim began having chest pains due to stress. I remember that the first one was the day we were in the Cancer Care Center with my mother, discussing her chemo and radiation. He began seeing a therapist and taking depression meds then, but I began noticing glitches in his memory that seemed abnormal. I began journaling them in 1992-3. Could he have the beginnings of Alzheimer's disease (AD)? At first I didn't disclose my fears to Jim. Unknown to me, Jim also had the same fears but didn't want to frighten me, so we kept quiet for about 2 years! I didn't feel that we would gain anything anyway, because there was no cure. One night, sometime in 1994, while in the hot tub, where we had many of our heart to heart talks, Jim confessed his fears and I confessed mine. We both cried, but decided we would work together to find out what was wrong. Jim was in his mid-40's and it was very uncommon to see someone at that age being diagnosed with Alzheimer's in the mid 1990's! Jim's paternal grandmother spent her last days in a nursing home with hallucinations and senility, and his dad was presently in a nursing home in Florida with AD which began in his early 60's. What made it even more confusing was that Jim also had Attention Deficit Disorder (ADD), diagnosed in 1993 after Kip was diagnosed as having ADD. Jim suspected he was ADD all along because he had problems in grade school similar to Kip's, and he saw kids every day with that 'learning difference.' Were Jim's problems with his memory typical of an ADD adult? At the time he was tested for ADD, they had run a full gamut of tests and knew his IQ was very high (133). Was Jim able to compensate for some of his problems because of his high IQ? Was it just from anxiety and depression over managing his ADD? Which came first, the chicken or the egg?

During this early period, we obviously saw his regular physician and she checked Jim's level of Vitamin B12 to make sure it was O.K. It was a bit low, so he was prescribed nasal B12 until his level became more normal. Low B12 can cause memory problems if not rectified, but the B12 had no effect on his memory. The male physician's assistant in the office thought all my journal symptoms were 'typical male behavior' of tuning out the wife.

Because of Jim's family history, we asked for a consultation with a genetic counselor (1997). At that meeting we pleaded for genetic testing, mainly the APOE4 marker (a late onset gene which might explain his history.) They don't usually concede to testing because there is no cure, having the gene doesn't guarantee that you'll get the disease, and some people find life not worth living if they know they have the gene. Even two genes don't guarantee expression of the disease. We assured the geneticist that we would be more at peace knowing the genetic results. If Jim had the gene(s) we could begin to live our lives differently (taking our vacations now that we would have put off until retirement.) The doctor acquiesced. We were referred to the University of Rochester Geriatric Neurology Clinic where they met with us, looked at Jim's prior psychological testing, and eventually drew blood for the testing of the APOE4 gene. They also drew CSF for Tau protein, an experimental test to detect the increased levels of a protein derivative that is responsible for the tangles formed in the brain that prevent the neuron's normal function and transport of messages. We liked the doctor and he seemed to take our concerns seriously. We felt as if we were making headway. We were told in the interim (these tests were sent away to other laboratories and would not be back for weeks) to get life insurance, long term care insurance, etc. now, because if these results came back positive, there were no laws in effect to prevent these tests from disqualifying eligibility for such policies. Even though there was no sure test to identify AD, these tests would be used prejudicially for the denial of those policies. Just Jim's concerns and my journal notes on Jim's behavior were in his medical charts, but that was enough. Jim could get a long term care insurance policy, but his lungs (he had asthma), brain (the memory problem notes), kidney (benign enlarged prostate), and skin (squamous cell carcinoma) were restricted from coverage. Why pay for long term care insurance when most of your body is not covered, the most important being brain, heart, and lungs! It was too expensive a policy for too little coverage so we didn't get it.

Two months later we made an appointment to hear the news. Unfortunately, the doctor we were seeing had moved on to greener pastures, and we were assigned to another doctor. He told us that Jim had two APOE4 genes (we had no idea that Alzheimer's might be lurking on his mother's side,) so that was an unbelievable bit of news. Jim's Tau protein in CSF was elevated too [>400 was elevated and Jim's was in the 600's.] This doctor with the test results, his history, and his psychological testing looked at us and said, "You are too young to have AD. Go home and live a good life." We were fuming! All we wanted was someone to say, "Well, it's not very common, but let's treat you as if you will develop the disease. We will follow you every year, and see what happens." We needed someone to take us seriously.

We went home and convinced Jim's psychiatrist (seen for depression and anxiety) to prescribe Aricept. Aricept has a very low incidence of side effects and was worth taking in case Jim had AD. We waited a little over a year, had another psychological evaluation, and then went to see the head of the Neurology Clinic. This was now the year 2000. We told him our dissatisfaction with the previous doctor. Now Jim's testing revealed a drop compared to the old tests showing he had some Minimal Cognitive Impairment (MCI). The doctor was warm and personable, and said that with Jim's MCI he would follow him every 6 months. It doesn't prove that it is AD, not all MCI patients progress to AD. Some stay at the same level, called benign MCI. He would treat Jim as if Jim were going to develop AD, and recommended that Jim up his dose of Aricept, and take other vitamins such as vitamin E and a few others, get plenty of exercise, and have plenty of sex! Close personal contact is important. The doctor had a big smile on his face, and that made Jim and I laugh. Jim pulled out a ten dollar bill from his wallet and offered it to the doctor as a joke. We could not have been happier. We weren't crazy after all! Jim would be studied by the head of the department, and eventually they would find the answer. We could now plan our lives a bit differently and make more of today in case our 'Golden Years' ended up being 'Fools Gold'. We were ecstatic!

APOE4 is a late onset gene, usually expressed after age 65. However, if a person has two APOE4 genes, it can be expressed much earlier, hence Jim's symptoms at age 45. Although research has made leaps and bounds since this time, and other genes are being discovered that play a role in the development of disease in general, no one knows what other genes Jim carried that helped to exacerbate the early expression.

A year or so after the meeting with the head of the department, Jim's diagnosis progressed to probable Alzheimer's. Jim let his close peers and his supervisor know of his diagnosis. They made some concessions for him that helped Jim to better handle his job: they decreased his work load of clients, purchased a recording system so he could tape his sessions for further study, gave him a speak/type program on his computer for reports (unfortunately he couldn't learn it,) and allowed Jim to go home for lunch and take a short nap to recharge his batteries. They were wonderful. Jim crawled to the finish line, June 26, 2002, when he qualified at 55 for his pension, and he retired.

During the next seven years we made the most of our time together while Jim was still functioning well. We began working out and walking at our local recreation center. This was especially helpful for Jim because working out would help to alleviate Jim's feeling of a 'sunburned brain' and 'brain fog' for a short time. I joined an Alzheimer's support group, and after retiring, Jim began facilitating the Alzheimer's Association's support group for care-partners with memory loss. He continued in that position for many years. He also accompanied staff from the association on many trips to lobby representatives for more funding. We were participants on numerous panels for public awareness of AD, and were interviewed on film for both local and national network television. Jim also was part of the first Public Television series called *Second Opinion*, addressing Alzheimer's disease. The Alzheimer's Association gave Jim a second career of sorts, getting word out that people are living with the disease, not just dying of it! He was so lucky to have those opportunities. Lastly, we knew we would not be able to travel later on, so we went to those places we most wanted to visit. Although I worked part-time after 2004, I retired from work as a Microbiologist in the fall of 2009. Jim needed me at home because he was getting lost more and more.

The most important thing that I have done for myself was to join the support group. It was in this group that we met Ann and Ralph Henderberg, and became devoted friends. We started meeting once a month for lunch besides attending support group. Then our lives required more frequent feedback, and we began e-mailing each other. When Ann was 'up' I was 'down', vice versa, or we would commiserate together. No explanation needed. E-mailing was the communication of choice because we were caregiving 24/7. That way we weren't talking to each other about things our spouses might overhear. This book chronicles the final three years of our husbands' journeys. Most pages are the e-mails we sent to each other, some are from journals, and some meetings/phone calls from doctors, etc. were written in the e-mail format to preserve the style of the book. The final section of the book is a collection of things we have learned along the way that would be helpful to other caregivers traveling this same journey.

Living with something so undefined and uncertain is definitely an unsettling feeling. What happened when Jim didn't show up on time to pick me up from work? Is he just a few minutes late, did he forget, did he have an accident, has he gotten lost and doesn't remember where he is? My emotions played with me...it was absolute panic and fear mixed with anger and worry. My adrenalin kicked in and each minute seemed like an hour. We didn't have cell phones then, so there was no way for immediate contact. I waited where Jim always picked me up, but periodically walked back to my lab to see if there were messages from him.

That first instance Jim had gone to our local supermarket, and when he came out he couldn't remember where our car was, nor the color, or make, or model. Somehow he managed to call our next door neighbor. Our neighbor picked Jim up, then called me through my work number, and I described the car so my neighbor could find it. Once found, Jim was O.K. to come pick me up.

In a narrow perspective, I was angry because of the extra hours I spent at the hospital when I could have been home, but in the broader view this was the beginning of a life where nothing could be counted on. Everything was uncertain. Some days were uneventful, and then just as you began to trust again, Whammo! An event would shatter that comfortable feeling, and life would be turned upside down.

Chapter One

2009

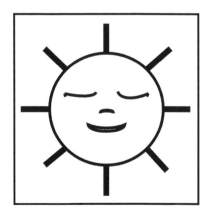

A Bit of Denial:

I think it's natural, even though the diagnosis is basically a sure bet, that we go along in our lives, taking one day at a time, and slowly getting used to thinking a little bit about the future and acting like we used to do before the diagnosis...we pretend the disease isn't there even though it shows us every day that it is! That's what helps us to get through every day and every week; a healthy bit of denial!!!

03/15/2009
Vicky to Ann
Scary Moment

Today, we went to a neurologist to inquire about an ongoing neuropathy problem with Jim's foot. As part of the exam, the doctor administered a MMSE (Mini Mental Status Exam.) Jim's score hit me like a blow to the stomach. It was 15 out of 30!!! Mind you, I did not know his most recent scores because he has been participating in clinical drug trials, and they test him behind closed doors. Ages ago, Jim scored almost too high to be in some of the Alzheimer's studies, and now a 15. That really woke me up.

04/06/2009
Vicky to Ann
My Birthday

Jim was never repetitive until now. About a month ago Jim started asking me the date of my birthday. I knew he didn't know, and that didn't bother me. It did become annoying, however, when he started asking me multiple times a day, every day. He didn't want to miss it because this may be the last birthday he will share with me, and he wanted to give me a BIG present for that reason. He was surprised that I didn't want a fuss or a party. I didn't want anything, not even a dinner party. All I wanted was a trip to the Canadian Butterfly Conservatory so that I could take some good photographs. Jim wanted my friend to be there when I opened his gift, and then we'd all go out to dinner, which we did. It turned out to be a good but quiet birthday. I really didn't want to celebrate. I, too, felt that it might be my last birthday with Jim, and that made me sad.

So it's now over, and I can relax and just look forward to each new day. Oh, by the way, we never got to the conservatory because that morning, Jim took sleeping pills that were meant for the nighttime and he had to go to bed 'til noon to sleep them off. By then, there wasn't enough time to go. Hopefully, we'll go tomorrow.

04/24/2009
Vicky to Ann
Working Dilemma

Today, I went to work as usual. Lately, Jim and I have been quietly vying over my wish to hire a companion to fix him lunch, take him places, etc. He adamantly said, "No."

I left a printed note for Jim, asking him to wash and dry the screens. I brought them up from the basement and put them in the garage with a bucket, a brush, and two towels. I also verbally told him the screens were in the garage (stupid me, why would I think that he would remember any of it?) Towards the end of the day I got a call from Jim saying he's not sure what to use to wash the screens. I told him the dish soap under the sink in the kitchen. He said "OK." When I got home, the screens weren't in the garage. Some were out on the deck, but the way they were positioned, I don't think he washed any of them. Then I found the rest of the screens in the basement, unwashed. Jim couldn't figure out how to wash them. He must have forgotten that we have a hose outside, and that we have always washed them outside in the past. While he got ready to go out to dinner, I washed all the screens. When we came back from dinner, I realized Jim must have tried to cook something on the stove, because two burners were lit and had been burning for at least 6-7 hours! The house could have burned down. Because I can't be with him at home, I made him promise ages ago that he would not try to cook anything on the burners. So much for promises. No more knobs on the stove. That was really serious.

We are truly at the cusp of decision making. I hate to insist that he go to senior care, but I'm getting awfully close!

06/30/2009
Ann to Vicky
Get-together

I've been thinking of our next lunch and had an idea. I know how much Jim loves kids, and wondered how you felt about each of us packing a picnic lunch. Ralph and I will pick up Brian's two children (Hassan and Aisha, our youngest grandkids) and meet in Mendon Ponds Park or someplace like that? Ralph and Jim could play with the kids, and you and I could have some talk time. Anyway, the kids are really well-behaved (even if they're mine,) and I think Jim would get a kick out of them. What do you think?

Not much new. Just slow, steady decline. Little things, but sometimes bizarre. What's more bizarre is that it's beginning to feel normal to me when he asks if someone is sitting next to me, or he'll ask where so-and-so went, because they were there a minute ago. I know I should enjoy each day because today is as good as it's going to get, but it's getting a little harder. I'm sure you know what I mean.

We went to a Just Friends (support group spin-off) picnic yesterday and while they're a great bunch of folks, I get the feeling we're all whistling in the dark. Strange mood I know, but I'll feel better tomorrow.

Vicky to Ann

That sounds great to me! And you are right; Jim does love to watch children play, and he likes to interact with them. As long as we aren't sitting under the shelter watching it rain! In a way I'm glad that the bizarre things are feeling somewhat normal. That means that your stress level is a bit lower. But that doesn't mean that you are necessarily 'at peace and happy.' Sometimes I feel more like Jim's mother or caretaker than his wife. I definitely don't feel we are equal anymore. I can share things with Jim, but he usually can't take in the whole picture of what I am trying to explain, and he remembers none of it. It's almost like I'm talking to myself! Even the sex is on its way out the door.

We can be comfortable with how things are if the declines are slight, but that doesn't mean we don't grieve for what was and is no more. The sharing is gone really, and each time something major strikes us as a big change, it sends us spinning again, and we get depressed. At least I do! And nobody understands like you, someone else dealing with it. We can't tell people who ask how bad it is sometimes or we'd really turn them off!

I made Jim promise that he will go to senior care in September. I haven't looked at any places yet, but I'll probably send him where he knows some of the folks from support group.

Anytime you need to talk (or type) just call or e-mail me. Jim usually goes to bed at 8:30 or 9.

07/04/2009
Ann's Journal
Holiday

Ralph and I, Brian, and the kids drove to the lake for a day with Nancy and Lou (daughter and husband) at his sister's cottage. The cottage is on a hill on the opposite side of the road from the lake. There are many, many steps down to the dock. Ralph was only able to make the trip once. It's almost harder to watch the physical changes than the mental because it's all so unexpected. It was difficult maneuvering the steps and once it was dark, he seemed afraid to walk down. It was still a great day though, the kids were so excited, and we had much food and many laughs. I got off the beaten track on the way down and Brian got way off the track coming home. We didn't get home until 12:30 AM.

07/06/2009
Ann's Journal
Alzheimer Association Event

We went to the first Social Club meeting of this 3 month session. Some staff from a local bakery did a cake decoration demo and we all decorated cupcakes. Not terribly exciting and Ralph was lukewarm about attending, but we met some new folks. It turns out we had met one of the couples at a party many years ago. He and Ralph hit it off, and I think the next meeting will be a little easier. Brian and the kids came over later and we made 'Grandma Friendly's Sundaes.' A pretty good day all around.

07/15/2009
Ann's Notes
Side Effects

Ralph didn't fit the normal symptoms of Alzheimer's, so Lewy body disease was considered early on in his journey. In addition to increasing hallucinations throughout the course of his disease, there were other physical problems as well. Constipation was a side effect of the drugs used to alleviate his symptoms. This sounds quite benign but it can lead to the more severe problem of bowel impaction, in which the bowel becomes partially or completely blocked. In addition to the pain, it can result in urinary blockage also. Ralph suffered with this problem many times during his illness. Usually, I could treat it at home, but once I had to take him to the Emergency Room. These sessions often led to more confusion and exhaustion because of the trauma involved.

LEWY BODY DISEASE

While many people are unfamiliar with Lewy body disease, it is a common cause of dementia in the elderly. Lewy body disease happens when abnormal structures, called Lewy bodies, build up in areas of the brain. The disease may cause a wide range of symptoms including:

Constipation

Changes in alertness and attention

Hallucinations

Problems with movement and posture

Muscle stiffness

Confusion

Loss of memory

Lewy body can be hard to diagnose, because Parkinson's disease and Alzheimer's disease cause similar symptoms. Scientists think that Lewy body disease might be related to these diseases, or that they sometimes happen together.

Lewy body disease usually begins between the ages of 50 and 85. The disease gets worse over time. The lifespan from diagnosis to death averages 7 years. There is no cure. Treatment focuses on drugs to help symptoms.

07/15/2009
Ann's Journal
Unwelcome Side Effects

The day started out well. We ran some errands and went out for lunch. The weather was great. Ralph was feeling and doing well until evening, when he had another impaction. We tried everything but nothing worked. We were both up most of the night. I finally gave him an entire bottle of Citrate. He finally had relief after 24 hours of much pain and bleeding. Bad, bad two days. Dr. H. (his GI Dr.) will see him Monday. We can't go through another one of these episodes. His dementia increased greatly as did the hallucinations. Friday, he felt somewhat better but slept most of the day. The hallucinations have stopped for the time being. I may cancel the picnic we had planned with Vicky and Jim. We'll try for next week. Vicky tells me Jim is also going downhill more rapidly. He was doing so well. I don't share much of what she tells me with Ralph as it bothers him too much. He thinks a great deal of Jim. We'll see them at support group on Tuesday.

07/17/2009
Ann to Vicky
Picnic

It's me again. I know you're working today, so I thought e-mailing would be easier than phoning this time. I got thinking about Tuesday and perhaps it's too much to do the picnic and support group the same day. I know that I'll be tired (especially after the kids) and can only imagine how Jim and Ralph will feel. I know they both like to be as sharp as possible for the group. Do you agree? The following Monday or Tuesday would be better. Ralph is feeling better physically but this last impaction did a number on his head. Still somewhat confused but not seeing as many visions as yesterday. I hope the GI doctor can help with this ongoing problem. Then I suppose I should get in touch with Dr. D. about the hallucinations. Probably nothing he can do except increase the medication. We'll see. We have an appointment with him in September. . . . Talk to you soon.

Vicky to Ann

Yes, I think for the guys' sake and ours, it would be more restful if we don't get together 'til the week later. I'm glad that Ralph is feeling a bit better.

I turned in my resignation today. I feel good about it. Jim can hardly use the TV remote to change channels now. For some reason he doesn't understand the number 10 anymore, and has a lot of trouble dialing the phone. Also, he can no longer tell time using a regular or digital clock, so that's one reason he gets agitated if I'm gone a long time. If he wakes up after a nap before dinner, he thinks its morning, not evening. He's having a lot of trouble with clothes and doesn't get the hanging up part anymore, so when I come home stuff is all over the place. I am more of a maid than I ever was! But he is such a sweet man, and I think how scary the world must be for him. It's time for me to be home.

One funny thing...Jim speaks more confidently about himself and what he can do even though he is failing more. His memory of the hard times he is having is not there.

We wish you both well and we'll see you Tuesday night.

07/20/2009
Vicky's Journal
Proof That There is No Denying Mid-Stage Disease

No patient with dementia can be exactly like any other patient as far as symptoms or behavior. Each patient is unique and their symptoms/behavior depends upon what parts of the brain are being destroyed by the plaques and tangles. Here is how Jim's disease is reflected in his behavior.

Visual agnosia (loss of visual comprehension by the brain) appeared ages ago when I gave Jim a card with two yellow labs on the front and Jim could only see one of the dogs. Now it has progressed to not being able to pick a specific item out of a group of items on a table. For instance, Jim is not able to pick out his wallet when placed on a table with eye drops, 2 pens, a magazine, and keys. In regard to meal time, Jim cannot discern what is on his plate, or where one food ends and another begins. Because he doesn't recognize what he is going to eat, he doesn't know how to approach the eating of it. I think this is why he tends to cut up everything and eat it with a fork whether it is a club sandwich, a hamburger, or meat loaf. If I show him how to pick it up, he becomes angry with me and asks me to let him eat his own food the way he wants. My immediate thought about my response was that I was making it easier for him by showing him how to eat it. I am also worried about how messy his plate will become if he tries to cut everything up. To me, by cutting it up, he would lose the essence of a particular food, because they would all be mixed together. My input is an affront to him. I'm telling him he doesn't know how to eat his food! It also takes away a little of his independence. It's totally my problem, not his! But it is so hard to sit there and say nothing! To help with his visual agnosia at home, I retired all my placemats and covered the table with dark green vinyl to help make the plate pop out for him.

Eating out with his friends can highlight problems too. Once he ordered chicken wings. When they came, he complained to the waitress that he couldn't eat them because they had bones! He also didn't like them because to eat them he would have to pick them up, and that would get his hands dirty. The order was returned to the kitchen. Taking Jim out to eat is a dicey proposition.

Reading a laminated menu is impossible because of the glare reflection. I usually have to suggest items that he might like from the menu.

When visiting a bed and breakfast, Jim could not tell who the owners were, even though they were the ones serving breakfast to the other people seated at the table.

Jim keeps getting out a new can of shaving cream when he needs it. He doesn't see the can that is already on the shelf with his razor, even though he puts the new can on the shelf in front of the old can!

Jim doesn't remember which towel, tooth brush, etc., is his, so I find my towel continually damp when I go to use it, likewise my tooth brush. At this point, telling him his error won't change the behavior because he won't remember, so I need to put my towel and tooth brush some place where Jim would not look. It took me a while to internalize this, but with frustration comes invention.

As a couple we did a lot of biking. Jim also did quite a bit by himself. Unfortunately, when Jim would take off his helmet, he would unthread the straps from the clip instead of separating the clip. In order to rethread it, I would have to look at my helmet and mirror that to get his helmet straps rethreaded.

It is near impossible for Jim to make a phone call, because he can't keep the number in his head long enough to execute it. But he also doesn't read well and so programming numbers into the phone won't work either.

Jim now doesn't remember where I am if I am not home with him. He used to know that if I were not at home, I was probably at work or someplace safe until he saw me later in the day. Now, he gets a bit panicky when he doesn't remember where I am. I used to have a pad on the dining table that told him the day and the date. I replaced it with a sign that said, 'Vicky is at work' with the work phone number.

Jim has a lot of trouble turning on and off the TV, and can no longer select Channel 10 because he doesn't remember that the number is created with a 1 and a 0.

Jim dresses completely for his comfort. He has put on 3 shirts all with collars...or just an undershirt, and gets mad at me if I suggest he put on something else. He doesn't care how he looks to others. I feel as his wife and caregiver, how he looks is a reflection on how well I care for him.

Jim trimmed his eyebrows today and he almost shaved them all off! He also trimmed his toe nails straight across so that they are very sharp at the corners. He doesn't think they need fixing and doesn't want my help. Aaaahhh! Later he asked for my help.

Clothes are left exactly where he takes them off, because he doesn't remember that he was the one who took them off. They stay there until I put them in the closet/dresser, or laundry. I am constantly opening his drawers to find the clothes balled up, because Jim didn't want what he pulled out, but didn't know how to fold it. I also find some clothes discarded on the floor of his closet.

Jim can't read a traditional clock or a digital clock anymore. Because he has nothing to measure the passage of time, he is starting to become anxious when I am at work, worrying that something bad has happened to me.

When we are grocery shopping, I get the items and Jim follows me with the cart. I have to keep turning around so Jim can see my face, otherwise he doesn't know where I am. He has no clue what I look like from behind or what I have on. Sometimes, I have turned around to find that he is following someone else who is 15-20 years older than me. That hurts! To think that he thinks that person is me!

Jim's temperature regulation has been abnormal for a while. It seems that when he started Aricept he felt cold all the time. This summer, however, he has started sitting around in his down jacket and the temperature is 74 degrees. I am always having hot flashes, so 74 is hot for me! Sometimes I come home and the thermostat is set at 80 degrees, and Jim complains when I want to turn it down!

I notice Jim can't listen to directions and follow them. If we are driving and I ask him to look at the green house on the left, he will be looking right at a red house and agreeing with whatever I say.

Jim still recognizes my voice but doesn't recognize his sister's (he doesn't speak to her as often.)

Many times Jim will walk out of the house with a key in his hand, even though he has not been driving since 2007, probably thinking it is our house key. So, now I will have to hide all the keys or they will end up who knows where!

One task Jim was always responsible for was blowing the deck and driveway with our leaf blower. Now, however, he usually can't start it because he forgets to switch it to 'start' from 'stop'. One by one the tasks that he once performed are falling away.

With all these changes, our relationship has changed as well. I feel more like his caretaker than his partner. He is very loving and demonstrative, but if he regrets something, it stays in his head and he apologizes over and over not remembering that he has said it before. After a while I begin to feel smothered. Sex isn't much fun either. When you are 'mothering' someone, it's hard to switch roles and become their lover. I think to be a lover you have to feel equal (at least in a woman's mind) and I don't think we are anymore.

07/21/2009
Ann's Journal

We had a fairly good weekend. Ralph continues to have dizzy episodes, and is very tired. He had episodes right after breakfast on Saturday, and again at the farmers' market. No hallucinating this weekend, but a few sightings on Monday. On Sunday, we went to Nancy and Lou's for dinner. We took Aisha with us and we all had a good time. Ralph still does well with people as long as he doesn't get overwhelmed.

On Monday we saw Dr. H. for Ralph's GI problem. The Dr. suggested Miralax daily. He will see him in a month, and then we'll discuss a colonoscopy.

Tonight was support group. We had a small but productive group. Ralph is hallucinating again, which I shared, and a couple of the other caregivers were relieved to hear that's a fairly common occurrence.

07/28/2009
Ann's Journal

Ralph is doing well with the Miralax. Good results and I've cut back on the dosage. There have been no hallucinations. They appear with any kind of trauma or illness. At least Ralph isn't telling me if he's seeing things. He told me he's afraid to tell me for fear Dr. D. and I will 'put him away.' So sad. Before dementia became a subject we could actually talk about, people thought that if one had dementia they wouldn't be aware of it. Not true. Ralph and others in his stage are very aware of their symptoms and feel fear and frustration over their disappearing abilities.

Ralph is walking every day but I know he's having more trouble seeing. Objects just don't seem to register in his brain, and I find he needs more and more help when we're out. Because of the visual perception (or lack of) he has difficulty eating. He has broken a number of drinking glasses in the last couple of months which bothers and frustrates him, so I'm looking for some nice plastic glasses. That will help. We'll still have a lot of spillage to clean up, but no broken glass to worry about.

On Sunday, we went to Alan's and Christine's (grandson and wife) to plan our annual Henderberg camping weekend. We took Hassan and Aisha with us. They were good, but I was so tired I couldn't wait to get home. I got a decent night's sleep and on Monday, we picked up the kids again and met Jim and Vicky in King's Park for a picnic lunch. The kids were on their best behavior, and Jim and Vicky enjoyed them. Ralph had a syncope (fainting) episode when we first got to the park, but recovered fairly quickly. Beautiful day all around.

08/05/2009
Ann's Journal
Ups and Downs

Things have been going well for the most part. On Friday, we went to a rehearsal of the RPO (Rochester Philharmonic Orchestra.) One of the events the Alzheimer's Association offers us is the opportunity to sit in on RPO rehearsals. Ralph loves any kind of music so he benefits from this type of stimulus. A good day with no incidents.

The following Tuesday, Brian took Ralph along while Hassan had his horseback riding lesson. Ralph had an episode there in the paddock and was confused and dizzy for longer than usual. Brian told me his Dad was feeling dizzy most of the way home. Today, he couldn't walk more than two houses without feeling strange and dizzy.

I'll spend all day tomorrow getting ready for our family camping trip. So much work for just a weekend. Hope Ralph handles it OK.

09/01/2009
Vicky's Journal
Was the Timing Ever Right

The summer of 2009 I was having increased anxiety about leaving Jim alone while I worked 3 days a week. The previous spring I had tried to coax him into agreeing to hire someone to be his companion for at least the days I worked. His days alone must be exceedingly long and boring, and he is losing his enthusiasm for facing each day. He just didn't have his normal 'get up and go.' Every time I brought up the subject, Jim refused. I had suspicions that Jim wasn't eating lunch and I know he hadn't taken some of his medications, but forcing him wasn't the answer. At the end of July, I awoke in the middle of the night and began mulling the problem over in my head. I decided then and there that it was time to quit work. Jim's disease had prevented us from amassing the retirement funds we would have wanted, but my decision was the right move. I immediately felt at peace. After reviewing my decision with the benefits staff where I worked, I handed in my resignation effective August 29. One month to go. As it turned out, there were numerous things that happened that next month to verify my decision:

1. Jim got lost while traveling on his bicycle to our rec. center to lift weights via the Erie Canal path. He never got there even though he made the journey many times before. He ended up at a senior living center and the head of the Alzheimer's Unit brought him home, bike and all!

2. Jim was going out with his two buddies and locked himself out of the house. We never locked the door to the house because we locked the garage door, but this time Jim locked the house door. Luckily, I was prepared and had a spare key hidden in the garage for Jim's pals to use.

3. A week before my final day, I took Jim to the rec. center to work out and swim while I ran some errands. When I came back to get him, he was accompanied by a gentleman who asked if I was Jim's wife. He explained that Jim had some trouble finding his clothes. I thanked the man for his help, and began scrutinizing Jim's clothes. He had on his own shirt, and

his swim trunks (that were not wet.) I pulled open the waistband of his trunks to see if he had underwear on. He did, but they were grey! Uh Oh! They weren't Jim's underpants, nor were the white socks or the white sneakers he was wearing. I took him back to the locker room, but I couldn't accompany him to the lockers, so I had to have Jim go in and ask someone to help us. He found a young man who was willing to help find Jim's clothes. I described to the man what we were missing, and then they went locker to locker looking for the misplaced items. I could hear slam, slam, slam as the lockers were opened and closed. They returned with Jim properly dressed. I asked the man to leave the other clothes folded on the bench for the owner to claim. It is kind of surprising, but every person Jim has ever asked for help has come through with flying colors! They have always been patient and caring. Before leaving, we stopped at the desk and told the attendant that if someone complains that his clothes were removed from his locker, that it was a man with Alzheimer's who accidentally went to the wrong locker. It was a partial truth, but we thought better of telling the owner that Jim actually wore his clothes! Jim has always been the cleanest person, so no harm was done. Looking back on that day, it was kind of funny seeing Jim come out in someone else's clothes!

4. Two days before my final day, I came home to find Jim very upset. He was so relieved to see me that he almost cried. He couldn't remember where I was, and got extremely worried. He used to assume that if I wasn't home that I must be at work. Not any longer! His days must be terribly long since he can no longer tell time, and he thought something terrible had happened to me. I made a mental note to call him a couple times a day to remind him that I was at work. I did that the last two days, but he was still in a tizzy by the time I got home. One day he must have dreamt that I decided not to quit after all, and another day he dreamt that I said I was going to place him in a nursing home. Neither was true!

5. Lawn mowing was one thing that Jim did fairly well up until now. He finished the lawn, and when I looked out it actually

looked like a blind man had done it ... no pattern, rhyme, or reason. There were also lots of un-mowed pieces sticking up here and there. I couldn't let it go ... it was just too bizarre.

6. I'm not sure, but I think Jim was starting to experience hallucinations. On several separate occasions he asked me if the children that were here today had left. He also woke me up in the night saying that there was a man knocking on the door. I had followed him out into the living room, because Jim's dad on several occasions started peeing in the closet or on the front door screen, and I wanted to catch Jim before he did something like that.

It is unbelievable that Jim could suffer such deterioration in a month's time. Was I just blind to these things happening before? I didn't think so, because I wasn't working full time – only three days a week. I was home four days. All I can say is 'was the timing ever right!'

09/14/2009
Ann's Journal
Looking Back and Ahead

Where did the summer go? The camping weekend was fun. Ate, drank, made camp fires, traveled around, and celebrated Aisha's 4th birthday. Marissa (great granddaughter) loved fishing in the catch and release ponds. Ralph did well during the day, but became somewhat disoriented at night. It helps to have our wonderful family support group surrounding us. I heartily recommend early disclosure so that even the youngest family member understands that Grandpa needs help. Speaking of grandchildren, Marissa stayed with us all of Labor Day weekend, Hassan and Aisha the next weekend, and Marissa back on the third. I was able to pick up a used sewing machine for her and we both spent the time happily learning how to use it. Marissa inherited her Grandpa's creative and artistic talent.

We saw our neurologist this month and he wanted Ralph to start using a cane. His balance is compromised and that along with his dizzy episodes make walking a bit dangerous. We got the cane and Ralph is good about using it, except...he carries it horizontally and the tip is never anywhere near the ground. I try to explain and show him how to carry it, but I might as well talk to the cane.

One of the Social Club programs was a 'show and tell' day. Ralph took a number of wood and marble pieces. Everyone was impressed with his work. He gave a presentation and answered questions. There was no hesitation in his speech which surprised both of us. He was truly his old self again for that brief time.

We finished our three month program at the Social Club with a boat trip on Canandaigua Lake. It was a gorgeous day and everyone (caretakers and partners) had a great time. Because the program has been so popular, we must wait three months before we can apply again.

We've started an exercise program at the JCC (Jewish Community Center). We meet three times a week and it's another Alz. Assoc. offering. We also go to the Memorial Art Gallery once a month to review and critique paintings and/or current exhibits. I never have to ask Ralph twice if he wants to go, and he really comes alive when he's in his element.

Ralph also had his eyes examined this month. His sight if fine, the macular degeneration is minimal, so his vision problems have to be cognitive.

Now, we're getting ready for a trip to South Dakota in October to visit our friends, Will and Launa. Will was our late son Craig's best friend growing up, and he has become one of the family. We're both excited about going, but I'm a bit worried about flying and going so far four years after diagnosis. Ralph seems to be worrying about the same thing.

09/20/2009
Vicky's Journal
Description of Behaviors—I just want my old husband back!

Jim is much more confused getting dressed. Sleeves trouble him. He does not know where they go...on the legs or on the arms...and how to get them there. In the same vein, he can't figure out which is the front or the back of the garment. Tags are no longer a cue of the back of the neck. If he tries to hang them back up, many times they're put upside down.

Cutting down limbs with a pole saw is equally confusing. First he can't accurately see the limb that needs cutting or where it needs to be cut, even though he has performed this activity for years. I thought maybe he could do this with some coaching and it would boost his pride, but it was so labor intensive for me to keep going over and over the directions, I finally gave it up as a very bad idea.

While mowing the lawn this summer, Jim left significant patches un-mowed, and in the process has lost the gas cap for both the mower and the gas can again. Usually I would go out and 'finish up' what he didn't complete. One thing I didn't know until the fall Jim died was that my neighbor also used to sneak out and finish some of the spots Jim left. Our neighbors have been so amazingly kind hearted and helpful!

Shaving is Jim's nemesis! Jim used to start shaving with his shaver and a short time into the task I would hear him complaining. He said it was broken. The shaver kept falling apart while he was using it. I put it back together and tried it on my legs. It didn't fall apart once, but it was poorly designed. The 'release head' button was directly below where Jim held it. Evidently he had changed his hand position just a little and was always hitting that button! Jim said it was not possible that he was hitting it because he had been shaving for years, and he would certainly know how to do it by now! I finally gave up and said I would use his shaver for my legs, and would buy him a new one. It took me a while to find one that did not have that button right below the hand position. Sometimes you just have to give in to the argument and spend more money to stop the behavior from happening.

Jim thought it was a neat idea to save on paper bathroom drinking cups by pouring the water from the cup into his mouth without touching it to his lips! Then he would let the cup dry out on the counter. The problem with that was, the next time he needed a cup he didn't remember that the cup on the counter was his. And so it goes.

By the end of the day there would be 4-5 cups on the counter. This drove me insane.

Chewing ice is Jim's favorite pastime. He swears it hasn't hurt his teeth, but when he went for his last dental visit, they called me in and showed me that Jim's teeth are all worn down. They look like tree trunks cut at almost ground level as if I could count the rings in them! Jim has been complaining for months that all sorts of things I or a restaurant serve him are full of gristle, and yet my same dinner was fine. Now it makes sense. I don't know how many times he has complained to the waitress about his 'poor cut of meat.' It's so bad now I don't want to take him anywhere for fear of what he might say or do.

Lastly, I took him to see *Cirque du Soleil*. I was amazed at how little he perceived when watching the show. He would be watching the ring where nothing was happening, and I would have to point out the amazing act in the other direction.

Let Them Do Things For Their Self Esteem Without Any Criticism:

- *Vacuum*
- *Dust – the items dusted were moved all over and I would silently put them back where they belonged*
- *Wash and dry dishes*
- *Clean the tub*
- *Clean the dish drainer*
- *Pick-up sticks with his long tongs*

Be generous with your praise.

These may not be done to the caregiver's satisfaction, but that doesn't matter. Pretend it is as good as you would have done. If you must clean some areas that were missed, do it when your care-partner is not around!

09/22/2009
Ann to Vicky
Lunch

As it turns out, we're not going away this weekend as planned. Would you and Jim still like to get together on Monday? I'm thinking we should go back to Jine's because the guys tend to do better in a more familiar place. However, it's up to you. Anyplace is fine with us.

This past week has been up and down. Some days, almost normal. Other days, confusion reigns. Ralph can no longer figure out how to put the dumpster and recycle bins out at the curb. Taking his pills is a major struggle even though I lay them all out for him. Can't figure it all out. I feel so bad, but at the same time I feel so frustrated. Hope you know what I mean. I'm just hoping he stays stable enough for our plane trip in October. I'm a little shaky about it but figure, why not? What do we have to lose? If he (or I for that matter) has a meltdown, the crew is getting paid for taking care of us. Right?

Anyway, let me know how it goes with you and Jim, and I hope to see you Monday.

Vicky to Ann

Monday is fine with us. Whatever restaurant is easier for Ralph.

I know what you mean about Ralph forgetting how to put out the trash. Jim now has his shaver 'fall apart' every time he shaves because he keeps pushing the 'open for cleaning' button which is right under the head! He has used that shaver for years, but all of a sudden he must be holding it differently. Anyway, to stop the complaining we went out and bought him another razor that doesn't have a button anywhere close, and now I have an electric razor to shave my legs. Sometimes you just have to throw away money to 'make things right with the world.'

It does get tiring orchestrating their entire day, doesn't it? From 'take your pills' in the morning to laying out the clothes to getting the breakfast... Jim doesn't recognize the Raisin Bran box...he says they change the box all the time and he can't recognize it. Well, it is always PURPLE and has big RAISIN BRAN letters on it, but then, we don't know what's going on in their heads.

Jim is golfing tomorrow morning so I will have at least three hours to get some stuff accomplished.

Go NOW on your trip...you probably won't get another chance and Ralph seeing Will's woodworking will really be good for him.

10/04/2009
Vicky To Ann
No Connections - Safety, Safety, Safety

In the last two months Jim has gotten more protective of me. He doesn't want me to do things where I might get hurt...like climbing on a ladder (even safely) or doing anything where he can picture bad outcomes. It is frustrating, but I can understand his viewpoint. I am his caregiver and if anything were to happen to me, he would be toast! He wants to protect me at all costs.

Jim likes to help out by getting the drinks for our meals. This morning, I told him that I wanted OJ for breakfast. He gets two glasses out, puts ice in the glasses, and then asks me what I want to drink even though I just told him I wanted OJ (no lasting memory.) He looked in the refrig. and picked up apple juice. He said, "Is this OJ?" I said, "No, it's apple juice." He said, "Isn't that the same?" The connections aren't happening.

When we go to the rec. center he doesn't remember whether I dropped him off or whether I am there walking the track. I have to be sure I am not late or who knows what would happen.

He hovers behind me even when I am on a small step ladder and only 2 feet above normal. If I turn around fast I run into him! He also transfers his fear onto others he notices. If a young person is riding his bike safely on the side of the road, Jim says that the person is crazy to be doing that in traffic (even if they are far to the right.) As parents, we all know our kids do crazy things at times, but this was not out of my comfort zone. However, it was definitely out of his. Everyone needs to be very safe in his eyes. He doesn't want me to go out after dark in the car. What does he think I am going to do when he is gone? Ugh!

My idea is to do things he would bug me about after he has gone someplace with his buddies, or while he is taking a nap so I can't make him nervous. The other day I cleaned out the gutters requiring me to climb on the roof...after he went off golfing with his buddies.

10/13/2009
Ann to Vicky
Quick Note

I just need to vent for a minute. Please think of us tomorrow as we leave for our trip. I'm exhausted and both of us are close to tears. Ralph just went to bed. He is so confused about this trip. I've done all the packing but he wanted to help get a few of his things together like shaving gear, etc. It took him hours just to get those few things ready to go. I can't imagine trying to do something like this again. A short car trip, maybe, but I'm afraid he's going to be frantic by the time we reach the airport. He can't remember where we're going. I tell him over and over.

Last Sunday we went to our grandson Alan and Christine's house for their daughters' birthdays. It's a half-hour drive and we talked normally all the way. As we pulled into the driveway Ralph turned to me and said, "Is Ann coming later?" He said it again as if it made perfect sense. I said, "Look at me. Who am I?" He said, "I guess I didn't recognize you with your sun glasses on." To top it off, when we went inside he interacted with everyone in a perfectly normal way. I think you and my friend who lost her husband to Alzheimer's are the only people who really understand how I feel. It's all so scary.

I'm still having trouble sleeping (last night, 3 AM). I just set the alarm for 5 AM, took two Tylenol PMs and if I'm not asleep by midnight I may have to try a glass of wine. Probably not.

Take care and I hope you're both enjoying Jim's sister's visit.

Hugs to you both.

10/20/2009
Ann's Journal
Trip

The trip to South Dakota went better than I could have hoped for. Before our first take-off from the Rochester Airport, Ralph asked me where we were. I explained that we were waiting for take-off and calmly explained what to expect. Lay-over in Chicago, transport by wheelchair, etc. I assured him that Will and Launa would meet us at the airport in Rapid City.

Everything went smoothly and we had a wonderful time. Ralph was stable and oriented during the entire visit. We travelled every day, and while tired, he was very content. I think part of the reason was that Will and Launa gave him loving support and attention, and I was also able to relax and let someone else take charge. A win-win altogether.

I never realized how scenic and interesting South Dakota is. We visited Mount Rushmore, Crazy Horse Memorial, Mammoth Cave, and the Black Hills, and Ralph kept up with all of it. (I didn't know it at the time, but that trip was the last for Ralph and me together.)

10/31/2009
Vicky's Journal
Angry Arguments Happen

This is the first really angry argument that we have had in some time. I had taken Jim to have blue light therapy on his face for precancerous skin damage. Afterward he has to stay out of the sun for 2 days or it will exacerbate the irradiated, damaged skin. It will heal from the inside out and the damaged skin will slough off. The next day Jim said, "That bastard!" I asked who he was referring to and Jim said, "That guy who did something to my face!" I told him the symptoms of tingling and pins and needles would get better each day. Jim said, "No, this has been going on for a while." I explained that I just took him a day ago and that sometimes he misperceives what happened because of the Alzheimer's. Then he got really mad at me. I thought he would think of me as a steadying force, a caregiver and wife who wants the best for him. He doesn't remember it that way and thinks I am lying to him. I probably shouldn't have had the procedure done.

How many times have I been told that you don't win an argument with a person with dementia? Why do I keep trying? I bet Ralph would have understood. I walked away and let the subject drop. Hopefully, in a few minutes he will have forgotten about it all.

11/11/2009
Vicky's Journal
Today's Entry

Over the past two weeks I have noticed a big change in Jim. If he asks me for directions, if I offer them, he will be lost from the beginning. Today we drained, cleaned, and filled the hot tub for the winter. Giving him one thing to get from the basement or garage was impossible. He would lose where he was going and for what. If he was in the garage right next to the deck, I could give directions slowly and he could still not follow them. I saw it over and over today. It was frustrating for me, but I didn't learn the lesson the first time, the second, or even the third. Jim would repeat, "I have done this many times before and I know what I am doing!" There was no easy way out of it because the hot tub needed to be thoroughly cleaned rather than Jim's attempt at it, or the hot tub would get too dirty before March and we would have to do it again in the dead of winter. So I couldn't trade places with him. He did carry the buckets of water to the driveway when we got to below siphoning levels, and that was a big help.

Jim didn't know:

- what a towel was

- a pink towel from a burgundy towel or a yellow sponge

- I asked for a green brush and he brought me a yellow sponge

- I asked for a bucket of water, he brought me a yellow sponge

- I asked him to dry off the clean part of the cover, he did the dirty part

While I was away this morning getting the car's undercoating checked, I asked Jim to vacuum the room my sister would be staying in this weekend. To my surprise, he vacuumed the entire house! That was wonderful (except those parts were already vacuumed) and I thanked him. The unfortunate part about it was that when Jim vacuums he moves furniture but can't remember where it belonged before he moved it. So everything was out of place and needed to be moved back in place before tackling the hot tub cleaning. With company coming, I didn't act frustrated, but I didn't shower him with praises like I should have. He is trying the best he can and sometimes I feel like such a shrew! I have to make him feel useful and needed...that is my goal from this day forward. I truly am going to try harder.

12/06/2009
Vicky to Ann
Watch Out For Crowds

Finding a Christmas tree to cut down out in the fields of a Christmas tree farm is one of my favorite winter memories. That is what we did today in 40 degree weather with the sun shining. We went with a friend and her son. When we found our trees, we left the guys with the trees and we went to pay and bring the cars up to where the trees were waiting to be bound. My friend's son was carrying their tree to her car. I looked around for Jim and he was standing with a bunch of other people, as if he belonged with them. He was standing in the background and looked like he was trying to keep up with the conversation, as if he were part of the group. It was as if he 'adopted' those people because he couldn't recognize us. I yelled to him, and he barely could recognize me from a distance of 5-6 car lengths. It was so sad to see him like that. Life can be really cruel.

I have to have his visual perception measured. How do they measure how strong his glasses need to be when they can't assess whether the vision is the acuity of the eyes or the translation by the brain? At this point I don't know if he even knows his letters anymore.

Chapter Two

2010

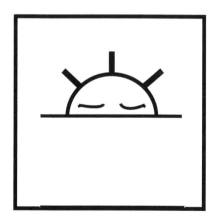

01/01/2010
Vicky's Journal
I Think the Disease Has Stopped

Jim came to me last night right before bed with a happy look on his face and said, "I think the disease has stopped! I did so well with conversation and everything and I'm still going strong. Seventeen years, it must have arrested!" (We spent the evening with friends celebrating the New Year.)

I didn't have the heart to tell him that it has not stopped, it's still progressing! So sad.

01/22/2010
Ann to Vicky
Laughter in a Straight Jacket

Your notes about the hot tub cleaning have blown me away! I feel we are living parallel lives. (I'll be quick, my computer's typing is very slow if at all.) The part about the towels and the sponge made me laugh out loud... also the locker room story. Other parts make me want to cry. Are you sure you don't mind me printing some?

Today, going to and from dance class, I composed some stuff of my own. I'll probably write in longhand until I get this glitch with the computer fixed. I will send or bring you a copy. Gotta stop now. This is taking forever.

P.S. Must get back to journaling. I read some of my e-mails in your folder and I had already forgotten how I was feeling at the time.

01/22/2010
Vicky's Journal

Jim is sitting on the couch. "Can I do something for you?" he asks. "Yes, you can get the drinks for dinner," I reply. He rises and goes over to the dining table... knowing the thought was something to do with that. He looks confused, and I tell him as if it were the first time,"

Would you get the drinks, Dear?" He sits at his place and looks up as if to say, "Where's the food?" The meal proceeds.

We are going to the rec. center to exercise. Jim needs his punch card for payment. The punch card is not on his dresser where it normally is. I checked yesterday's shirt, and it's not there. "Jim, where is your wallet? I gave it to you this morning before we went to the doctor. Is it in your jacket pocket?" He looks... "Nope." After much searching I find it in the kitchen by the refrigerator. It has his punch card in the pocket. "Do you have your eye drops?" We get jackets on and get in the car. "So you have your eye drops and your punch card?" "No, I can't find my punch card." I get out of the car and go in the house. The punch card is on the dining room table... right where he picked up his eye drops. Need I say more?

01/22/2010
Vicky's Journal
Bouts of Anxiety, Fear

A few days ago Jim asked me to take him back to where he had worked as a school psychologist and a family therapist. He created a family therapy program for parents and their troubled children, because seeing the entire family made more progress than just seeing the child. He also taught parenting programs to enrich the parents' skills in dealing with their children. Jim has been lamenting since he retired that the people he used to work with were no longer offering the parenting classes anymore. He knew that getting the parents to change the way they interact with their children was more than half the battle. He wanted to talk to the head of the department about some idea he thought would be helpful, that they were not presently implementing. Right away, the idea made me nervous. I didn't want him to embarrass himself in front of the department head. I imagine they dropped the parent groups as part of a cost cutting measure. Could Jim clearly express himself? Time marches on, and would they lend an ear to someone who has been retired for 8 years and is coming in to tell them how they should run the show? I told him that I was nervous about his going there... that time had moved on. Jim remained very insistent, and so I conceded and drove him there. When we pulled into the parking lot, Jim looked very confused. I asked if he wanted me to accompany him to the department. He looked at me appearing very flustered and said, "Is this it? It looks different to me." I said, "This is where you used to work, and where you asked me to take you." He said, "Is this where I exercise?" I said, "You mean the rec. center where we go every other day to lift weights?" He said, "Yes." He was starting to hyperventilate and get upset because he was so confused. He didn't understand how things were so mixed up! Jim said he felt stupid because he made me drive there, and was very apologetic. I then drove to the rec. center and tried to act as if it was a little ripple in our day. I was glad, actually, that the 'mix-up' happened because I wanted to protect him from getting hurt emotionally. We didn't stay at the rec. center as long as usual, because the confusing experience made him tired.

Jim's days are always filled with frustration. He loses his wallet, his rec. center card, his gloves, the gas caps, etc. It just rolls from one thing to another, and I can't really make it all better. I try to make his day rewarding by taking him places that please him, but the disease always gets in the way.

01/30/2010
Ann to Vicky
Why I'm Tired

Wednesday I did all the laundry. Today (Saturday) I did all the laundry. I just folded 5 pairs of Jockey Shorts and 4 pairs of briefs (3 days). Not because they're dirty, but because he takes them out of his drawer and leaves them all over. Only you know what I'm talking about.

I've invited Nancy and Lou (daughter & son-in-law) over for a soup and salad supper tomorrow night because they have us over a lot. Then I invited Brian, Shino, and the kids 'cause they haven't seen each other in a while. Today my guilt kicked in and I called our grandson Alan and invited them (5 if Brittany brings her boyfriend.) I made chili today and I'll make soup tomorrow, and wonder why I'm tired Monday morning! Seriously though, we'll have fun and I have to do these things while Ralph and I are still able to enjoy it all.

Vicky to Ann

Yes, I do know what you are talking about. Yesterday alone Jim used 3 pairs of briefs... and since I'm not sure if he had them on or not (look for wrinkles)—in they go to be washed!

I will type the notes on the NH tonight or tomorrow (note: Ann and I have started visiting nursing homes together so we will be able to choose the one(s) we like beforehand.) I finished taking down the wallpaper in the den and painted the cubicle where the computer is. I didn't remove the computer and all its' wires, so when we move I'll have to do what I couldn't get (10 years from now if I'm lucky.) That's why you got no reply earlier, because stuff was all piled up and covered.

You will find this funny though... today Jim walked out of the bedroom with a bright yellow highlighter and yellow lips! He said the Chapstick wasn't very good! It's like having a three year old! I just looked at him and had to smile. I washed off his lips and told him it was highlighter. I asked him if he knew what highlighter was (he was the highlighter king in college... by the time he was done every word was underlined, just about.) He said, "Not really."

Hope that highlights your day!

PS. We are waiting to see if the time around the support group winter party is when Kip wants us to come to New Hampshire. He was supposed to call us tonight but hasn't yet. There was something else I wanted to tell you but I don't remember now what it is. Oh, yes. You are amazing for having so many people over! I always disliked having big dinners... and now I hate it more. I do it... but only when my guilt gets the best of me.

02/04/2010
Vicky's Journal
Relationships

I know I am supposed to bolster Jim's self-esteem and make him feel useful, but sometimes it backfires! Today I sent Jim out to shovel our neighbor's driveway. They were away on holiday but will be back tomorrow. I thought it would be nice if they came back to a cleared driveway! I point to the house that needs the driveway done and send him off. The next thing I know Jim has the snow rake out (the aluminum rake that is used to get snow off roofs.) He has fallen in love with the snow rake. The other day I found him out in the front yard moving snow around with it. Jim was presently 'combing' the snow behind their 2nd car in the driveway and then moved off onto the snow in the yard, not accomplishing anything. I brought the snow shovel to him and said that it might work better than the snow rake, but he disagreed. I ended up shoveling with the shovel and Jim messed around with the snow rake.

Next week we are off to see our son in New Hampshire. Hopefully there will be sticks or something that Jim can gather to keep him busy!

02/07/2010
Ann to Vicky
Jewish Home

Looking at my calendar for next week, it looks like Friday would be the best day to check out our next nursing home. Even though my friend will be back, we can just take separate cars. Our dance class will be out at noon. That will give us a little more time to talk before a 1 PM appointment. Then, we should have plenty of time to pick up the guys and get to the Life Center by 4 PM. Busy day, but sometimes easier to do a whole bunch of things in one day. What do you think? Otherwise, with your trip and my March shows we should probably put it off until late March or early April. The shows will keep me busy until March 19th. Hopefully, we can get an appointment on Friday. I'm not sure when their Sabbath starts. I think it's Friday evening. Let me know.

PS. Just had a thought. If you call tomorrow morning and they can see us tomorrow afternoon that would be OK too.

Vicky to Ann

I will try for Friday at 1 PM. Tomorrow I am supposed to have my hair straightened again...a 4 hr. appointment and I have my ultrasound tomorrow afternoon at 3:30 PM, but I don't know if that will all come off. Jim accidentally put herpes fever sore ointment in his eye this morning. I washed it out twice and I washed around the eye with soap and water, and he put eye drops in all day long. The eye doesn't seem any worse for wear...It's not red or tearing, but he says it feels irritated. I explained that it looks fine, and I didn't really want to take him to ED for that. He couldn't accept that the eye doctor's office was not open today no matter how many times I told him. He was frightened, but would not accept anything I said, and said that I was not listening to him or believing him. Unless he wakes up tomorrow and forgets what happened, I will have to make an appt. and wreck my own. We will see. I'll let you know.

02/08/2010
Ann to Vicky
The Usual

I'm thinking that for your sanity I hope you can talk Jim into day care before spring. Did the eye irritation clear up so you could go to your appointments? It sounds as if you're going to have to put meds and such in a hiding place somewhere to protect Jim from himself. It's easy with a child because you can just put them up high, but a 6-footer can reach pretty high. I suppose it sounds funny in a way but he's liable to harm himself at some point. You just don't need all that worry.

Going along with our parallel worlds, I decided this morning to re-paint the bathroom. We did it a year ago, but I wanted it a little darker so I got the paint a month or so ago, and have been putting it off because I hate to paint. I thought it would be a breeze because I was going to put on one coat. It wouldn't have been too bad, but poor Ralph wanted to 'help'. The rest of the day was a nightmare. I'll go into detail on Friday but after all was said and done, he told me he was sure 'someone else' was here doing the painting. He tells me this while I'm trying to peel the paint off my hands, because I not only hate to paint, I'm a messy painter besides! Oh well, tomorrow is another day and I already see some spots I'll have to redo and then get some smudges off the ceiling...and the toilet...and the vanity...and the floor...etc. etc. etc.

We'll be in touch about Friday and especially, let me know how the ultrasound went.

03/05/2010
Vicky to Ann
A Bit of a Tiff

Well, the last two to three days have been tough. We went out for a quick bite to eat last night with some friends and Jim was trying to put catsup on his fries, but the catsup bottle was a wide mouthed one. It wasn't coming out, but I knew eventually it would end up all over, so I suggested he stick a knife in the mouth of the jar to get it started. Well, very loudly he said, "Would you just leave me alone!" Even our friends jumped. I know I probably tend to 'help' him too much, but I was really mad at him for doing that in public.

I told him that he fights me every step of the way, and that I would like to leave for at least a week and see how he did by himself! I would like to take him to senior care one day a week even though he thinks that he is fine by himself. So I said, "So what happens if you stop up the toilet or you have the bathroom faucets running full force, and you can't figure how to shut them off?" I also told him of his walking out on top of Kip's above ground pool when the water was frozen, and that he could have fallen through. I even explained why he shouldn't be out there, but he still went back on the frozen pool three times! We made peace, but I am still upset. And I am not very lovey-dovey, to put it mildly. I went for my mammogram this morning and luckily booked a massage this afternoon. The time away was nice. Jim was upset, and I think I scared him a little by saying that I would like to leave for a week. He was remorseful. I know he is frustrated with me helping him, maybe embarrassed and ashamed? But it is a fact of life and I wish that he would accept it. That's a selfish way to talk, but it is where I am right now. I am resentful.

This afternoon he went outside in the late day sun with the roof rake and was raking the snow that was at the top of the driveway down to the bottom (our driveway is dry blacktop) but Jim was pulling the snow from the garden and the grass to the street so it would melt. Our neighbor across the street was looking at him as if he was loony, as was I. It embarrassed me to see him out there doing that, but I was good and didn't say anything. It hurts sometimes to see him so nonfunctional. And yet we are so lucky in some ways.

Don't know how your life is going right now, but I know you've been there. Hope you are getting a breather, and that your hand is feeling better.

Well, I am done talking your ears off...am going to go out and walk around the block. Maybe tomorrow I will be more productive. Today was a lost cause, except for the massage!

Ann to Vicky

I wanted to get right back to you when I read your note last night, but was too tired to get my thoughts in order. I know just how you feel. Some days I think I'm devoting my entire life and thoughts to Ralph and dementia and I still feel guilty when I want some 'me' time. I swear we live parallel lives, you and I, because last night Ralph went out and started doing dishes. I knew he was trying to help and I knew how tired he was, because we had a full day with haircuts in the morning and Aisha the rest of the day. I already had a half load in the dishwasher, so I told him I would put plates and such in the washer for him and he could do up the pots. He got angry and stalked off and didn't speak for a while. Then he said, "Why can't you just let me finish something instead of taking over?" I told him I was sorry, but the main problem lately is when to step in and when to let him struggle. When he does the cleaning up, I find food and dishes in the strangest places, but he resents my mentioning it, so it's easier to do it myself. I know you know what I mean.

I was thinking about your letter when I went to bed last night and thought: I should appreciate this time we have because I know it's going to get much worse. Then I thought: Maybe now is the hardest because it's such a juggling act trying to help without hurting their feelings and maybe when they go further down the path we'll just take over and lead them in everything. I really don't know anymore. This week I've been rehearsing more hours and so I'm feeling guilty over leaving him, and guilty with my dance group because I don't want to let them down by not knowing the routines. The dancing is another decision I'll have to make. If I brought it up to the support group, the facilitator would just tell me to get respite care for him, but he's not ready for that. Even Brian said today that he sees what I mean when I say Ralph shouldn't be left alone for very long.

On another note, Tuesday we went to Voices (a get-together of dementia folks who answer pertinent questions for the quarterly newsletter for the Alzheimer's Association.) While there, a staff member came into the library and asked if Ralph and I were still going to 'Meet at the MAG' program that afternoon. Then she asked if we could come an hour earlier so the Director of Education could film a video with us about the program. They want to distribute the 'arts and Alzheimer's' idea across the country. We agreed and shot the video. Neither one of us were prepared so there was no time to get nervous. The Director of Education said it would be on their website as soon as he could edit it and then would go to YouTube. I didn't even have time to check hair and make-up, but you know what? Stuff like that doesn't matter anymore.

On a lighter note: When we caregivers were gathered for Voices, Ruby was saying that her husband still insists on driving and it drives her crazy. She worries constantly but she said that every time she calls him he just says: "I'm fine, I'm in Henrietta (a nearby suburb)." She said he says that every time. "Don't worry, I'm in Henrietta." Always Henrietta. At that, Jay very gently said, "Maybe Henrietta is his girlfriend." Well, I think they could hear us laughing on all three floors.

Guess that's all for now. Hope things have quieted down for you. It's so scary not knowing what part of the brain is going to be hit next. Thinking of you often.

Vicky to Ann

Yes, I have quieted down, and it is so amazing that our lives are so similar. We do have parallel lives, I think. It's nice to know that someone understands everything! Sometimes I do feel selfish, and then how really lucky we are, but then sometimes I say, "Now wait a minute...some of our friends are going to Florida in a week for two weeks and then lazily making their way back home and here I sit. Our lives are ticking away!"

At least neither one is violent. Today Jim brought up that a few weeks ago I wanted to put him in a nursing home. I said, "Now wait a minute here. I never said that." I explained our looking at nursing homes for the future AGAIN, maybe even for me, and I told Jim that he manufactured that in his head, and maybe before he gets all upset about something that he should check his facts with me. He could have dreamt it. I said, "Do you really think that I would put you in a nursing home now? What kind of a wife do you think I am anyway, Honey?" But our day ended on a better, calmer note. I am not looking forward to the years to come, that's for sure.

03/16/2010
Vicky to Ann
Wood Piece

Please convey to Ralph that I loved his wood piece he brought to support group. He did such a great job on that. It's too bad he can't still do some of his hobbies in some form...it would help keep him occupied and fulfilled.

Ann to Vicky

Thanks. Ralph was pleased that you liked it. I feel so sad that he has no other way to convey his gift of creativity any more. I try to find ways but he seems to have lost his inner spark. Simple ideas (like birdhouses and that sort of thing) would bore him and he probably couldn't do it anyway. Good group tonight. I think we were all surprised. A lesson to me to be more compassionate with everyone in the group. We're all in pain and just expressing it differently.

Hope Jim was OK when you got home, but I hope he was lonesome enough to come next time. Take care.

03/20/2010
Ann to Vicky
Saturday

Whew, glad it's Sat. night and this week is over. I did 3 shows as scheduled. Ralph went with me Monday and Wednesday.

On Thursday he said he didn't really want to go again, and that he would be fine on his own. However, he didn't want me to go alone (he worries about me more these days) so I carpooled with 3 other dancers. Ralph seemed fine when I got home, but shortly after I got in the house he wanted to know why there was a group of people in the side yard. Not only people, but a dog and a goat, too. Now, what do I do? He was really happy to be home, and was able to work out in the yard and sit on the porch, so I know it's not as lonesome for him as the winter indoor scene. I know he's not ready for respite care and Brian keeps assuring me he doesn't mind doing his computer work here. I guess that's how we'll work it for now. Ralph's been out walking every day and getting back home fine, and doing well except for his speech and occasional sightings.

Today Brian came over and helped me paint the woodwork in the kitchen (I'm keeping the wallpaper for now). Tomorrow he'll help me put up new wide rods and I can finally hang my new curtains.

I got a kick out of your airport control visual (note: Vicky simulated putting Jim to bed to the support group by putting on a navy vest, ear protectors, and 2 orange hand lights, and pretended to be a ground crew person who direct the planes into their gates.) It's perfect but not many people would understand how accurate it is. I think the only thing that keeps us sane is our sense of the ridiculous.

I just bought a new dementia book. I'll let you have it when I am through. It's written by a son taking care of his mother. It's interesting and at times humorous, but I think caregiving for a spouse is more stressful than caregiving for a parent. What do you think? You've been in both situations. I've also gingerly taken a look at the book you loaned me. I've been reading parts and it's not as morbid as I thought it would be. That's it for now. Time to turn in. Hang in there.

Vicky to Ann

Got a lot of work done in the yard these last few days...our garbage cans for outside refuse are full. Can't do any more until they get emptied on Tuesday. Jim has really been 'dopey' these last few days. I don't know what else to call it. I'm afraid he's reached a new low and that he'll be this way from now on. He didn't know how to turn on the shower vs. the bathtub water yesterday, and also couldn't open the sliding glass door. He doesn't know where anything is in the kitchen anymore, or anywhere else for that matter. He's like a lost puppy. Jim also worries about me when I go out by myself. He doesn't want anything to happen to me.

I took him golfing yesterday...I know you must think I'm nuts! I tried to stay calm and not to hurry him too much, but it was hard because he is so slow. He doesn't use the correct clubs anymore or stand so he can take the shortest line to the hole, but it was nice just being out there. I was so tired when we came back that I took a nap. Directing him the entire way was exhausting.

Jim doesn't want to go to day care but I'm going to try to push him into going about May or June. I will need the time to do things around the house. Thank heaven that I contracted with a lawn guy for this summer to mow the lawn and I will trim. There is no way Jim could mow even though he thinks he can. Not only is he losing his speaking (word finding), now he is losing the meaning of words and that's even worse.

I do think caring for a spouse is worse than a parent. We didn't have Jim's parents for direct care...Jim's mom took care of Jim's dad until he was nursing home ready. After he died, then Mom immediately started showing signs. So Jim's sister went from arrangements for Dad to arrangements for Mom: prescriptions, doctors, and emergencies. She is glad it is all finally over. Now it's our turn.

03/23/2010
Ann to Vicky
Coffee Break

I think the next time we meet we should start at the coffee shop and forget about running errands. After I got the call from Brian about Ralph, I was so distracted, I forgot a lot of the things I wanted to talk about. Ralph was still confused when I got home. Then he asked me a couple of times, "Do you know where Ann is?" I said, "Honey, look at me. Who am I?" He looked at me blankly and then went out in the kitchen and had a melt-down. He kept saying, "Please don't get mad at me. I made a mistake." I feel so bad for him and today I'm walking around on the verge of tears and a feeling of dread in the pit of my stomach.

I hope we can continue our coffee meetings. I know I need it. I just think we should make every minute count. I can't imagine how Ralph feels (and Jim, too) when they are completely alone in their foggy world. Meanwhile have a good trip, stay safe, and I'll talk to you next week.

03/23/2010
Vicky to Ann
Rain

Don't worry about running around the sewing store with me. I didn't mind at all. Would it be better in the future to meet somewhere really close to your house for coffee? Jim seems to be doing OK alone so far. I went to the hospital after coffee and dropped off some mold pictures (I take photos of molds under the microscope for identification purposes.) I said "Hi" to everyone and left. Got home 4 hours after I left and Jim was fine. I called in the interim to let him know. It was a rainy day, and he wasn't about to go outside.

Today was really interesting. We were watching it rain all day (after going to the podiatrist to get Jim's ingrown nail cut out,) and all of a sudden late in the day Jim noticed that the deck was really wet...all except three boards closest to the house. They were dry because they were under the eve. Jim interpreted the scene as the water starting to come from the edge of the deck and had reached to within 3 boards of the house, like a wave was coming. He was afraid that the water would eventually spill in the house and wet the carpets! He was thinking of the rain coming from below like water was rising instead of coming from above. He went downstairs and started getting plywood out to help divert the water, but I insisted we didn't need them because what he feared wouldn't happen. What I did say was that we needed to take some boards to Kip's in N.H., so Jim forgot about the flood! (We are going to N.H. to help Kip move into his new house.)

The docs are still deciding what to do, if anything, about Kip's irregular heartbeat. He has a bad cold now, probably from lack of sleep.

Hang in there and try to remain positive. Jim didn't know me once last week...I think I told you that, but maybe I didn't. At least when they look at us they aren't alarmed that someone strange is with them...that would be really awful. I think they realize we belong, but may not remember why. Once when we were in bed in the morning, Jim asked me if we ever got married. Also today Jim asked if Kip had been married before or if he had any children.

Ann to Vicky

Thanks for the reinforcement. I really needed it. I do remember Jim's asking you if you were married. I left Ralph again today for a couple of hours and met friends at a restaurant just 5 minutes away. He was fine, and then he went with Brian and Hassan to Hassan's horseback riding lesson in Lima. Hassan is going to be in a show in May.

Can you stand 2 cute kid stories from an obnoxious grandma?

1. Brian picked up Aisha from pre-school today and while walking home Aisha said, (and this is an exact quote) "Well, Dad, I've got a boyfriend." Brian said, "You do?" Aisha said, "Yes, and the last thing I needed was a boyfriend in <u>preschool</u>, but he says he loves me." She's four.

2. Brian, Ralph, and Hassan stopped at the American Hotel in Lima for a bite of supper. It's a very old landmark hotel that serves all kinds of soups and sandwiches. Very old, full of nostalgia. Hassan asked the waiter for hot chocolate, but added that there was something else he'd rather have but couldn't think of the name of it. The waiter left and then Hassan ran after him saying, "Excuse me, sir, I thought of what I wanted. I'll have a non-fat cappuccino with just a little sprinkle of cinnamon." The waiter looked at him and said, "You're getting hot chocolate." I don't know where he came up with cappuccino and I'm sure he's never had it...but I told Brian it sounded like Niles on Frazier. These are the little things that make it easier to bear this upside-down life.

Ralph just came out with his shaver and was looking for the end of it. He thought it was his electric tooth brush.

Tuesday or Wednesday next week would be fine for our monthly lunch with the guys. I know Ralph looks forward to our get-togethers but I guess we should hang out for no more than an hour (the guys get antsy). Then, you and I can plan another coffee date. I guess I'm getting used to this disease...that Jim's concern about the deck makes perfect sense. It's getting easier to imagine what their world is like. Maybe that's what the latest book meant by going where they are.

I've got to go set up our pill dispensers for the week. I always forget until I give Ralph his night pills and realize the box is empty. Tomorrow I have to do a good pick-up and cleaning because the person from Alzheimer's Assoc. doing a safety evaluation is coming at 4 PM. Again, have a good trip and I'll talk to you next week.

04/07/2010
Vicky to Ann
Birthday

Ann, hope you are doing OK. All is 'well' here...being a slug for a day or two. Thank you for the birthday card...I had a really nice day. An ortho visit, out for breakfast, out for dinner...and a nap in between.

04/09/2010
Ann to Vicky
All is Well

Hi. Nothing wrong with being a slug. I'm going to be one tomorrow and skip dance class. The past week has been so hectic. Our Easter party on Saturday was a big success, but I've been pooped ever since. Aisha was here for her usual Thursday today. We went to the bank and got groceries, and spent the rest of the day watching Barbie videos and playing.

Ralph is having his usual ups and downs, and I'm having a little more trouble dealing with the downs. I feel guilty, but lately I tend to feel annoyed when he's confused. You're the only one I'd share that with, but there it is. I hope you understand, but I guess I'm a little tired of hearing about what a good job I'm doing. I don't think I earn that accolade. I'm just trying to get us from one day to the next without either of us falling apart.

Guess I'll do a little escape reading and hope I feel more loving tomorrow.

Vicky to Ann

I know exactly what you mean. Being married to a psychologist, Jim is always sitting me down and asking me, "How about we both try not to yell at each other." #1 he means me, and I don't think I yell. I just raise my voice some when I get frustrated. Like when he makes all the excuses after asking me for help, then says "Oh, that's exactly what I was going to do" when it was not at all! Sometimes I would just like him to say, "thank you" instead of making excuses.' I know it makes his ego feel better, but hey, how about a little truth here. I am really not trying to punish him, but it is frustrating. Jim, too, has his ups and downs. We did some straight talking on one of his down days, and I was trying to explain to him that some days he thinks that he is well, and that the disease has stopped its progression. On the other hand, he's always telling me how lucky he is. If he kisses me once, he kisses me 4 times when he goes to bed. I know he is grateful, but sometimes it's a bit too much!

Being a slug is better than going insane, I guess. Hang in there.

04/10/2010
Vicky's Journal

The day before my birthday I took Jim to the Hallmark store to buy a card for me. I had already ordered my present and received it a week before: a Dyson Ball vacuum. I told Jim that I didn't want anything else. He reluctantly agreed, although he preferred to get me a 'surprise' gift. In the store he asked the sales clerk to help him, disclosing that he had Alzheimer's. I could hear her quietly reading verses to him as I searched the store for a card for Jim's brother-in-law. When he picked a card, I proceeded to the cash register, paid for them both, and the clerk put them in a bag for Jim to carry. At home he would remove the card he picked for me, and give me the other card to mail.

The next day, my birthday, I told Jim he had a birthday card for me in the top drawer of his dresser. I asked that he remove the card, sign it, put it in the envelope and give it to me. A bit later he came out with the card and laid it on the dining room table. I let it stay there for an hour and then asked Jim again to sign it and give it to me. He took it in the kitchen and worked on it for a while, and finally brought it out to me, but he brought only the card. I showed him the envelope in the kitchen and asked that he put the card in the envelope and give it to me. He did. When I opened the envelope, it held another card. My card was somewhere in the kitchen. Jim found it and gave it to me. It was a beautiful card with a wonderful verse. He signed it on the opposite page "wth all mmy love, ttthis card exp expresses howh much love you". He made multiple tries at the wording and it was almost illegible. So-o-o tragic.

Five days before my birthday we were taken out to dinner by two of our close friends, because they would be away on the actual date. At a crepe restaurant, Jim ordered a Reuben crepe. Wherever he goes if they have a Reuben on the menu, Jim orders it. After the meal, our friend asked Jim how he liked his Reuben. Jim said that it wasn't so good. He never would have answered so truthfully before, for fear of making our hosts feel bad. Jim felt no embarrassment.

We went to a restaurant for my birthday with another friend. I realized then that Jim wasn't wearing his glasses. He has been forgetting them a lot. Usually he would realize that he didn't have his glasses on because he would notice his poor vision. Now, however, I think his perception is so bad that he doesn't miss his glasses. I found him studying the menu upside down. Why didn't I notice that Jim didn't have his glasses when we left? I tell myself that remembering Jim's glasses is another task I have to take on.

A few days ago we went to an ice cream parlor on our bikes on the Erie Canal. Mistakenly, I ordered both of us a triple scoop cone. Jim took his and was waiting for me to pay. Jim was holding his cone, but not really watching it, and had the cone tilted to the side. It looked like the leaning tower of Pisa. I called out to him that it was going to fall, and just as it did, the manager caught the two scoops that fell off into a plastic cup! I have seen him tilt ice cream before, so I don't know what possessed me to order a 3-scoop cone. From now on I will order 3 scoops in a cup with the cone stuck on top. Sometimes the symptoms have to hit you in the face before you recognize a problem and make a change.

04/10/2010
Ann to Vicky
Better Days

I'm out of the current slump for now. Ralph has been more alert, less confused, and I'm sighing less. We watched the new movie *Sherlock Holmes* with Robt. Downey Jr. and Ralph seemed to 'get' most of it. I was really surprised. He's always loved to figure out whodunits and I guess he can still do that. His motor skills are down and so is his cognition as far as reading and writing, so it's good to see the real Ralph shine through from time to time.

What really sent me into a tailspin this week was: We went to the Alz. 'Meet Me at the Mag' (Memorial Art Gallery) on Tuesday and there was a lady there who didn't speak, just let out a yelp or a laugh from time to time. It was a bit eerie. I was talking to her daughter after the tour and asked if she had Alzheimer's or one of the other dementias. She said that her mother was originally diagnosed with Alzheimer's by her neurologist, but then was seen by Dr. D. He thought she had 'primary progressive aphasia' which is one of Ralph's possible diagnoses. That was a little hard to digest even though I know the outcome, as you do. Anyway, on the way home Ralph asked what was wrong with that lady. I said, "She has Alzheimer's, she's just a little bit farther down the road."

I can't wait 'til we go to the sex seminar. What's with the guys and their constant kissing? I know I should appreciate it but I can't pass him by without ending in a clutch. Do you suppose they're just afraid we'll leave them without support? Or, are they really that horny? I keep getting hints about 'what he really wants' but it's so hard these days. It's so tough switching from caregiver to lover. What to do? I hope we can get together either before or after the session for a talk.

Well, we just got back from a mile walk around the trail near here, supper's cooking, Ralph's napping, I have a glass of wine, and all is well for now. Love to you both.

Vicky to Ann

Jim constantly kisses, but he doesn't ever ask for sex anymore because he knows he can't perform. It seems like the testosterone has gone out of him. I don't know whether he feels like sex but just doesn't ask, or that the interest isn't there. Is not doing it at all better than trying and failing?

Seeing the woman at the MAG would depress me, but not everyone is the same, right? Keep your hopes up! At least we have each other to complain to about our troubles. It really does help me a lot to know I can whine or growl to you when I am annoyed. It seems there's always something wrong too...the dry eyes or the ingrown nail, or something else.

But today was beautiful and I gardened for a bit (while golf was on) so that satisfied me. Also coffee Frappuccino ice cream with chocolate chunks lifted my spirits too. Hugs to you both.

04/11/2010
Ann to Vicky
Eden

This afternoon we went out for a ride and ended up around Buffalo Rd. and Union St. There is a new senior campus there based on the Eden Alternative Theory which is supposed to be the next best thing for senior care. We toured one of the 4 houses. It's quite lovely. A large living room, dining room, huge kitchen, and 12 bedrooms. No long hallways. There is always staff for meds, baths, and general care. Food sounds good and you can have access to the kitchen to do your own thing if you want. There is a large central courtyard, and patios for each house. Lots of room to walk and garden, if you wish. They accept couples, dementia and non-dementia alike. Trouble is, I can't imagine the non-demented (me, for now) hanging around as much. There is a lot of obvious dementia there. Ralph would be free to come and go as he wished as long as I was with him. Just like now. He asked a lot of questions and seemed interested but on the way home he quietly said, "I'll commit suicide before I live like that." Oh, boy. I told him not to worry, I didn't think we could afford anything close and when he needs more help, I'll hire it like Jane did. Of course, that makes tons more work for me, but I'm sure he wasn't thinking of that.

So, we stopped for ice cream, came home, had supper, and now I'm so depressed I'm going to watch *The Diary of Anne Frank* on Masterpiece Theater to cheer me up. Love and hugs.

04/12/2010
Vicky's Journal
Camaraderie Among Caregivers

Having someone who knows and who has been there is a very important thing. You immediately bond because they know what you have experienced, how hard it is, and how you just have to keep going. Even if your marriage is VERY strong, as I feel mine is, there are still times that you would like to scream at the top of your lungs! None of us really has the choice of opting out of the situation.

I attend support group every month for an hour and a half. Each person generally gets a chance to speak as to how their month went. Sometimes if one person has a problem and needs more time to talk it through and get input from the group, others have to sacrifice some time, but not everyone needs time to unload. Some months are just 'the same.' These sessions are not gloom and doom. We laugh a lot about things that have happened to each other. Somehow being all together allows us to step back a bit and laugh at tragedy…it's a 'sick humor' society that we all understand.

A relatively new caregiver of our group was talking with me, and I was describing how Jim doesn't know what he is eating or how to eat it…she said to me…"Great! Feed him something inexpensive and keep the good stuff for you…and you'll save on the cost!" She didn't really mean it, but you have to laugh because if you don't, you'll cry or get depressed. It makes these new behaviors more trivial, and helps us move on and not dwell on them. It helps to voice them to someone who knows. It's beneficial for those of us who have not experienced something yet, because when we do experience it, if we do, we can accept it as par for the course and not something earth shattering.

In a way, support group is 'doing our homework.' You join when a loved one has just been diagnosed, and stay until you no longer need support or can't leave home to come. Attending lectures and reading books about people with Alzheimer's also helps. It gives some peace, staves off anxiety, stress, and fear about what might happen down the road. Getting knowledge beforehand helps prepare me for the future, gives me confidence, and allows me the ability to put thoughts on the back burner and focus on today. It helps me to live each day the best that I can. Doing as much as I can beforehand helps me to deal with the unknown. I have read a lot of Alzheimer's books, attended lectures, prepared our legal papers, and have even interviewed the major nursing homes in the area so that I already know which ones I would want to use, if necessary. It is well known that with this disease, you think you are OK, and all of a sudden you are in a tail spin and the person with the disease has to be placed. At that crucial time when there is no time to conduct interviews, it's nice to know which one you would choose. Even less urgent decisions about needing senior day care or getting help in the home can be made more thoughtfully by listening to what others in the group say about places they are using.

04/14/2010
Vicky to Ann
Possible Title and Why I Chose It

When thinking about writing a book about our experiences, I came up with the title Laughter in a Straight Jacket. It was a mental image that I had of a caregiver in a straight jacket...the jacket preventing her from laughing uncontrollably and out loud, she was just quietly shaking as she laughed silently.

Many of us have situations where, if you take a few steps back, or maybe you don't even have to, the situation seems quite funny. But you don't laugh, you hold it in until you are with people who are dealing with the same disease...and then you share. And laughter comes quite easily instead of tears or the dread that you felt when you were in the circumstance. You laugh because you've all been there, and those of you laughing don't mean to be cruel and uncaring...but the whole scenario is so 'out there' and absurd that you can't help but laugh. And laughter is certainly better than crying. It's a cathartic experience. Laughter and tears are very close together on the emotional scale, and one can lead to the other.

There are many serious sides to having Alzheimer's or one of the related dementias, and it certainly isn't all fun and games being a caregiver. It is one of the hardest things you can do in your life. But if you can do it the best way you know how, and utilize the advantages in your community, you can make it through and have no regrets. You did your best.

What do you think?

Ann to Vicky

I like your analogy. It says it all but I wonder if anyone other than a caregiver would 'get' it. I know we've talked about this and I also wonder if a book will ever be a reality. I know we're gathering a lot of data.

Nothing much new here. Days start out pretty normal but anything out of the ordinary throws Ralph for a loop. He was fine this morning so around noon I decided to leave him here and go food shopping. I was almost ready to check out when Brian called and said he had just called his dad and Ralph sounded quite confused. When I got home it took him 10 minutes to tell me about some phone call that he didn't understand and didn't know what to do. That's all it takes to screw him up. Anyway, Brian took him to Springwater and then to Hassan's horseback riding lesson (I kept Aisha) and all was OK again. However, he told me tonight that he's been seeing more people lately, but was afraid to tell me. I have a feeling Dr. D. will want to put him on a higher dose of Seroquel, and that's going to knock him out. He's been out walking more and I hate to see him sleeping a lot again. What to do? These apparitions don't seem to scare him but he is bothered by them and well he should be. It's funny. You talk about your 'new normal,' and that's how I feel about all our visitors. As I was pulling out of the driveway today, he said he thought there were two people in the back seat. I asked if they were male or female. He said female and I said, "Too bad." Later, I thought how odd to be so blasé about hallucinations. Again, the new normal. Where will it end?

04/15/2010
Vicky's Journal
The Long Haul

Early on in the disease, I thought that I would escape this terribly long and lonely journey. I thought Jim would end his life as he had talked, and that I would be able to go on. I knew after it was over that I would be deeply saddened to be without him, truly alone in this world…my life's partner gone. (Jim and I are proponents of euthanasia for those people going through this disease when they feel that the time is right. It is such an awful disease for the afflicted to know and see their losses as they happen. We have watched enough family die of this disease.) But I wanted to try living a life on my own. Jim told me recently he wouldn't be able to commit suicide.

I wanted time to myself to read a bunch of good books, or go shopping for an entire afternoon, to go for a long walk, to feel the cool air again and the sunshine and be at peace. But it seems I am doomed to spend the rest of my life being a caretaker to someone who is disappearing day by day. He is someone who can't interact with me…who can't challenge me in a positive way, or share in the things that I love to do. Although I love Jim and am devoted to him, my life is becoming so alone. At night I wait for the time when he goes to bed so I can do what I want to do…sit and watch my types of programs on TV as much as I want. When Jim is up, he is bored with the shows I watch. So I let him watch what interests him. I want to travel and see the places in the US I have never seen. I want to see the Grand Canyon, Bryce, the Rockies, Cape Cod, Maine. I don't want to spend the last 20 years of my life, or 10 anyway, taking care of him instead of living. It's so confining. Jim is so healthy even though he has lived 17 years with the disease, he could live another 10 easily at home…and how much money will we have in the end? I just don't know and it's scary!

Now, it's April and the 'suicide' thing is on…travel is off…except to go visit Kip in New Hampshire. Jim is such a sweet man, though. I love to think about the days when we were first in love, how exciting it all was. I would not change anything about marrying him again, except that it would have been so much fun not to have the disease around…or would it? Would we have become as close as we are now? We share our feelings more now.

04/17/2010
Ann to Vicky
Nothing Much New

We haven't e-talked in a while and I'm wondering if you and/or Jim are going to support group on Tuesday. We'll be there. I don't know about Ralph, but I need it. I feel things are changing too quickly and I'm not dealing well with it all. I find I'm more angry and I feel guilty about it because I know he can't help the decline, and I finally figured why I'm so pissed off. There were many things I wanted done around the house and now it's too late. He's trying to clean out and moves at a snail's pace, and I can't stand to watch. He'll ask me what he can do for me, and I give him the simplest task and he screws it up. I want to smack him and I can't. Now that I've written it down I realize I don't want to share this with the group. Just you for now.

This week hasn't been a total loss. We took Aisha to the zoo Thursday. We were there for 4 hours and Ralph was good about pulling her in the wagon, but he was awfully tired when we got home. Aisha had been asking for an overnight so I figured Thurs. was good because she was tired from her big day. It worked out well. She never moved all night. Yesterday, she went to dance class with me but, of course, wouldn't talk to everyone who was fawning over her. I told her on the way home that even though she's shy, she must answer people when they ask her a question: name, age, siblings, etc. She said she didn't mind answering one person at a time but "I don't like to be surrounded." I love her use of language and she is my sanity saver. I'm beginning to realize it's easier to chat with her than with her grandpa. How sad.

I got an e-mail from Grace from group yesterday. She said the doctor put her husband on Namenda and he's a changed person. Much more alert and interested in life in general and is excited about a trip they plan to take. She said it's hard to believe the difference. I have to tell you, I felt a little jealous and, of course, felt guilty about that. Maybe I'm just a small-minded person and am just realizing it.

Right now the laughter has been minimal but the straight jacket's looking pretty good.

04/17/10
Vicky to Ann
We've Had a Down Week

If you're an awful person, then I am right there with you! I've been meaning to write, but I needed some peace before I started. Earlier in the week I brought up the argument Jim and I have been having forever…I need his acceptance that in the future, when he gets worse (I see almost daily changes) that he agree to have someone in the home with him…and/or his going to senior care 1 day a week to give me time to get things done. He says absolutely not. He asked me to show him how to get to the rec. center on his bike so he would remember. He used to make the trip all the time, but now he can't. I said his perception isn't getting any better, it's only going to get worse, so learning and making proper decisions on his bike was probably not going to happen. He says he sees things exactly the way I do! Here we go again. At least Ralph says he sees things that aren't there. He admits he has problems. I ended up going into another room and calling the Alz. Assoc. to sign up for Caregivers Connect, a grant where they assess the home for safety and do an assessment of Jim, have 5 free therapy sessions…so I can get Jim to agree on having a companion. I decided to scare him about therapy, and he actually got on the phone while I was talking, which was awkward. Today Jim sat me down and said he wasn't being fair to me…so I said, "What does this mean? Did you change your mind about allowing someone in or going to Senior Care?" And he said, "No". So where are we?

His left eye started bothering him today and he insisted that we go to the eye doctor. Of course, it is a weekend again and it's closed. We did a number of things including drops, cold peas compress from the freezer, etc. and then he went to bed (the 6th time the eye has bothered him but there is never anything wrong other than dry eye…it maybe looks a little red…I suggested allergies.) I feel bad that I have been pushing him…I really feel sad and crushed, and asked myself if this all went away and I was by myself, would I want it that way, or would I be devastated because Jim was gone? I don't know. I think I would be unhappy either way. I just don't want to make the choice.

We had company for dinner last night and neither had a clue what we're going through. The husband started explaining how Jim could use a GPS for hiking, or to go to the rec. center...not realizing that he wouldn't even be able to turn it on! The wife asked when we were alone what I do with all my time now that I'm not working! Ugh!

04/18/2010
Ann to Vicky
Eden

I have the card for the person in charge of the Eden style living place in Chili. Do you want me to give her a call and get an idea of costs? I'm sure there will be other 'Edens' popping up perhaps further east. There's also a new concept called 'Green House'. I looked it up and it's the same premise, but the homes are mixed in the community (like group homes) and they try to place the person near their familiar neighborhood. Problem is, I didn't see anything about dementia care, just regular nursing home care. I'll look further when I have a chance. I suspect there's quite a bit on line that I didn't see.

PS: Wouldn't it be funny if all four of us lived together in Eden? The guys would be taken care of and we could go out and carouse all day and come home to a nice dinner someone else fixed. Now, that's what I call Eden!

04/18/2010
Vicky to Ann
He Just Came Home

Earlier today I was gardening in the back yard, and Jim came out of the garage on his bike and told me that he was going to ride his bike to the rec. center by way of the canal, and there was nothing I could do about it. I knew I could not talk him out of it so I reluctantly let him go...as if I could stop him in some way? What was I to do...throw myself in front of his bike? Anyway, he just came home. I was beginning to worry but he said he didn't have any trouble at all. That doesn't mean he won't have trouble in the future. I am so glad...I was worrying about having to call the police or go out looking for him!

Ann to Vicky

I had my computer unplugged so I could take it to Nancy's, but couldn't get online there. I just read your e-mail about Jim on his bike. I'm glad I didn't know. I can picture him riding right into the canal! It's funny because I just had a talk with Ralph at breakfast about his walking any distance. His vision is so poor around the house, that I asked him if he had trouble when out on the road. He said he thought he was seeing and perceiving well outside. I told him that he shouldn't go on West Side Drive, because it's very busy and he shouldn't even think about crossing that road. He went into a long story about where he crosses WSD and how easy it was and he could see oncoming traffic, etc. I gave up. Like Jim, he's going to do what he wants as long as he's able to do it, and I guess we should just let them go, like we did our children. I hope there's a guardian angel specially trained for dementia duty. I really think we're living parallel lives. Rather comforting for now. I, too, think about 'after'. I'm too old and tired to start another relationship. Who wants an old man in their lives? You, on the other hand, are young enough to go on to a new life. I'm sure this sounds cruel and heartless, but it's true. I continue to hope 'after' is a long way off, but what I see day to day tells a different story.

One more thing and then I must get busy and clean this sty. Yesterday, I was diplomatically trying to tell Ralph about the seminar on Thursday. He asked me what it was about. I said "Um, aw, well, it's about spirituality and, er, intimacy." He said, "Great! Maybe they can give you some pointers." I could have throttled him!

04/19/2010
Vicky's Journal
Picking Your Battles

They always say with this disease, as it progresses and behaviors get harder to deal with, pick your battles! Jim has been an easy person to deal with for the first 16 years of the disease, so I really can't say I've had to 'pick my battles' until now. This past winter Jim was feeling cold more than ever. I bought him 2 pairs of silk long underwear that he could wear under his clothes, because even with the thermostat set at 73, it was too cold for him! He graduated to flannel pants that many men wear as pajama bottoms, only Jim would wear them under jeans. He also wears an undershirt, a shirt, and maybe even a sweatshirt, and then sits on the couch in his down vest. More recently, he has insisted on going to bed in his clothes, belt and all. I have tried to encourage him to let me get him some more comfortable clothes for bedtime, but he insists he is comfortable. So I give in and say, "Suit yourself." It's not worth arguing about and making him upset. It won't hurt anyone, so I let it be. The problem is when he doesn't want to shower or take a bath the next day. Then he continues to wear the same clothes. If he showers or bathes, I make sure to lay out all clean clothes. At least it makes me feel better. If I don't get clothes out for him, he gets all confused what clothes are his and what are mine, what goes on first, etc. When I lay his clothes out on the bed, I always have them laid out so underwear is on top, then outer clothing and socks last. Sometimes he goes in my drawers and when he puts on my stuff it's always good for a laugh. If I ask him what he wants to wear, that is too broad a question. Instead, I give him a choice of two shirts and let him pick which one he wants to wear. It gives him a sense of control.

Jim's appetite is not very strong lately. Sometimes he doesn't want to eat. I want lunch, so I go ahead and eat without him. I am watching his weight and he is not suffering. Besides, he likes to eat a pint of cookie dough ice cream every day and after dealing with Alzheimer's, I say he deserves it, so go ahead. Heart disease risk or no...his blood pressure is below normal and his cholesterol is only a little high but not that bad, and if he dies of eating ice cream so be it! One day he came to me and said, "I know a great way to commit suicide". I said, "How?", and he said he would eat ice cream until he died. I said that would take a long time and when he got so fat that it would kill him, I couldn't lift him anyway...that way is not so quick! I don't think that is the way to go.

You Will Never Win an Argument with a Person Suffering from Dementia:

You can't rationalize with them. Don't even try to explain why things are...just agree with them. It saves a lot of energy. That's called "going where they are." If they ask why they don't see their mother (and she passed away years ago), just say that she is on an extended vacation and won't be back for a while. It is less cruel. Jim's mom used to ask us why she didn't see her husband anymore. If we told her that he was dead, she would mourn all over again and, of course, it would be quite upsetting for her. If we told her he was on a big business trip and he would be gone for a few weeks, she accepted it.

Don't try to hurry a person with dementia. It's not possible and just gets them more upset and agitated!

Jim told me recently that he doesn't want to go to support group. His excuse was that his buddies might call and want him to go out...at 6 PM-7:30 PM on a Tuesday night? Not likely! But I should just accept the fact that he didn't want to go and the underlying reasons don't really matter. He may not be able to put into words why he doesn't want to go. I had a hard time listening to his excuses. Mainly, it's because I was worried about leaving him alone. It's almost as if you feel you will be arrested for husband abuse if someone finds out you are leaving him alone and he has dementia. You can have a more fruitful session if you don't have to worry about what your husband is or isn't doing, or if he has wandered away from home while you are out. At that point, for your peace of mind, get someone to sit with him.

04/21/2010
Ann to Dr. D.
Keeping in Touch

Ralph and I will be in to see you on May 26th. However, some things are easier addressed beforehand. While I have done fairly well at arranging our financial affairs and making some order out of our many years in this house in case we have to move, there is one big item still on our 'to do' list. We haven't made what they refer to as 'final arrangements.' I'm going to have to do that while Ralph is still capable of understanding our decisions. We have often talked of anatomical donations to the U of R. It is certainly the easiest and most practical way of handling it. However, Ralph wants to donate his brain at his death. He feels it's important to help in any research that's being done, especially with frontal temporal dementia. We found that we cannot designate that through the U of R program. Could you send me a note or letter stating what should be done at that time to insure you are notified immediately? I'm not putting this well because it's not the stuff I like to think about, but I need something to put in our papers, especially if I should become disabled, or let's face it, dead. There, that wasn't so difficult!

In general, Ralph continues his slow decline. He is having more trouble dressing and he struggles with language. Some days he is more fluent than others. He is walking a lot and Brian, Nancy, and I keep him as active as possible. He enjoys the younger grandchildren, goes to horseback riding lessons with the 8 year old, and he and I recently spent a day at the zoo with the 4 year old. He was very tired from hauling her in the wagon, but it was a good tired. He still hallucinates from time to time, but that has almost become our new normal. He'll ask me if there are people in the front yard, I tell him no, and he's fine with that. I suppose we could put him back on the morning dose of Seroquel, but he has so much more energy without it. His distant vision is fine, but he is having more trouble with near vision, and reading is almost impossible and very frustrating. I will have his eyes checked again before we come in, in case it is the visual acuity. On the positive side, his personality remains intact and he has yet to say or do anything inappropriate. We are all so grateful for that. We're still active in the Alz. Assoc. and even helped make a video for the Memorial Art Gallery about the MAG/Alz. program. As for me, most days I'm OK but tired, and always tell myself to enjoy the day. It's as good as it's going to get. However, there are days when I just want to go outside and scream or, at least, find a Tea Partier to kick.

Thanks for any help you can give us and we'll see you next month.

04/21/2010
Vicky to Ann
Things Are Happening Fast

Wow, things are happening fast! Jim took a walk 'around the block' today while I was washing up the staining brushes for the deck, and later he arrived home in a gold car. He had walked down our street, and ended up three streets away. He saw a man outside and asked him to take him home. And yet he still insists that riding his bike is a different story and that he knows how to go on his bike! Now, does that make any sense at all?

He asked me the topic for the talk tomorrow, and I told him, "Spirituality and Intimacy." He asked if he could go, and I said "NO." I said when they talk about intimacy, and I want to ask a question, I don't want my partner to be there ... I would feel funny. I told him I would fill him in when I got home.

He's much more repetitive with the questions. I will answer and not 5 seconds later he asks the same question again. We went to supermarket today after going to the rec. center to work out, and when we got to the parking lot he just sat there and opened the window. I asked if he was going to come in as he usually does, and he said, "Oh, I thought we were home." So he came in and shopped with me (pushed the basket.) While I was putting things on the conveyor, he said he would walk around and meet me at the other side of the cashier. I finished putting things up to be scanned and looked up and there was no Jim. He must have walked right out of the store. I thought, gee maybe he went home with some other woman! Then I went out after paying and he was in the parking lot looking all over (at the opposite end to where we parked) for the car. I yelled to him and he didn't really know it was me because I had my hair pulled back. I had to yell a number of times to get him to come to me. See, if you want to lose your husband, just change your hairstyle. No one has ever brought that up in support group.

Ann to Vicky

It's amazing how I can smile while feeling so sad about our guys, but you're right. It's easier to lose a husband than we ever thought, and no, that won't be talked about at support. I do feel, though, that you and I brought a lighter note to last night's proceedings.

Now, let me tell you how my Wednesday went. It started off as a pretty good day. I met a friend for coffee in the morning and Ralph was fine at home. In fact, a friend called and when I called her back later she said she had a great talk with Ralph and he talked with no problem at all. Of course, she couldn't leave it at that. She added that perhaps he got nervous when talking to me because I talk and think so fast it might intimidate him. I was speechless and just said, "Well, do you want him?" which was stupid but I couldn't think of anything else ... Anyway, at 6:00 we were leaving to meet Brian and his family at the rec. center. Shino and I had signed up for a yoga class and Brian, Ralph and the kids were going swimming. As Ralph opened the passenger side door, he misjudged the space and the corner of the door caught him just below the eye. It didn't look as if it needed stitches so I ice packed him and we took off. Shino and I took our class, the kids swam, and Brian took care of his Dad. When we got home, I realized one lens of his glasses was almost out and the frame crooked so we're going to have to get them fixed before the seminar. I think I'll make it O.K., but keep your phone on. Meanwhile, he's been a bit disoriented since we got home. I gave him a couple of Tylenol and he's sleeping. I'm sure he'll be better in the morning but it's amazing how traumatic a relatively minor event can be.

04/22/2010
Vicky to Ann
Spirituality, Intimacy, and Sexuality

[Setting the Stage] Ann and I went to this seminar held at an assisted living home for people with dementia. We walk in and we are the only two people there. We wait for others to arrive, and no one else comes! We introduce ourselves, and the speaker immediately assumes we are mother and daughter. There are 14 years between us, but Ann looks very young for her age. We correct him, gulp. Then we discover we are the only two (we thought we would have others to help us broach the subject matter) and say in our minds, "Aw hell, we are here to learn about all this, so we might as well take advantage of the situation."

I was impressed by the seminar leader. I think because it was just the two of us, we received a lot of attention, and although it would have been good to hear other people's problems and possible answers, at least we had our upper most questions addressed. In the next week I will have to write a summary of the things I need to work on like quality unpressured time with Jim, and trying to make him feel good more often. For example: use of cologne, buying some updated clothes, etc. I buy things for myself online, but he always says he doesn't need anything.

Perhaps an earring or a tattoo? What do you think?

Sorry I couldn't spend some time after the talk with you ... It's the story of our lives, isn't it?

Give your Ralph a pat for me!

Ann to Vicky

Dear Daughter,

I liked him too, but I can't forgive him for that hurtful remark. I guess this disease is aging me more than Ralph. First, the woman in the bagel shop calling me Mama, and then the speaker. Seriously though, I thought I would be uncomfortable but I wasn't. I didn't feel ill at ease at all, but imagine if you or I were alone with him. That seems a little creepy. All in all, I thought it went well and when Ralph got home the first thing he said was, "Well, how did it go? Tell me what you talked about." I pretty much covered it as best I could and talked about the non-sexual intimacy ideas which I, too, will try to work harder on.

Don't worry about having to dash off. I was going to stop at Nancy's, but when I called she was still at work. She said she had errands to run before going home but then decided to do them another time, and we met at the Italian restaurant in Pittsford Plaza for a glass of wine and an appetizer. Then I went to the bookstore to browse to my heart's content. It was heaven, but I was happy then to spend the evening with my loved one. A little respite goes a long way.

Earring maybe. Tattoo, no. I think they're such a turn off. Time for bed. Aisha tomorrow. Love and hugs to you both, even if Jim doesn't remember me. I think he really does but was a little distracted the other night.

PS. The more I think about it, the more surprised I am that we were the only ones. I thought a lot of folks would be interested, unless most couples dealing with dementia are a lot older.

04/22/2010
Vicky's Journal
Intimacy, Sexuality, and Spirituality

We all discuss a lot of things in support group, but one thing that never seems to be discussed is sex. Our support group has both men and women in it, and many would find it uncomfortable with a mixed sex group. The questions linger though, and so finally I decided to 'present my case' and see if there were others who would be willing to share who had similar problems in support group. It is also important to present it here in the book, because I have not read one book having to do with Alzheimer's that broached the subject!

Jim and I married in 1969, right in the middle of the sexual revolution. Our parents were very conservative, and sex was not talked about in our house much. I learned where babies came from at about age 8 when a friend told me, while on the swings at a local playground. She had read it in an article in Readers Digest. I believed her, but I thought the whole idea was utterly disgusting. I'm never going to do that!

When I was old enough to be taught about menstruation, I watched a movie in Girl Scouts (with our mother's permission) made by the manufacturer of sanitary napkins. Mom didn't really sit down with me to explain everything. She just asked if I had any questions. After that, some prior incidents that I caught a glimpse of became clear. A few

Thanksgivings prior, Mom was looking for more dinner napkins and having seen the sanitary napkins in the bathroom closet, I brought them out to show her. Although she must have been surprised, she kept her cool and said she didn't want to use those, to put them back. I think it was before company arrived though!

The week before Jim and I were married, Mom tried giving me the marriage-sex talk, but by then I knew as much or more than Mom would have told me. Despite being in the middle of the free love era, Jim and I didn't have sex until we were married. Of course, I didn't find out Jim was a virgin until Kip was a young adult. I guess Jim wanted to maintain the aura of a man who knew what to do.

Jim is now 62 and is in his 17th year of Alzheimer's. About a year and a half ago we started having trouble having sex in the traditional sense. At 61 I am post-menopausal, and so vaginal dryness may be of concern, but even with lubricators, things weren't working. I felt it was the effect of Alzheimer's. Jim just couldn't put the 'car in the garage' so to speak. I had the feeling that he didn't quite know what to do. We decided to please each other manually, and continued without much problem until about 5 months ago. Jim began to have more trouble reaching orgasm and sometimes couldn't maintain an erection. We then mentioned the problem to our family doctor.

After doing blood tests for testosterone etc., everything came back normal. She had us try a manual pump that creates a vacuum around the penis, thereby allowing the capillaries of the penis to fill with blood to make it erect. A synthetic band is placed at the base of the penis to maintain the erection while having sex. Then it is removed to allow the penis to deflate. This device has to be used daily to start to get the penis used to the feeling of erection again in order for it to get hard enough for penetration. I must say, that using that contraption with a dementia person takes a real 'hands on' approach by the caregiver. You have to have a good relationship with your spouse to do this! By the time we were ready for sex the 'atmosphere' was just too clinical and the arousal had all but dried up. Besides, when I placed the ring on ... Jim complained that it hurt too much no matter what size we tried! We decided that method wasn't for us. It was cheaper to try this than to use pharmaceuticals. Later we did try three different prescriptions, but to no avail.

Jim was disappointed, but he didn't seem as bothered as I thought he'd be. I do know for Jim, his penis was one of the things about his body that he was most in awe of ... when asked once if he had cancer of the penis therefore making removal a must, he said he'd rather die of cancer.

He offered to please me if I wanted, but most times we would just lie down together, hold each other close, and reminisce about the past ... So here we are, two people who love each other, not having sex anymore, but trying to preserve some closeness anyway. I think that is so important for both of us. Each feels loved, and it reminds me why I am in this caregiver role. Jim is so utterly sweet and loving, attentive, and cares for me. Even now, he tells me many times a day how much he loves me. And I try to do the same for him.

No one could say for certain, but I felt that his inability was linked to his dementia. Sex is 50/50 physical and mental. We all tell ourselves things while having sex, and if you don't have enough memory to fantasize how can you possibly be successful? Our neurologist thought my ideas made sense.

So as you know, we signed up for the program, and ended up the only two there. What we learned from the discussion was helpful in directing me towards some areas of our relationship that I had let slide, with so much of my time taken up by caregiving and housekeeping. Both Ann and I expressed that being in the caregiver or 'mother' role so much of our day and facing the declines in our spouses from knowledgeable, capable, independent beings makes it hard to then switch gears and change to the lover role. It was more than just being tired. I see my husband in a different light now and part of lovemaking was relishing the protector, proficient lover, the virile man that embodied him. The memory loss gets in the way and the spontaneous abandon isn't there.

The presenter encouraged us to work on increasing the self-esteem of our partners. At a time when each step of life is so difficult, it makes sense that they need and crave some feelings of self-worth. They want to feel needed and valued. Some ways to boost their morale is to make sure they are well groomed ... showered, shaved, dressed nicely, and have a haircut periodically. We should complement their appearance, and their choice of clothes for the day (even if we picked them.) I thought of putting some cologne on Jim occasionally because I love to smell cologne on men! That would help me to focus on the man/woman relationship rather than the caregiver/care-partner one. I do like to see Jim look handsome when we go out, but I have to get him ready with some aplomb, or he becomes resistive about changing his clothes for something more suitable for the specific occasion. He expresses that he doesn't care how he looks. So I must make a more concerted effort to dress him well and compliment the image.

Besides setting aside tasks that they can do for us, we need to show that we are glad they are here ... by physical contact. A touch of the hand as we go by, an unexpected hug, or just sitting next to each other and stroking a hand, or holding hands. All throughout our marriage Jim would tap me on the rear as he went by or as I passed him, and I would do the same. We called it a 'love tap.' That has not stopped with the dementia. Since I had 3 discs fused in my neck a number of years ago, Jim has been giving me neck rubs to ease my muscle tension. Over the years, he has developed into quite a good masseur.

If we have a leisurely day ahead, I may crawl in bed with him (we have 2 twin beds pushed together and covered as a king) and we will hold each other and reminisce about how wonderful our dating years were, how we were so attracted to each other, and how we wanted to spend every waking moment with each other. During those times I would always tell Jim that even if I knew he would get Alzheimer's later in life, I would still make the same choice again, I would marry him. I know that made him feel more secure, and Jim always seemed happier after those mornings. That replaced sex for us.

I know it is important to do activities together that we both like. It serves many purposes. I can be Jim's memory and remember what we have done together, but also I naturally act as Jim's liaison to whatever we are doing or with people we meet. Jim and I have been fairly active during our marriage: hiking, camping, water skiing, scuba diving, snow skiing, and biking), I always try to provide Jim with two activities during the week. Now these include golf, bowling, canoeing, and hiking. We once biked together on the Erie Canal path, but that is a bit risky for Jim now because of his perceptual problems of where the path is and who may be coming in the opposite direction or passing from behind. Golf is becoming more difficult, but we have a 9-hole golf course near us where we can go at odd hours and progress on our own with little worry of holding up the other golfers. (It's very labor intensive for me because I have to remember where his ball is every moment). For other activities I have to do the planning and packing if that is required, but it's worth it to see Jim have fun! Most of our activities are outside, and so they connect us with nature which is soothing and peaceful. Nature is our religion in a sense. Although we were both raised as Presbyterian, we have grown away from organized religions. We like to say that we are AWEIST (a word brought to our attention by Ann) after the words of Phil Zuckerman. Aweism is the belief that existence is ultimately a beautiful mystery, that being alive is a wellspring of wonder, and that the deepest questions of life, death, time, and space are so powerful as to inspire deep feelings of joy, poignancy, and sublime awe ... in his words. This is our form of spirituality. We believe in the goodness of the human being, and that we should help our fellow man. If we live right, then we will live well with a sense of satisfaction and peace. For us, there is no reward of heaven when life is over.

Most people probably believe in God whether they practice religion or not, and if they belong to a church, that is one of the most wonderful support systems they can have available to them. It refreshes them and provides them with helpful parishioners, and a reason to keep going. Religion helps people to feel connected and have social support. It fosters respect and compassion, and allows them to be a contributing part of something greater than themselves.

While we are on the subject of sex, I'm sure many have heard that some people suffering from dementia may elicit bold sexual behaviors such as fondling themselves or exposing themselves in public. This is not a common occurrence, but it can happen. The person still feels the excitement of the act but does not have the filters that stop such behavior, because the plaques and tangles may have destroyed the area where the inhibition resides.

05/23/2010
Vicky to Ann
Shavers and Other Drama

I forgot to tell you that Friday I had to go out and buy Jim another shaver! He says he can't use this one anymore because every time he uses it he coughs, like he's breathing in the whiskers. It could be, because I do hear him coughing when he shaves. I clean and empty the shaver daily, but that doesn't stop the coughing. There was nothing I could do but agree to buy him another shaver ... a different brand.

Also, I printed some pictures of the people we would be calling for the picture phone including myself, Kip, and the two friends that take Jim out weekly. I presented the pictures to Jim (the size they will be on the phone) and he didn't recognize any of them including me! I forgot to tell you that while we were in Florida and at the pool (I had a scarf on my hair,) I walked into the pool towards him and he said, "So where do you originally come from?" And I said, "Look closely, I am your wife!" Then he made some poor excuse as to why he doesn't recognize me.

I was very good today. This morning, I made French toast and I asked Jim to pour orange juice for both of us. While pouring, he dropped the carton and it splashed all over the counter, toaster, and upper cabinet. But I just said, "Bring over the waste basket", and I cleaned up with paper towels, and said, "Want to pour that glass again?" I'm slowly learning to bite my tongue!

Jim's birthday dinner went well tonight, but he was exhausted by the time everyone left (9:45). He told me our friends talk about things he doesn't understand. It's not that they are insensitive. It's just hard for them to realize when he has lost the gist of the conversation. He said there were too many people (3).

Ann to Vicky

What do you suppose is up with all the shaver drama with these guys? Ralph still thinks we should take his shaver back and get it fixed. I reminded him that we did take it back and the salesman said it just needed cleaning. I discovered that he was using some kind of cream that clogged it big time, so I took it all apart and soaked the top parts in water and detergent and now it works perfectly. Do you think maybe Jim is using some kind of lotion that makes him cough?

It's been a fairly quiet weekend. Friday night we went out to dinner at a nearby golf club with another couple. Things went smoothly until we went up to the soup and salad bar. I got my salad, took it back to the table and went back to help Ralph. He was OK 'til we got to the end and he tried to take the crouton bowl back to the table. When I got that away from him he did the same thing with the bowl of bacon bits. He doesn't even use either item. The whole event made me decide for sure that we're not going to the posh Baltimore wedding for my niece's son.

I was going to write a letter to Dr. D. (neurologist) but as I reviewed my notes from last time I realized nothing has changed, they're just a little worse. I mainly want to know how he feels about Ralph staying alone. Maybe I don't want to know.

I'm off to watch an Agatha Christie mystery with my dear, confused husband.

06/01/2010
Vicky to Ann
Companion

I am ecstatic! Brian M. (the companion) says that he was doing computer work with his Dad and got tired of no human contact so took on working for a home health agency. He seems really nice and responded well to Jim. They went to Mendon Ponds Park for a walk, a long chat, and a trip to Ben and Jerry's for ice cream. They had a really good time. Jim was so happy that I called the owner and Jim told him how great Brian M. was. Jim is so pleased, and he's all excited about going to the gym next time.

How quickly my mood can turn around. After they left, I felt like yelling to the roof tops that I was free! Call me Helen Reddy.

Hope things are OK with you. You probably had a busy holiday weekend so maybe you're tired. REMEMBER to take care of yourself!

Ann to Vicky

I was going to write to you last night but I was too tired. I was going to give you heartfelt sympathy after your note about Jim slipping. Now I can rejoice with you about the turn-around. I have to go to an extra rehearsal this morning so I'll keep this short. Dr. D. said that Ralph should not be alone for more than an hour at a time. Brian can't be here until noon today and I'll be gone from 10-2:30 so he'll be alone for at least 2 hours. I'm already worrying and I'm probably going to stop doing shows.

Glad things are looking up for you.

06/02/2010
Vicky to Ann
Ups and Downs

Today, Jim held the ladder while I got up on the roof to hose down all the blossoms from the locusts and get everything cleaned up for the summer, cleaning skylights, gutters, etc. It took me quite a while and Jim disappeared. I spent at least 10 minutes beating on the metal helmet guard for the gutters so he could come hold the ladder while I climbed back down, but no show. I know he heard me because I heard him trying to get the lock undone on the sliding door, but he never came out to check what the racket was! I finally climbed down by myself, and went in and yelled at him for not coming to check what the racket was all about. I thought he would be mad at me or hurt because I yelled at him. After cleaning up the debris from the roof, I went inside and Jim was just sitting on the couch without the TV on, and looking off into space. I asked him if he was mad, and did he want to talk ... and there was no answer so I said, "Fine, I'm going to shower." So I did and came out and sat down and asked if he wanted to talk now ... and he looked straight at me with a slight smile on his face and still didn't say anything. After I went into the kitchen he said quietly that he wanted lunch and wanted to go to the rec. center. But he acted in slow motion, dopey like. I think this is going to be the new norm. I gave him two Ritalin and off we went to the rec. center. He seemed better tonight, but he was the worst I'd ever seen him. He couldn't even figure out how to put his shoes on. He wore one shoe and one slipper. I am glad I got the companion, but I'm going to have to get a sitter to be with him too. Going out to the movies is no longer possible without a sitter.

By the way, while we were eating lunch, he asked what the other people were doing in the house. I said, "Where are they?", and he pointed to the other side of the living room. So I guess the hallucinations have started too.

Ann to Vicky

Oh boy! We're going to have to start taking Dramamine. All the U-turns and ups and downs are making me dizzy. And how come you thought he was mad when you were the one taking a risk coming down that ladder? It's so easy for us to feel guilty about everything these days, isn't it? I sometimes feel I'm not doing anything right and yet, deep down, I know I am. Is that making sense?

I went to the dance studio this morning (I belong to a performing tap group) and luckily Brian was here by 11:30. Everything was OK, but I hate to depend so much on Brian even though he seems to want to help. I'm very lucky to have a supportive family to rely on.

Dr. D. is trying to find something to help the hallucinations. He says there is a new drug that could help, but Ralph would have to have blood tests every week, and then every other week and so on. He thought out loud for a while and then decided to try an additional Namenda mid-day. Now, Ralph is giving me a hard time about taking it. He can't understand why he needs it and insists it's already causing some itchy spots on his face and arms. I've seen three and I think they're mosquito bites. Good grief. How come Job didn't have Alzheimer's along with his locusts and boils? That would have cured his patience. Or his wife's. While Ralph was insisting tonight that he didn't need any more meds, I went into the living room. He hollered in to me, "Is Ann in there with you?" I replied, "Yes, she's here" and let the matter drop.

We went to 'Voices' yesterday and then to a bed and breakfast tour in Mumford. (Another outing sponsored by the Alz. Assoc.) A very nice day. The Voices partners chatted in the library. I can't believe how many dementia folks are still driving! Very scary.

I'm so sorry your high didn't last very long. Do you think Jim will be OK for lunch next Monday? If you think we should cancel, let me know. Trouble is, will things be any better next week? Let's hope Monday is a go.

06/04/2010
Vicky to Ann
Easy and Quiet

Today I could pretend that life is what it was a few weeks ago. We are taking things easier. Pretty soon we will be sleeping all day, getting up for dinner, and going to bed.

Jim is anxious for Brian M. (his companion) to come again...a good sign. Still have to make some calls about senior sitting but don't want to do it in front of him or where he can hear me. Will have to wait for a better time.

06/06/2010
Ann to Vicky
More Normal Day

I know what you mean about easy and quiet leading to a more normal behavior. Yesterday, we went to an American Craftsmen show at an art center in Lockport. Ralph was fine on the ride out. After walking around the center for an hour and a half he was a bit confused. He was able to rest on the way back, but when we stopped about half way home for supper, he was totally befuddled. He kept asking me when the rest of our party was coming, who was that driving the car, and who was in the backseat. It was obvious to the waitress because he had so much trouble deciding what he wanted and how to eat it when he got it. She was very sweet and patient. When we were leaving, he started to go into another room instead of out the door and she said to me; "It must be very difficult." I was taken aback because I didn't know it was that obvious and said something like, "I wish people could see him as he was." She said, "I know, but you are doing a wonderful job." I thought I was going to cry. I was so stressed after driving 150 or so miles and dealing with the delusions, I treated myself to two glasses of wine when we got home.

Anyway, I slept until 10:00 this morning. We have just been relaxing all day and he is like his old self. I know what you mean about sleeping all day, getting up for supper, and then going to bed. It may be boring but it makes for calmer dementia folk.

Ralph still wants to travel a bit, though, so I'm going to look into some short overnight jaunts. He needs shorter days and even though I'm doing the driving, I think it's all just too much stimulation for his compromised brain.

He's taking a nap now so I'm going to pay the month's bills and start supper.

Hugs back atcha and we'll see you both tomorrow at 1:30.

Vicky to Ann

Thanks for the note. At least today was better for you.

Jim gets bored at home, but gets very tired if we do too much. My dream is to go to Nantucket or the Florida panhandle (before the oil spill) by myself or with a friend after all this is said and done and just go out for meals, read good books, walk the beach and collect shells, and look in shops. And have wine every night looking at the shore. That's what keeps me going. I fantasize about that. I know in reality I might get bored, but then that would be a change of pace. Right?

06/12/2010
Ann to Vicky
Please Pass the Dramamine

Nothing spectacular is going on but I want to dash off a quick note while Ralph is at the market with Brian and the kids.

Ralph was calm, stable and alert on Mon. Tues. and Wed. Then, on Thursday everything changed. Total confusion reigned. Yesterday, he insisted he was OK staying alone while I went to dance class. Then, he was doing something that I thought would embarrass him. He was trying to put two almost dead roses in a plastic bag for me to give to Marion (one of my dance buddies). I said something about it not being a good idea and he flew completely off the handle.

Shouted to me that I never give him even an inch of independence and why do I have to butt into everything. He was hurt and I was hurt because I had spent the morning trying to make sure he was in touch with someone (neighbor, Brian, etc.) while I was gone. We were both very upset when I left. I cried all the way to class and started to turn around twice, but decided I should go and hope all would be OK while I was gone. He was OK when I returned but said I had really hurt him, and I said I was sorry but he had hurt me too. I can't let it all be about him and his feelings. As it turned out, Marion was thrilled with her roses. After Ralph had stalked off, I put a wet paper towel in a baggie with the flowers and then I noticed there were four little buds ready to open. I guess he wasn't being silly after all. Don't know why I'm going on so but you're the only one who would understand.

Also, it got me thinking that it's true I may be worrying too much. I've got to give him a little more independence, i.e. staying alone and if something happens, so be it. I'll still do the best I can to keep him safe, but I can't keep taking away his feeling of normalcy. I think you know what I'm trying to say. I guess I have to go where he is. Like, ignoring the fact that he can't figure out which toothbrush is his. I tell him it's the green one. Now, I have 3 green toothbrushes in the holder (I'm not sure where they all came from but the dental office gives us new ones every time we visit), my yellow brush, and Aisha has a pink brush with a cover on it. So, of course, last night he used the pink one. I threw it out and didn't say anything.

Love to you both.

Vicky to Ann

I know exactly where you're coming from. The last few days Jim and I have walked around the neighborhood and he keeps noticing that the street is all 'alligator' cracked in many places but the surface has not yet cracked up enough that big chunks are missing. He said that we should go around and get signatures to force the town to resurface the road. Yes, the road is cracked, but since there are no pot holes I said they probably have worse streets to do before doing ours. The cracks were caused by the heavy logging trucks that they've used for the ice storm and the Labor Day microburst. I told Jim I was not going to spend my time drawing up a letter and going around to neighbors' homes, when I had other things to do. So he said he would walk around and speak to the neighbors. Well, I was really worried about this because I thought he would look foolish, especially since his language skills are not the greatest lately. I didn't want to tell him that, though. I keep hoping that he will forget about it. Friday, he said he wanted to walk around the block by himself, and I said ... "Don't go door to door about your paving idea, because people are at work and you won't find most people home" ... so he came in. I don't want people to think ... "Who is this guy?" Not everyone knows him and knows he has Alzheimer's. He gets on these kicks and won't let them go! He also knows our friends are going to Alaska for two weeks and he says "Why don't they ask us to go?" I said, "Because you have become very anxious when they've asked us to go previously, and we had to back out" (this was years ago.) Then he obsesses about why he reacted that way, that he's better, and wouldn't do that now.

Jim is also much more emotional. If he watches *Dr. G. Medical Examiner* he cries for the dead person. He turns off a program if it has any swearing, and he won't watch *Law and Order SVU* because of the abuse. And he complains incessantly about the news continually covering the oil spill, and wants to change the channel all the time. Ugh!

You are not the only one who gets dumped on emotionally. We try to protect them, but they don't know that is what we are doing. They only see it as stifling their independence, and yet we don't want them to be hurt.

I look more and more to the days when I won't have to go through this anymore, but I know I have a long, long way to go. I also know having my independence and being alone won't be so great either ... waking up and having no one to cook for or eat meals with or watch the news with...even though they don't answer or comment much ... it's still a being you share things with.

Jim is coming to support group Tuesday, to complain about how come there are no new programs about Alzheimer's lately. He wants to make sure people don't forget. He's getting to be a little old man who complains about everything!

Note the time. (3:07 AM) ... I can't sleep ... don't know why.

06/16/2010
Vicky to Ann
Emotions

Discussing emotions and outbursts in group yesterday makes so much sense when looking at it after the fact when no emotions are in play. But when I am in the thick of things it's terribly difficult not to let my emotions enter into the 'battle.'

And I'm not really sure that therapeutic fibs will work because Jim may 'call me' on what I say that might not really be true! How do we know they won't have a 'flight into reality' and know the real truth when we try to smooth over the falsehoods?

Jim gets mad at me frequently because I am demeaning to him in my tone of voice ... and it's hard for me to catch it. I feel that I'm trying to be patient, and I almost never pick up on my tone before it's too late to change it. I feel so conflicted sometimes that I welcome his loud snoring so I can go and sleep in Kip's room rather than be in the same room with him. It's like my little haven away from it all. But then I feel guilty because our marriage is basically sound and I don't like what it means when someone tells you that they are sleeping in separate bedrooms. I don't even sleep in the same bed with Jim like you and Ralph do. We have separate twin beds pushed together with a king spread on it.

Emotions, emotions, emotions! Why is it we are not supposed to have any but they can? And why is it we have to adapt to their idiosyncrasies? I know ... because they can't. Ugh.
Going through a lot of changes.

- Scheduled the putting in of paddle fans in two bedrooms and they are purchased.

- Went today to price bathroom cabinets, new sink, and counter top.

- Tree guy is coming any day to take down our big tree by our bedroom.

- Plumber is looking for a comparable pipe stack to replace out leaking one.

We have decided to sell/give away our hot tub so I am cleaning and staining that, then will list it on Craig's list ... too much to handle at this point. Paring down, getting ready for the hard part. I'm really not as depressed as I sound ... just disgruntled!

Hugs big time.

Ann to Vicky

Re: Support group ... I think the most caring thing the facilitator said was that when she was taking care of AD folks, they were already in the midst of their disease and that's all she knew of them, while we are constantly reminded of how our loved ones used to be and what they did. We are subconsciously comparing that to where they are now. The part where you mentioned how much we hide our emotions in order to function is so true. Maybe that's why we sometimes end up laughing hysterically at some ridiculous thing they've said or done.

We're getting the emotions out one way or another and laughter is the easiest way. Of course, too many times there's absolutely nothing to laugh at. I can't tell you how many times I've had to stop what I was trying to do this afternoon and help Ralph with the simplest things. But, oh so important to him. Like you said, when is it our turn?

Ralph has been OK the last few days but the mythical 'she' is around us most of the time, especially in the late afternoon and evening. It's constantly, "Where is she, how is she going to get home, she picked up our supper things and now I don't know where she is," and on and on. I hear him talking when I'm not in the room, too. That's somewhat new. Yesterday was a good day all in all, and we even had some fairly successful 'play time' when all of a sudden I thought, "OMG, I wonder if I'm in the middle of a threesome!!!"

Forgot to mention this. Last week Ralph saw the optometrist again. He's the one I used to work for, and he spends so much time and shows such patience with Ralph. He couldn't find any big change in acuity but then he dilated him again and found some 'bubbling' on his lens implant. The Dr. said that it is easy to correct in the ophthalmologist's office so we'll be seeing him in July. It's done with a laser and shouldn't be traumatic.

Guess that's it for now. Hugs and love to you both.

07/24/2010
Vicky's Journal
Revelations

Two days ago I was getting Jim ready for bed (getting night time pills, asthma inhaler, dry eye drops, Exelon patch, and eye gel) when he asked me to sit beside him on the bed and talk for a bit. He said that our relationship has changed in the last few weeks. He remarked that we were more like two roommates than husband and wife. He was definitely correct. That is exactly what it felt like to me. I disclosed that we were making a number of necessary changes to the house, all occurring in this last month. As I am sitting here trying to figure out how long this stuff has been going on, I am shocked to realize that the time frame is that short. Wow.

I am in a dilemma also. I am not getting a full night's sleep every night. Due to the most severe hot-flash filled summer I have ever experienced, and adding in the warmest and most humid summer on record, my sleeping pattern has drastically changed. I used to go to bed about 10:30 PM and would sleep until morning, no problem. Now I go to bed about 11 PM and wake up at around 1:30 or 2 AM and can't go back to sleep. I know staying in bed is not a good idea because you associate trouble sleeping with the bedroom, so I get up and read for an hour and then return to bed and sleep until 8 AM. Sometimes I have to get up multiple times at night (hot flashes as well as wakefulness.) Consequently, I don't wake up refreshed, and in some instances I go back to bed for an hour because I feel like a slug and can't wake up.

Because of brain fatigue, Jim will frequently take a late afternoon nap at about 3 PM. When he does, I join him and have no trouble sleeping. I know that naps are troublemakers for a good night's sleep, but I can't resist them in favor of working while Jim sleeps. It is an escape as well as a refresher. I have also done what I can to reduce my night time hot flashes.

Jim has had more speech problems lately. He attempts to express a thought, and if he has trouble at the very beginning because the right word won't come, and I can't help because I don't know what he is about to say, he aborts the conversation. He will get angry at me... or himself if I start to play '20 questions' to find out what he is trying to say. So, if I'm not reasonably sure, I let it drop. I'm sure his speech problems contribute to his lessening conversation. If it's too frustrating... don't do it! He talks less while watching TV and changes channels more... probably due to an increasing lack of comprehension. Jim is quieter when we are out with other people because he has trouble keeping up with the conversation. I need to include him in things that I say to try to engage him with others. We are not talking rocket science, but to Jim we might as well be, because he can't follow the context well enough to add anything.

The long and short of it is that we are talking less to each other. Jim likes to listen to the news while we eat, so that decreases our interaction even more. We should probably stop doing that, but I hate to restrict something he loves to do. I also feel less like a wife and more like Jim's mother, and I know I hover too much.

I am very conscious of Jim's growing boredom with his world. It is shrinking smaller and smaller. He can no longer go off by himself riding his bike on the canal path to the rec. center, or go see a friend, or play golf, or go to the mall to buy a present. He has gotten lost 3-4 times in the most recent months (either someone has brought him home or I have been called to come pick him up.) I now accompany him for his workouts every other day so there's no sense of independence anymore. I include him in grocery shopping (he pushes the cart while I find the items ... I tell him his accompanying me makes it easier to shop ... a therapeutic fib) so he will feel useful. I try to plan a couple activities every week that are fun to get him out of the house. I have also hired a companion for 3 hours a week to take him out to bowl, walk, get ice cream, or even fly a kite. He finally agreed to that as long as the companion was male. I got him from a local agency and the agency did a great job of pairing the companion to Jim. They enjoy each other's company. Despite this, Jim feels that I am out of the house a lot while he is in the house. Yes, I am watering the grass seed, trying to clean up the gardens and edging them (I have the lawn cut) or doing laundry in the basement. I get together with gals from our old scuba club once a month for dinner, go to the pharmacy for meds, or talk to a neighbor in the yard, and Jim is in the house ALONE! I do try to plan as many outings as I can while Jim is with his companion, but even though I am really not gone that much, it feels as if I am to Jim. It's a no win situation.

Jim has no time awareness anymore and doesn't know when he gets up from a nap whether it is the same day or a new day... even if it is light out. Thus, he has no real grasp of time and how much I am gone. His connection with the world is getting weaker and weaker, and more isolating, and he feels it. Trying to please him as well as getting household chores done is stressful, and to tell the truth, after a full day, I don't always feel like a wife either. I feel like his mother or his landlady. Stress gets in the way of the expression of the love that I feel for him. This 'volunteer' job doesn't have a lot of perks! I love him with all my heart, and I would give anything for him not to have the disease, but my emotions are shutting down. Not feeling helps to get me through. But it is taking a toll on Jim. He notices the change, and doesn't feel as loved.

We both admitted that part of this difference is our separate reactions to the disease. Jim suggested that we see a counselor. I am willing to do that, but I asked for 2 weeks for us to see if we can make a difference ourselves. I want a chance to try to bring more of our old relationship back, be more conversant, and talk about the little things. I have to make a big effort to show him how much I love him in lots of little ways ... a hug here ... a pat there, and openly saying I love him every day. He is an innocent bystander who happens to be involved in this awful mess. I want to keep him at home as long as possible for a multitude of reasons, the best being that I will know he is getting good care and love. So we will revisit the subject in two weeks, see how we are doing, and go from there.

08/01/2010
Ann to Dr. D.
Ralph

You last saw Ralph on May 26th and at that time you gave us a sample pack of Namenda which Ralph was to take mid-day for 5 weeks and report back the results. You suggested it might help with his hallucinations. I haven't written sooner because I honestly don't know if it helped or not. He was seeing things while on the additional Namenda and is still seeing apparitions on a daily basis. I have a feeling the additional meds were just an exercise in futility.

The ironic thing is: his actual vision has become worse, but his visions are very clear. On the plus side, he doesn't seem threatened by them. Sometimes there are folk dressed in Amish clothing. Sometimes he sees a choir dressed in robes standing in the road, and the other day there were two women in wheel chairs by the front door. He even described what they were wearing. He was concerned about them but then saw a paramedic tending to them. As to the choir and the endless parade of people in our back yard, they never speak to him. He tells me he sometimes asks them what they want, but they don't answer.

Other times he tells me he was speaking to a woman sitting next to him, but she has disappeared. When he tells me what they were talking about, of course I realize it was me. This happens if I leave the room for a few minutes. He will discuss their conversation in perfectly lucid terms but insist it wasn't me.

I'm not sure what, if anything, I should do about these fairly new events. He remains gentle and loving and only occasionally flares up in anger and frustration, and then feels badly about things he has said to me. At least that tells me he is still empathetic and feels the sorrow for both of us. I'm trying to take it all in stride, but it feels as if I'm Alice in Wonderland. The family helps and I don't know what I'd do without their support.

If you have any pointers about the meds, let me know.

PS. Do you ever get the feeling we know absolutely nothing about the brain and our place in the cosmos?

Dr. D. to Ann

If there is no clear benefit I would suggest that we stop the extra Namenda. As disappointing as it is, we do not want to use medications that are not helping. If the visions become more of a problem, we should try to control them with low doses of Seroquel. I know that we do not understand how this all works ... which is why I am at my desk at 1:30AM. We are making progress.

I am not sure about our place in the cosmos, but I am continually inspired by the courage and character I see in people every day, you and your husband being prime examples.

Let me know if new issues arise.

Ann to Dr. D.

Thanks so much for your prompt reply. I'll let you know if the hallucinations become violent or threatening. I suppose we could try the ½ Seroquel again but it tended to make him too sleepy during the day.

I want to apologize to you for the remark I made about no one knowing how the brain works. I was just being flippant. I know that you are probably the hardest working researcher out there and if there is an answer, you'll find it, if not for Ralph, then possibly our children or grandchildren. Sometimes it's easier to take a step back and ponder the grand scheme of things, if there is one, than focusing on my own small world and problems.

Thank you again for all the care and concern you've shown us both. Knowing you're there if we need you is so reassuring. Stay well and try to get some rest.

09/15/2010
Ann to Vicky
A Puzzlement

Why is it that when we go to the doctor we wear our best underwear, and then take it off and hide it under the rest of our clothes before the doctor even comes in the room? I could be wearing a thong made out of crepe paper and no one would know. The same goes for bras and mammograms. Is it just me or are we all so silly?

Anyway, the scraping and smushing went well, at least I haven't heard anything negative. Ralph had an appointment at the VA at 9:00 AM yesterday and I woke up at 4 AM and he was washed, dressed, albeit his shirt was inside out, and was asking me if it was time to leave for his appointment. I convinced him to go back to bed but it was under protest. He was so confused. I had to leave him in the middle of the appt. to run over to my mammo appt. and then back to fetch him. They still won't pay for his Namenda so I've pretty much given up on that. They did give him a new cane, a quad, so now he has two canes to carry around with him as neither one will ever touch the pavement.

Do I sound a bit discouraged and bitter? You bet I do. I can no longer remember what he was like 5 years ago, and when I started talking to him like he was a kindergartener. People are now beginning to notice the problem sooner. When we were with Nancy and Lou I thought he was acting OK and then the waitress quietly said to me, "would you like a couple of extra napkins?" When she brought them Lou tucked them into Ralph's shirt and he didn't seem to mind, but it was another clue to me that I don't always see the changes. I had to laugh when you were talking about food shopping and Jim asking people to move when he could have squeezed by, because Ralph doesn't ask people to move, he just parks in the middle of the aisle and stands there while people struggle to get around him. I try to leave him at a cross aisle and tell him I'll pick up what I need and bring them back, but he insists on trudging along so he can 'help'. I can understand perfectly why you envy some folks who have their freedom. I'm not ready to let him go. I just want the rest of him back.

Enough of that. Are you going to share some of your latest Life in a Straight Jacket stuff with me? I need to start sorting out what we have and try to put some order to it. I've given up journaling. Right now, I'm just keeping all our e-mails. That's it for now ... Love 'n hugs.

09/15/2010
Ann to Dr. D.

Ralph had an appointment at the VA yesterday with his new nurse practitioner. I explained about Ralph's decline despite the fairly high MMSE numbers. He reiterated what they've all said before. Keep in mind, this is the government we're talking about. Anyway, he told me there is no way they can prescribe Namenda to Ralph if his numbers are above 14. We talked about the delusions, etc., to no avail. He gave us two options: 1) He wondered why you didn't just keep Ralph on Aricept which they would pay for even though I said you thought he was doing well on the Namenda (I thought it was arrogant of him) or 2) Ralph could be evaluated and tested by one of their neurologists and then go through significant red tape which may or may not lead to an Rx for Namenda.

I really don't want to put him through any more testing unless you feel it would be beneficial and I don't see the sense of going back to Aricept to save a few dollars. My only thought on this was that I wonder if we should try the Aricept and Namenda together again. I personally think we'll just tighten our belts and pay the price until our insurance kicks in again next year.

Any ideas besides the ones you can't print?

Dr. D. to Ann

I am very sorry to hear that they are persisting in their unreasonable and unreasoned denial of appropriate care. I think the system is administered in a grossly inhumane manner. At least that is my version that I can print.

Mr. Henderberg should not be put on a cholinesterase inhibitor such as Aricept because of his history of life endangering side-effects (falls). He should have Namenda, on the chance that it might slow disease progression. If that is the case, the effects may be small and it is a personal and financial decision that you both should make. I apologize for the system's putting you in this position.

Ann to Dr. D.
VA

Thanks for your input. There is no way we will cut down or discontinue the Namenda no matter the cost. I have nothing to compare his frontal temporal dementia to, but it seems to me he's doing well considering it's been 5 years since his diagnosis. If nothing major occurs, we'll see you in December.

09/16/2010
Vicky to Ann

None of my underwear is presentable ... but then who wants to look at it anyway!

I am still here. Kip didn't want us to come just now... maybe sometime in October.

Last night I thought I made an OK dinner. Breaded fish (frozen) with tartar sauce, carrots, and beans. Jim said it was too bland! I told him he was lucky I made him anything at all! He said, "Well I guess I shouldn't have said what I said." So tonight I made baked chicken, baked potatoes, and corn. I cut everything up and buttered the potatoes...it's easier now rather than watching Jim try to cut stuff up and having it fall off the plate. That marks a new stage in our eating. When will the baby food jars be coming?

Today, Jim was thinking when we got up from a nap that maybe we should consult our friends who are sex therapists about his problem! I said we already consulted Dr. D. and he said it probably was the Alzheimer's. That's all I need is to consult with a sex therapist with a partner with no memory of even what to do! That's a REAL devoted caregiver, don't you think?

Ralph sure has some memory to be up at 4 and getting dressed! I feel sorry for you that early, although I know a little of what you mean. Sometimes Jim leans over and whispers to me it's time to get up... and I look at the clock and it's 6 AM. So I tell him the time and tell him to go back to sleep. Pretty soon I'm going to start him back on sleeping pills so he will sleep longer in the morning.

I really do hear your pain and frustration. It really is tragic, this damned disease, and I get feeling low every time I look at Jim and see how far he has declined. It was easier to ignore when they weren't so bad, but now Jim can't even talk straight. He goes around saying "I can't find my eyes"...meaning his glasses, or standing there not knowing what to do with his pants...or sitting in the bathtub with the curtain drawn and the water filling up because he can't figure out how to make the shower part turn on or pull the plug so the water doesn't accumulate.

Yesterday, he insisted he wanted to vote. Well, I took him and finally we gave up because he wrote his name on the ballot (which invalidates it) but couldn't read the printing on the form or see the dots to fill in, and I couldn't make him understand that he couldn't vote cross party in this election. That's the last time he will vote!

I don't know that I've written much except in something I call 'dateline' where I add a new date and document stuff that makes me upset. I save some of our e-mails too...if you want I can download Laughter in a Straight Jacket (LIAS) on a disc and bring it to lunch on Monday...Funny...by mistake I typed LAID instead of LIAS...but that's the last thing I need or want. Want me to give you a disc with what I have so far or don't you want to weed through it?

By the way...don't feel you should be writing stuff. It's an outlet and I only do it when I feel the need. Perhaps we won't feel like doing anything when this is all over. It should just help us cope with the present!

09/20/2010
Vicky to Ann
Letters to Juliet

To get Jim out of the house yesterday I suggested a movie...Jim can't follow difficult plots, but this movie was *Letters to Juliet* staged in Verona, Italy. An American girl and her fiancé travel on different paths, and the girl finds a new love on her travels while writing about an older woman trying to find an old love after 50 years apart. It was not a difficult plot, and it was beautiful scenery, and a very cute romantic story. In the past Jim has always appreciated those types of movies because he is a big softie. I thought the movie was great, and I cried at the end. When we walked out of the theater I asked Jim, "Wasn't that good?" He said that he didn't like it at all and that he couldn't get into it. I was so taken aback...he said maybe it was because of his eyes that were bothering him (dry eye problems), and he was cold the entire time and was miserable. He wanted to ask me to leave before the movie was over, but didn't have the heart.

I was so shocked by this, and it brought tears to my eyes. I could hardly keep my emotions in check while we were driving home. I guess I so wanted him to like the movie to prove to me that we were still the same couple who were in love as much as the characters. It made me realize (as if I didn't already know) that the man I was sitting next to in the theater wasn't the same man I married. He doesn't have the capacity to be, because Alzheimer's has stolen that from him. From now on we won't necessarily like the same things. True romance has left our lives forever.

Sometimes you have these epiphanies and they are a real blow. You go along in your daily routine and try to hide your emotions away so that nothing will hurt you. You take antidepressants so you can function without being a crying mess all the time. You try to pretend that things won't get any worse, or at least they will go slowly. You go along day by day and say that things are normal. Everything is fine. It's how we deal with the disease, by not thinking about tomorrow. And then something like a reaction to a movie will reduce you to tears.

Most of us on this journey feel that life isn't fair, that we have been cheated of the final years of our lives by this disease. To make me feel better, I think of what I will do in 2-3 years when it is all over. I will go to some beach somewhere and rest, walk the beach, pick up shells, and look in old stores for interesting things, and get myself ready to start a new chapter in my life. Dreaming about that feels really good. I say, "I can wait that long." But I know in reality it's been 17 years with the disease now, and Jim is quite physically fit, and can still express himself for the most part. So how many years will it be before he dies, will I spend most of my old age caring for him? What about me? Will I be too old to go to that beach by myself when the end has come? Will I be too poor to go? Will I be too scared to go? Too bad to think about, so I put my head down and just keep doing what I have been doing and get by...only trying to do it a little better for Jim!

09/25/2010
Vicky to Ann
Golf etc.

Golf was an absolute nightmare the other day. We had to walk off the course at Hole 6 because people were backing up behind us again. We had already let two groups play through after Hole 2. Jim now can't recognize the green from any distance, and I not only have to show him his ball wherever it is, but also stand there and point to the green. Even then he can't see it and may turn 180 degrees and start hitting back towards the tee. It took us 2½ hours to play 5½ holes. If I can stand it maybe I'll take him 1 more time. Maybe then the weather will be more overcast so other people won't want to go...or maybe go to the driving range.

The thing is, he asks about golfing all the time and keeps wanting to call his friends and ask them to golf. At this point I think it is a big imposition on them to take Jim golfing, and so far they have avoided it since spring. But I don't want to tell him that he is too handicapped to be playing. I don't want his feelings hurt. I am thinking after this next week of putting the clubs in the basement so that he won't see them day after day and maybe he will forget about them...I'm hoping.

I feel really bad about not inviting people over for dinner like I used to. We do a lot with various friends and they are always inviting us over for dinner but these days I don't reciprocate. It is hard to get motivated to even clean house let alone have people for dinner. I have to get out of my slump and, hopefully, if I can solve my poor sleeping hours I'll be better. I am going for a physical this Thursday. I have started giving Jim his sleep meds and he sleeps as long as I do now. I just have to fix my sleep problem.

I hope your week went well since Monday. Ralph's spells are really strange. It would be really nice to know what causes them! Tell Ralph that we received his 'Thank You' card two days ago and we thank him for that. Was it hard to have him sign all those cards? Jim can't really write his name anymore. [Ann's note: This refers to an 80th birthday party my kids and I held for Ralph. I knew he was declining and there would be a time in the near future when he would no longer recognize his family and friends. We rented a cabin in a local park and invited everyone we could think of. We had a great response. Family/friends came from near and far, and Ralph was oriented and 'with it' the entire day. I guess I knew in my heart it was his 'last hurrah.']

Our bathroom cabinets came in and they had to reorder the main cabinet because the head of the company didn't like the way it was done. So they put it on rush order. It will probably come in again when Jim's sister and niece come to visit Oct 14th. One time Jim's sister and brother-in-law and his aunt came to visit and we had no kitchen!

Oh well, that's all for now. I'm getting tired just thinking about how long this is going to go on…with Jim's health so good and all.

09/26/2010
Ann to Vicky
More Nightmares

I have to get this all down today and send a copy to my LIAS file before I forget the details. First of all, I started to write to you 3 times after you sent me the note about how you felt during the *Letters to Juliet* movie. I wanted to console you but damned if I could find the right words. I felt so bad for you and the usual, 'a day at a time,' 'it is what it is', 'enjoy the time left' just seemed like silly pat phrases that we all use to cover up the hell. Lately, for me, and probably for you, 'a day at a time' means another day of stress and fatigue, 'it is what it is' means that what it is is crap, and 'enjoy the time left' suggests "Why?" That being said, let me tell you about Friday. You mentioned Ralph's 'spell'. I think you were referring to the knee buckling collapsing that he did last Monday. I can deal with that. When I woke up Friday, I was so tired I felt like lead, and decided there was no way I could get dressed and go to dance class. After 3 more hours of sleep (noonish) we decided it was such a nice day we'd take a long ride. Everything was fine and we headed out towards Bloomfield and Sharkey's Ice Cream Parlor. Got there and they were closed. Seems they went on fall hours. No matter, we were still enjoying the day and headed up Rt. 64 towards Pittsford. I asked Ralph if he wanted to go to Aladdin's as we hadn't had lunch, and he said, "Sure." Then, all of a sudden, he said he wasn't sure where he was and his head felt 'funny'. I said, "Do you want to go home?" and he said, "Yes", he didn't feel like going to a restaurant. "Fine. Let's head west and stop at Byrnes Dairy and get ice cream to take home." He said that sounded good. Anyway, here is the dialogue for the rest of the trip as I remember it. Mind you, there are miles between each exchange.

R: What's your name?
A: Ann, what's yours?
R: I'm not sure.
R: Are you my wife?
A: Yes, and you're my husband.

R: Oh.

R: Where do you live?

A: Chili.

R: I think I live in Chili, too. I'm not sure.

R: What's happening to me?

A: You're just a little confused (went on trying to orient him.)
Remember Dr. D. said these things will happen and not to worry
about them.

R: (amazed) You know Dr. D? How do you know him?

A: He's your doctor and I take you to see him.

R: I can't figure out how you know him. I'd like to know what's going
on....

A: (As we went through Avon) I got a speeding ticket here once.

R: So did Ann.

R: Did you ever go to a support group that meets at MCH?

A: Of course, I go with you.

R: Funny, I've never seen you there. Why haven't I seen you?

A: Well, your group meets in one room, and my group meets in
another room. I take you there.

R: Take me? Why don't I take myself? Oh, that's right, I
can't drive.

After what seems like hours we arrived at Byrne Dairy. I asked him
what flavor he wants and he tells me, all very rational. When I came
out, it went like this:

R: Would you mind dropping me at my house?

A: Of course, we'll go home now.

R: (on the way) I think you're pretty cute.

A: I think you're pretty cute too. At this point, he starts telling me
which way to go, where to turn off Chili Ave., where to turn on our
street, and which house to pull into.

R: Would you like to come in?

A: Sure (I'm thinking, OMG, he's going to cheat on me with me!!!)

Oddest thing is, once we got into the house he kept talking about 'she'
and where did she go, she got out of the car and then just disappeared
and on and on. I gave him a dish of ice cream and he fell asleep. Things
were more normal for a bit and then later that night he came into the
living room and said, "It's eating at me that something's wrong with

you. Are you angry? What did I do? Why are you so quiet?" I tried explaining that I wasn't mad, that his confusion was upsetting to me as well as to him, and so forth. He started talking about 'she' again and how she was driving and stopped at a store, and then he proceeded to tell me exactly how we got home, which roads and so on like there was an accurate map in his head. But it was always 'she' who drove a little too fast and she turned here and there, and when I asked him where I was all this time he said he didn't know. I assured him (again) that 'she' was me, but he didn't seem to get it.

Yesterday, Brian (bless him) took Ralph for most of the day. I couldn't believe how much energy I had and how much work I got done. Anyway, Brian said Ralph seemed oriented all day and we had a good dinner, talked, all was well. We watched some TV and he went to bed about 10. I was just deciding whether I'd write to you or read for a while when out he came, said he couldn't sleep and that we had to straighten things out between us. He just knew something was wrong with me. Said we went out for a ride on Friday and had a good time, but he couldn't figure out why I suddenly seemed a little upset. He said he couldn't sleep until he straightened it out. So, instead of a little me time, we spent the next hour going over the day before, and as soon as I had him convinced the 'she' was 'me' he started in again about her driving and everything she said and how he still can't figure out how she knew Dr. D. I asked where I was while she was driving, and he said he guessed I was sitting next to him. I told him there isn't room for 3 people in our front seat and he said he hadn't thought about that. My personal guess is that 'she' is going to be in our lives, for better or worse, for a long time.

We're going to Nancy and Lou's for dinner and when she called to invite us, I started to choke up and she was concerned. I have to reassure her that I have to let go and cry sometimes. She shouldn't worry but I know she doesn't wholly understand. No one does, except you and a few other caregivers. I need to vent and let go, but I don't want to let her see it today. She and Lou are leaving for their Italy trip a week from Tuesday, and I want her to think things are more normal than they are. It's going to be a trip of a lifetime for them. So, this afternoon I'll put on my Academy Award performance.

That's about it. I know you have it as bad and maybe worse as I do, but I needed to share it all with you. Thanks for listening.

Vicky To Ann

I don't have it worse at all. Nothing hurts more than not being recognized and you did such a superb job being cool and giving spectacular answers! I'm sorry that this is happening to you. It probably makes you think you are not appreciated because he's always saying 'she'. I'm glad you wrote down the entire conversation because if we ever compile a book that would 'say it all' about the topic of not being recognized and how outwardly cool you have been when you are hurting so on the inside. It would make me feel that I was a 'ghost' in the house rather than a human being that has wants, needs, and feelings! I don't know whether you will ever get over it with time, as he refers to you as 'she' more and more often. You will have to let me know. It's something that even if I bolster myself to expect in the months to come, it doesn't hurt any less. I am giving you a BIG LONG HUG right now to help with your pain.

It is so weird that the directions part of the brain is so intact and he can recall everything you both said, and yet he can't make the connection that it's you. And yet Jim is so handicapped now with speech and he can't set the table. Today I asked him to get me a soda out of the fridge. I was gardening. He went to the freezer and was looking around...so I directed him to the refrig...and he's looking all over because he doesn't recognize what a can of soda (pop) is. Finally, I said never mind, and went in and got what I wanted. He said, "Well, there are so many things in there, how am I supposed to know what you want?" Always an excuse! I know that's unfair, but I wish just once he would say, "Honey, I don't understand what you want". Just once admit that it is the disease, but no, he always has an excuse as to why he couldn't do something. I'm not asking for him to be normal.

Lots of hugs...and know down the line I will be experiencing the same thing.

Ann to Vicky

Thanks for the big hug. It must have worked because I'm feeling better. When we were going to Nancy's he told me a number of times how much he loved me, so I think he's beginning to realize how 'out of it' he was. This morning he switched from 'she' stuff to telling me he is going to lose it if I don't start doing something about 'all the things' that need doing around the house. Keep in mind he does nothing to help. A number of months ago the ice cube maker in our fridge started leaking. Brian took it apart and ordered a part for it. It was little more than a hose. When it came to his house it was the wrong part and cost over $60.00 on Brian's charge. Well, one thing led to another, and Brian was busy with a million things and didn't get around to sending the part back. Meanwhile, I decided I could live with just using ice trays for the time being and kind of forgot about it. Not Ralph. He forgets who I am but can't forget the ice maker. He said he was going to lose it big time if I didn't get on it and get the repair done, because it was using a lot more energy without said ice maker???? So, of course, I called Brian and asked what he could do about that and a couple of other small repairs. I'll e-mail him tomorrow and explain how I was coerced into bugging him. We really need to have our bedroom re-done but he never mentions that. I figured today that it will cost over $2000.00 for just our non-generic drugs 'til the end of the year and that isn't figuring in the cost raises which sometimes go up $50.00 every 3 months. I can't share that with him but that's why I don't want to get into a lot of repairs right now. In spite of all the above, we had a good time with Nancy and Lou, and even had a lot of laughs.

I was thinking about your golf dilemma. One good thing about living in Rochester is it's almost October which means it will soon be snowing. You definitely can't let him think his friends don't want to play with him. Meanwhile, you'll have to bite the bullet, or in this case, the golf ball. Do you think the reason they don't want to admit they can't find things (soda in fridge) is because that would mean admitting they really have a serious problem? I think if I had my life to live over, I'd like to study the brain, because nobody really knows the first thing about it.

Let me know what your Dr.'s advice is on your insomnia. I was doing better until the last few days. Now I'm back in sleepless land. Tomorrow I have to be at the Geva box office by 8 AM to try and get sale tickets for *The Christmas Carol*. I want to take the great granddaughters (Brittany and Marissa) and the tickets range from 50-59 dollars for medium priced seats.

Time for bed, and hopefully sleep.

09/30/2010
Ann to Vicky
Jan's Story

Hi...How is your week going? Ralph had that sore throat/cough thing that's going around. He's feeling better and not contagious, so we will still be meeting you tomorrow. However, you know how the smallest trauma, e.g. flu, cold, whatever, affects their mental status so you can fill in the blanks. It's been a so-so week. Lots of confusion but so far he seems to know me. Don't know whether that's good or bad.

About *Jan's Story* by Barry Petersen: I'm bewildered. Jan was diagnosed in 2005 and was already in assisted living by April of 2008. I'm not saying she wasn't ready to be placed (although I questioned it) but he goes on to talk about 'years' of caring for her, and how it had been 'years' since they had any intimacy. Where are all those years? Then, he talks about his deep grief and depression, and then guilt about seeking another woman. These are all issues we may be facing too, but it seems to me he could have been visiting and hugging and caring a lot more than was let on in the book. She even went to dinner at her brother's house after Barry was seeing his new friend. So she asked her sister-in-law who that cute guy was? So what? I went through that last week but it didn't make me run off with another 80 year old (that last part made me laugh.) Anyway, I guess what really pissed me off was that I could understand if it was someone he already knew or worked with, but to go searching through an online dating service? Please. I guess I'm getting old, but that just seemed too bizarre to me. According to all the accolades sent his way, you and I should be receiving Nobel prizes. Would love to talk about it but it will be hard tomorrow.

Looking forward to our lunch. Love' n hugs.

Vicky to Ann

I agree about *Jan's Story* ... I was put off by that too, but then you have to remember that a lot of men are like that. Try 17 years (not saying I have been having hard times all those 17) but I would have a live-in boyfriend by now if I acted like him. His life as a reporter and his marriage is all about leaving and coming home to a loving wife that did everything...she had to or his absences wouldn't have worked. And when he had to start to make arrangements for her he probably thought that was a humungous job ... being that he was never home in the first place!

Jim's update: when he gets up in the morning he just sort of stands there in the living room (remember, he sleeps in his clothes.) I have to get the breakfast, set the table, turn on the TV, pour the juice, dole out his pills and his eye drops...and then say come and sit down and eat, and then he does. He's just sort of in limbo...convinced him to stay home for my physical because I told him I didn't want to tell our doctor how things really were with him there...that I would feel guilty about talking in front of him. She prescribed 10mg. generic for Ambien that I can either take at that dose or split it...yippee. Received a referral to a neurologist and otolaryngologist, because I have had 12 instances of choking on my saliva when swallowing since July. Don't know what that's about, but at this point I'm not going to worry 'til I hear something bad. I will just wait and see.

I finished James Patterson's book, *Sundays at Tiffany's*. Then I read *The Girl with the Dragon Tattoo* by Stieg Larsson. That book was good, but not great. The second got me hooked, though. By the way, I have book 2 and am going to get book 3 by that author and can lend them to you, but you have to get your hands on the first book and read them in proper order!

Looking forward to tomorrow.

10/05/2010
Ann to Vicky
Update

I'm going to get this started while supper's cooking. I didn't get much chance to talk to you at lunch the other day, but I think it was a good thing to get us all together again. The guys needed it as much as we did.

Why are you being referred to a neurologist? I can see starting with an ENT doc but I don't understand the neuro. connection. At least not at first. Anyway, when are you going? Let me know how you make out. If you've never had a laryngoscopy done it's no big deal. They use local anesthetic on the scope so you don't feel anything. You'll just feel a little numb on the way home.

Ralph and I have both had colds, coughing, and such over the weekend. I had already promised Hassan an overnight so we had him here from Friday after school until Sunday night. He's no trouble but I'm still not feeling great. Yesterday, we went to the Life Center to a reception for Nancy, the woman who ran the Social Club at Carter Street. It was nice and she was touched, but Ralph seemed so much more out of it than he did at the last get-together. I have to keep in mind that he's been coughing and feeling lousy too but still, things have changed lately. Sometimes I feel as if misery loves company and I enjoy talking with all the other caregivers, but lately I've been sick of the whole Alzheimer thing, present reader excepted. Dinner's ready. More later.

After the 'Social' we went to Nancy's and picked up Taylor, their golden retriever, and brought her back here. Robert was going to take care of her but he had to go to Washington for a Green Peace event. Anyway, we have Taylor for the time being. I'm coughing more and hope she's not giving me an asthma attack. She hasn't bothered me lately, but I was always very allergic to dogs. If I get worse, I'll have to ship her to Brian's but she seems content here and besides, Brian's ferrets scare her.

Vicky to Ann

I am going to the neurologist because I had three vertebrae fused in 2004, and more of my vertebrae could be growing spurs that press into my spinal column. It needs to be checked out. I'm not worrying about it right now.

It's really hard to keep Jim occupied...I really hate that he 'watches' TV all the time, and when it's raining all we can do is shopping or go to the rec. center.

Sorry you both have been sick...we just got our flu shots today.

My cabinets are in and I am waiting to see when they can deliver them...and when our carpenter can install them. I'm hoping it's before next Thursday when Jim's sister and niece come, but I'm betting it will be after that.

I'm hustling to get the PowerPoints for work done, so I can say I am finished for good. Almost there.

Take care and eat a piece of chocolate for me!

10/07/2010
Ann to Vicky
An Ordinary Day

First of all, I had to see my primary because my cold got worse. I couldn't stop coughing and as I had already figured, my dog allergy is kicking in. He said that even though the dog hasn't bothered me lately, you can't undo an allergy and I would probably keep getting worse. He said I didn't have bronchitis yet but put me on an antibiotic anyway. Brian picked her up this afternoon and took her to his house. He said tonight she seems to enjoy all the attention from the kids. I feel bad about it, but it didn't make sense to get sicker when I've got Ralph to take care of. I swear we'd starve if I ever got really sick. He just can't manage anything. I tried lying down this afternoon, and he asked if he could do anything to help me. I said he could take some bags and pick up Taylor's poop (mind you, golden retriever, hearty appetite.) I said it would be in a 10 foot semi-circle right in front of the porch door. Anyway, out he went to clean up. I looked out once and he was way out by the back shed. Next time I looked, he was looking in the front yard. After a while I just grabbed some bags and cleaned up, probably 8 piles of it. Ugh.

Now, since dinner, he's been really out of it. Wants to go home, wanted to know where he was, asked if he was married, asked if I was a shrink, and so on. Then he got really upset and said how scared he is. It's all so exhausting for both of us and he's such a dear, good man. He doesn't deserve this hell.

Meanwhile, I totally forgot about your upset kitchen and that you're having company next week. Would you like to postpone our lunch on the 18th? It's up to you.

Guess I'll go lose myself in *The Help* by Kathryn Stockett. I'm reading it, and loving it.

We'll talk soon.

<u>Vicky to Ann</u>

I'm sorry you are 'slogging' through life lately with your cold and Ralph's confusion. It's got to be so heart wrenching listening to how scared he is. And I know how tiring trying to let them help is...there really isn't much they can do...they just keep watching us work. I'm going to look online for some kids' games that maybe we can do.

Actually, it's my upset bathroom, but all is well. My cabinets came in and passed inspection and were delivered yesterday. The counter top was delivered today and it actually looks as if they are all the correct measurements! Our carpenter comes tomorrow to take out the old and put in the new. Perfect.

Nancy and Beth come next Thursday and leave on Sunday. They won't be here long. I have decided on menus and will shop Tues. or Wed. and will start cleaning and changing beds after the bathroom is done...should be done by Monday. So it will all work out. I probably mentioned that when I had my kitchen redone, we had Nancy and her husband and an aunt all together and had no running water or counter tops in the kitchen, and the refrigerator was in the dining room. We had a microwave in the basement and the grill. This will be piece of cake!

I have been mostly a slug lately saving up all my energy. Finished *The Help* and LOVED it. Now I am on *The Girl Who Kicked the Hornet's Nest* by Stieg Larsson, then after that I have Jimmy Carter's book to read.

I have the door off the bathroom in readiness for the carpenter... and Jim asked tonight; "How can I go to the bathroom?"... I said; "Well, the toilet is still here, you can just sit on the pot with no door. I won't look. He's now driving me crazy with: "When is Nancy coming? Today?"...every few minutes. I shouldn't have told him she was coming until next week.

The 18th is fine. The company leaves on the 17th so I will need a break...although I'm sure I will have fun. I just hope it's not too much for Jim. He's constantly trying to put on jackets and he pulls the sleeves inside out and can't put it on, then can't zip it or he tries to take things off over his head when they don't come off that way.

Today, he tried to go home with the lady that was parked next to us at the rec. center! She looked at him as if he were crazy.

Hang in there.

10/17/2010
Ann to Vicky
Update

I need my catharsis of writing to you and getting my feelings in print. Please don't feel you have to send a long reply because I know you have company. Just let me know if the Frog Pond (restaurant) is all right with you and Jim.

Last Sunday, Brian had to take Hassan to the doctor. He had an acute asthma attack. Dog, of course. Brian had to take her back to Nancy's and the next door neighbors said they would watch her 'til Robert got back. Meanwhile, I kept Hassan Sunday night and Monday so they could clean up the dog hair. We went for a ride in the afternoon and stopped at a Deli to pick up sandwiches. Hassan came in with me and then Ralph said he felt dizzy and went back out to the car. While I was waiting for our order, Hassan went to check on Grandpa and said he was asleep in someone else's car! The owner had to tell him it wasn't his car and to get out, but all was said in a nice way. I think he understood the problem. When you told me about Jim almost going home from the rec. center with another woman, I had to chuckle, but it didn't seem so funny when it happened to me.

Some friends from California that our kids grew up with came over Sunday evening to visit before heading back home. Ralph was very quiet and had little to say. He acted as if it didn't matter that they were there, and we hadn't seen them in three years! I guess it's what they call 'the flat affect.' I think they were a little shocked.

As you can probably tell, I've been a bit depressed lately (not sleeping among other things,) and Ralph is noticing it. I try hard to keep my feelings about his care locked in so as not to hurt him, but this morning he told me he feels as if I can't stand him sometimes. That did it. The dam broke and I cried and cried. I try to make him understand it's the disease that frustrates me so much, and I keep assuring him I want to take care of him. I don't want to be without him, and I love him and all the years we've had. I can't tell him I'm already losing him bit by bit, and that's not so much depression as grief. I probably need to increase my antidepressant but I'm determined to tough this out.

Two other reasons I'm in a bad mood. I'm having trouble with my foot. I think it's fasciitis but I can't get in to see the foot doctor until November 2nd. Because of the pain, I had to cancel out two shows this past week, and I'm not sure I'll be able to do the next one on October 28th. I don't think they can do much for fasciitis except rest it, ice it, and take ibuprofen. A cortisone shot is the last resort. The second reason I'm upset is I picked up two prescriptions for Ralph yesterday. The bill came to $999.04 and we have to pay it all, because we have fallen into the infamous 'donut hole' where we have reached the limit of our drug coverage for the year. Ralph knows it because he was with me, but he doesn't know it at the same time.

One good thing. While I was resting my foot I was able to finish *The Help* and loved every sentence. I was sorry to see it end.

Guess that's it. I hope you were able to have a good time with Jim's sister, and it wasn't too much stress for you. Can't wait 'til tomorrow. I just wish we could 'talk' more but I'm trying to be more aware of Ralph's feelings. If I'm down, he's down. We've been together a long time.

Vicky to Ann

Hugs first! Sounds like things are getting much harder for you. And to be hurting with plantar fasciitis doesn't help either. Boy, your pharmacy bill was a shocker! Are we stressing you by meeting for lunch? Money wise I mean?

It has been a long week but one well worthwhile. We had a great visit with Jim's sister, Nancy, and his niece, Beth. Both are so understanding and loving with Jim (and showing it,) but it's good to have the house to ourselves again. Jim saw the eye doctor first thing this AM for his ongoing eye problem. Also, our mower isn't working right, and I have to call to see what the turn-around time is for that. I almost couldn't get it going today...and got stung by another yellow jacket today on the back of my ankle!

So tired my head is going to roll off my shoulders. Tomorrow!

10/22/2010
Vicky to Ann
Coasting

Not much happening here. Doing laundry, Dr.'s appointment, food shopping, ironing, etc. Whatever, whenever I have energy.

Otolaryngologist didn't see anything wrong but he wants to do a barium swallow. The hospital will call with an appointment. He says there's probably nothing wrong, but why would choking on saliva start all of a sudden in July?? I'll see the neurologist next Thursday.

Hung pictures I had framed for the bathroom...water colors of violets. The bathroom looks much better now.

Jim has normalized to being even worse...as you know with Ralph. Now, when I'm getting breakfast he just stands there by his chair and sort of stares into space. It seems I have to orchestrate everything now. I'm going to mow leaves tomorrow with our neighbor's mower (ours is in the shop) and while I do that I will have Jim wipe the plastic chairs on the deck so I can put them downstairs. That should be interesting.

Last week, Jim shaved with toothpaste...most times he shaves with his old razor and no shaving cream, because he says it does a better job. I have shown him the shaving cream, but he doesn't want to use it.

He wants to close the curtains so it doesn't feel as cold in the living room. I told him I can't stand to be in the house in the daytime with the curtains closed, so he's just going to have to get used to the cold. I would go bonkers if I couldn't see outside. Also, he doesn't want to go out for a walk because it's too cold at 50. What will he be like at 22 degrees?

Just musing...sleeping pills working well...how about you? Do you think your doctor will prescribe them for you since it's not Valium?

10/23/2010
Ann to Vicky
Re: Coasting—Means Downhill, Right?

I was going to answer you last night but decided I was too tired, but then lay awake until almost 2:00. My doctor doesn't want to prescribe sleeping pills and I can understand that, but I need to get back to a reasonable schedule. I never opened my eyes until 9:30 this morning and then I beat myself up because I can't get all the stuff done that needs doing. However, I hate to go to bed the same time as Ralph because he's been in a very romantic mood lately, and I just can't deal right now with all that entails. I love the closeness, touching, hugging, and all but to go further just isn't in my psyche right now.

Anyway, nothing much new, no significant changes this week. We both had dental appointments Wednesday and just having his teeth cleaned exhausts Ralph these days. He slept all the way home and after we got home. The smallest trauma is too much. Yesterday we had to go to a wake for my cousin's husband, who died suddenly. We were there an hour and a half and Ralph did very well, talked to everyone. Of course, he had trouble keeping family sorted out, but so did I. My cousin had 8 kids and they all have kids so my cousin has a good support system going for her. We went to dinner on the way home, and by then he was getting really confused. I always try for a booth and in the back, darker area of this particular restaurant. We go there quite often and I presume they all know there's a problem, because they are extra nice to him.

My foot is a bit better, but I'm not going to cancel my appointment yet. We have a show to do Thursday. I think I'll try just doing our duet because it's a soft shoe, no taps. I'll forego the tap numbers for now. There's so many of us it won't matter if I'm in them or not. Then, we have no shows until the second week in December, so we'll see how my foot is by then. A minor ailment, all in all.

Have you read *10,000 Joys and 10,000 Sorrows* by Olivia Ames Hoblitzelle? It's another Alzheimer's book and a little different. It is written by the wife of an Alzheimer's sufferer after his death. The husband reminds me somewhat of Jim. He was a professor of comparative literature at Barnard and Columbia, but then became a family therapist. Both he and his wife were into meditation and Buddhist and Hindu teachings, spent time in ashrams and there's a lot of that in the book. I ran across a section that talks about how the stresses that a caregiver shoulders are, for the most part, hidden from others. I identify with that as well as the myriad of roles the caregiver plays, and the never ending demands on us. She talks a lot about losses and death, and how we want to deal with that. I thought you might want to order a copy for yourself.

Guess that's all the news for now. I hope all goes well with your neurology appointment. Oh, almost forgot; I so enjoyed meeting Jim's co-workers last Monday when we had lunch. It gave both Ralph and me a glimpse of the old Jim and why he is so special. (Some former co-workers stopped at our table.)

Vicky to Ann

Thanks for your note and the paragraphs from the book. I think I'll order it...sounds like a book I'll want to keep. I always enjoy...that's not really the correct word...your emails. It just helps me in knowing we are traveling together through this slow agony...one that doesn't show to anyone who is not dealing with the disease. Today Jim asked what he could do. I set him up on the deck with spray cleaner, paper towels, and three plastic chairs. He did one very well and I showed him where to put it in the basement. I reminded him that he had two more to finish...and I started mowing the lawn. He went inside and was watching TV. I asked him to do the other two chairs and he said he already did, which he didn't. Then I asked him again, as if it were the first time, and he said his back was hurting so he went inside and took a nap. So, I finished two hours of mowing leaves, then did the chairs and stored them in the basement. Then, when I went into the house he asked me what he could do to help??? You've been there many times. I wanted to strangle him but I just said, "No dear, but thanks."

I've been thinking all day...is there some kind of faucet you can have Brian install on your kitchen sink that won't move? (Ann: This after I told Vicky how Ralph turns the faucet around and pours water all over the counters.) Worries like that make us not want to leave our spouses alone. Yes, downhill all the way!

10/26/2010
Ann to Vicky
A New Wrinkle

I have a new phase to tell you about at lunch. I hope I can get through it without crying. Maybe we could sit in that darker, middle part of the restaurant. Whoever gets there first can ask.

We had an 'episode' last night. We were in a restaurant and it hit out of the blue. Total confusion and delusion. The worst of it is: Last night and this morning he can talk about nothing else. He's so aware of his unawareness if that makes sense. We had ordered and were talking, sipping wine, snacking on the bread, and all was perfectly normal. Suddenly, he didn't know where he was, thought there was a crowd around us, and pretty much panicked. The poor waitress hurriedly packed our dinner while I grabbed his jacket and got both of us out of there. He kept saying he didn't know how he was going to get home, didn't want to get in the car, because he said it wasn't ours. When we got home he insisted a stranger drove him, kept saying; "I don't live here, I live 2 doors down, and I want to go home. I tried calming him, showed him pictures on the wall that he photographed and framed, but he was determined to go 'home'. I called Brian, and he came over and told his dad; "Let's go for a walk." When they got to the end of the driveway, Ralph turned around and said; "I live here. Let's go in." And that was that.

10/28/2010
Vicky to Ann
Unpredictable Behavior

I hope things have calmed down a bit. I guess neither one of us has thought about our guys getting worse, and having unusual reactions every time we go anywhere. Slowly but surely our worlds are closing in on us ...the things we can do with our husbands and the things we can't.

Yesterday, Jim and I went to an Alzheimer's luncheon where there was a speaker. We were seated at a table with Ava and Pauline and two other caregivers. Shortly after we got there they served the salad and after Jim finished his salad he said to me; "Well, we can go now." I said; "No, we can't...they haven't served the main part of the meal and the speaker hasn't presented yet." So, the speaker started to speak and they served the main course. Jim took one bite and then he decided he was done...because he wanted to lose some weight! The meal was really delicious too. Anyway, he listened to the speaker for a few minutes, and then leaned toward me and said; "I really don't like what he's saying!" and he had this angry look on his face. I thought...Uh Oh...what's going to happen next? Well, he sat there with a really sour puss and sitting sort of sideways so others could see his reaction. When the speech was over, they had questions and answers. I was afraid of what Jim might say, and whispered to him not to say anything if it wasn't nice. He went to the microphone and commented on how much exercise has improved his progression. Boy, I was relieved. When we went outside after it was over I asked him what he was so mad about...and he said; "I was mad?" I explained how he looked etc., and he said; "I don't know what you're talking about, let's just drop it!" He didn't remember it at all.

But, I sure learned something. I am not going to take him to anything like that again just in case he embarrasses himself. So if I can't leave him alone and can't get someone to be with him, I just won't go. It's sort of the same thing with lunches. I never know whether he will dislike the food for some dumb reason or whether things will go fine. If I suggest something he should eat because it's relatively 'safe' then he will most likely say he doesn't want that. Suddenly I'm not dealing with this respectful gentle guy, but someone who could fly off the handle any minute!

Anyway, that's what I learned this week. By the way, Kip is definitely coming home for Thanksgiving. A good thing.

Ann to Vicky

I've been trying to get back to you since you wrote Thursday night. I was ready to write last night and then decided I was ready for sleep, after two Tylenol PMs. Wrong. I lay there debating about getting up and turning the computer back on until after 2 AM. Then I slept through two hours of the radio playing before waking up at 8.

You and I seem to be see-sawing in our moods lately. The past couple of weeks I was so depressed I was thinking of asking my doctor if I could increase my antidepressant. Then, I made up my mind to do the show Thursday, and I can't tell you how much better I feel. I know I must get out and do these things or I will go mad. Of course, after the show Thursday and class Friday my foot's been really hurting, but not much more than usual. I'll see the podiatrist Monday and try to convince her I can't give up dance. Matter of life or death.

Ralph has been O.K. since his episode on Monday. Hasn't talked about it lately. He had a chance to go out with a friend yesterday to Hamlin Beach area to do some trail clearing. He was gone from 8:30 'til 3:00 and it did him a world of good. His friend was very patient with him and I'm going to talk with him when Ralph's not around about doing this more often. Some folks might do well with a group such as day care with crafts, and bingo and such, but he definitely needs to do things outdoors. Of course, cleaning up the yard is beyond him, but that's OK. I think we both needed a day away from each other. Here's a good point I learned from you; Ralph was so anxious to be ready when his friend came, he was up and dressed before I woke up. I didn't have time to check him, but when I helped him get ready for bed he had on all his night clothes under his jeans and shirt. I told him it was no big deal, I was going to do laundry today anyway. I'm learning not to sweat the small stuff.

I had to go out today for a short while and he answered the phone when I called. Another victory!! Usually, he not only can't figure how to call out, he can't figure out how to answer. As you can see, I'm just putting thoughts down here without much organizing. I figure we'll both sort this stuff out at some point in the future. I was thinking about what you said about not realizing our guys are changing all the time. I think we both realize it and have chosen not to dwell on it. It's too painful thinking about what's next. Ralph can't even open the bed by himself without needing help. He can't understand how to get between the sheets, so I help with that every night now. It amazes me how 'normal' he can appear to friends. The women I dance with keep saying, "Ralph recognized me, and we had a chat and he seemed great." I know they think I'm exaggerating when I say that I can't always come to class because I can't leave him alone for long. It used to bother me but I don't have time to explain it all. Too complicated.

I know just how you felt at your luncheon. You must have been on the edge of your seat worrying about what Jim would do. I guess if he was going to say something off the wall, I can't think of a more understanding crowd. When Ralph had his episode Monday, I just concentrated on getting our food packed and paying and getting him out of there. I was oblivious to everybody around us. I just didn't care what anyone thought. In thinking about that night, there was a booth full of noisy folk right behind Ralph and I'm wondering if their shrill voices had something to do with his thinking there was a crowd at our table. His poor brain was probably overwhelmed.

I wonder how much longer we'll be able to do our monthly lunches. So far, Ralph has been eager to go so we must make sure the guys sit together even if it means we wait longer. I just checked my calendar and we're getting together the week before Thanksgiving so I assume that's still OK with you. I know you'll be busy with Kip coming in and I'm glad you'll have family with you. I wish for your sake Kip lived closer.

Hang in there and know I'm sending my love to you and Jim. So glad we're here for each other.

10/30/2010
Vicky to Ann
Another Bout of "Something Has Happened to Me"

Friday, I woke Jim up to tell him I was going to the car dealer to have the snow tires put on. I called him while there because they said my back brakes needed doing and that I would be about an hour longer. When that was done, I called him and said I would be home in about 20 minutes...was going to stop at Wegmans across the street for some staples. When I got home he was sitting with his head in his hands. He thought something had happened to me! He was very upset. I guess I should have woken him up and made him get up because he must have fallen back asleep, and then didn't remember where I was. But I called him twice and spoke to him!! Anyway, that day I got him to agree for me to have a companion with him if I'm going to be out.

I saw the otolaryngologist and he didn't see anything wrong when he scoped me, but I have the swallow test at RGH Monday with barium (Yum). The neurologist is having me get an MRI on Tuesday…I didn't know I could have one with a titanium plate and 8 screws in my neck, but the doctor and the imaging group say that I can. MRI of my brain? No weakness of my muscles to suggest myasthenia gravis or MS, so we'll see. I'll keep you posted.

11/3/2010
Ann to Vicky
"Sheeeeee's" baaaaaack

Yesterday we went to the "Meet Me at the MAG" (Memorial Art Gallery) program. Ralph enjoys it so much and the docents love him because he contributes a lot. The day went well (we even voted), but I was cleaning up after dinner and Ralph said, "Have you ever gone to the Mem. Art Gallery?" I should have just said "Yes" but instead I said, "Yes, I was there this afternoon with you." That confused him totally and he kept asking me what was wrong with him, and she said this, and she said that, and did this, and did that. I was hoping he'd forget about it, but he started in again this morning. Just now, he came into the living room and asked me who went into the bedroom a few minutes ago and said he should clean up his mess. I said I did, but I don't think he believed me. Life is changing big time. His vision is decreasing daily and I think that adds to his confusion. I just wish 'she' would come over and clean up my mess. His mess is that he's trying to clean out his dresser drawers and it's been over a week now. He won't let me help because he's afraid I'll toss one of his 'treasures'.

Meanwhile, I saw the podiatrist Monday, and I have plantar fasciitis like I thought as well as a heel spur starting. I have a lot of exercises to do and the night boot to wear. I'll see her in 4 weeks. She asked how you and Jim were, and she thought it was great that we had found each other. She said I could try dancing with it and that it probably wouldn't injure it further, but would make it more painful. I haven't decided what to do about that.

Now, do you know how your tests turned out? I've been thinking of you, but figured you might not know for a few days. I have a good feeling they won't find anything. Keep me posted.

Time to read for a while. Been sleeping better, but it's still hard to get up in the morning. I don't like facing what new challenges await me.

Love you, wish you lived closer, but then we'd probably both be a couple of winos. (Not really, but the wine does help to relax us both in the evenings.)

Vicky to Ann

Hi Pal, I'm feeling sad with you. I guess we should be glad that we have to take this a day at a time because we wouldn't want to see what's down the road. I've been thinking. Ralph seems pretty good when out at a restaurant (at least he doesn't make a mess like Jim,) but when things get too bad to be able to go to a restaurant, maybe we can meet at each other's houses and just bring our own lunches so the other doesn't have to do anything?

Recently, I came home from grocery shopping and found the bathroom faucet running quietly. At least he can't easily see the stopper and the faucet can't move so everything was fine. Then yesterday he left the kitchen faucet on and didn't know it, but he doesn't usually move that faucet so that was OK too. Things are changing. Every time I open the kitchen door to the garage he asks where I was or where I am going. If I'm out mowing leaves, even if earlier he was out blowing leaves off the deck, he will go inside and then he will think I went out some place. I came in from 2 hours of mowing leaves and he asked me if I had a good time, thinking I was out with someone.

Today Jim was having a hard time speaking and he asked me a "what would happen if" but couldn't tell me the specifics so I couldn't answer him.

It's interesting that Ralph could fill out a ballot. Jim couldn't at all last time so he said this time it would be better if he didn't vote, because he didn't know the people running well enough. I accepted that and voted on the way home from my MRI.

The swallow study didn't pinpoint anything in the throat or upper GI area, it did show why occasionally I have trouble with really dense foods going down. The lower third of the esophagus is wavy looking at the edge, which she said was due to arteriosclerosis?? So it didn't work as well...quite common and they don't do anything about it. She also said that I had a hiatal hernia which I know I have (they couldn't catch it on film 7 years ago.) I told them I suspected that I had one because of my symptoms. I sleep on a wedge and that works fine for me. They were surprised that I felt no GERD. I'm still waiting to hear the MRI results of my brain (I would have expected them to do my neck, not my brain)...anyway, it went well. I didn't sleep much the night before and was tired. I pretended I was at a luau with all the guys twirling fire batons, and I actually almost fell asleep! I have an appointment next week for the results.

Finally got around to cleaning our bedroom and dusted the living room. The place has been a pig sty.

I am thinking about contacting a college guy down the street and asking if he is willing to 'adult sit' for me and earn some extra money. Of course, Jim still says "No", but I think that will change soon.

I really like *10,000 Joys & 10,000 Sorrows*. I am reading that and *Away* by Amy Bloom, and Jimmy Carter's new book all at once. They each provide something different depending on my mood. Love Ya.

11/06/2010
Ann to Vicky
Same old, lots of new twists

Not much new, but Ralph has had a few bad days which gives me bad days too. I, too, am reading *10,000 Joys & 10,000 Sorrows* by Olivia Ames Hoblitzelle. I find that some pages leap out at me as if I just said them. Others, not so much. I'm probably closer to Buddhism than Christianity, but I'm skipping over a lot of that anyway. I'm usually in bed when I read and don't have access to a highlighter but I'm turning down the pages so I can go back over them...I noticed that we have our foursome lunch, support group, and gals lunch all in the same week. Perhaps we should change our lunch so it's not so crazy.

Ralph has been much more confused lately. We're also arguing more. He complains to me about me which really pisses me off. In his clearer moments we've talked about the fact 'she' isn't around except when I am. I suggested maybe he's seeing 'ghosts' or images of me because his vision is so poor. I do tend to scoot from one room to another without staying long in one place. He's also been more panicky and scared lately and worries that he's going crazy. I try to explain it's a physical, not mental illness, but I don't know how much he gets. I said to him today, "Do you think Jim is going crazy" and he said "No," that he knows it's his illness. I said that Jim is going through the same difficulties. Don't know if that helped or not. Brian, thank God, called this morning and offered to take him out for lunch. I thought of all the things I could get done around here but decided to call my friend Anne and meet her for lunch. The dust can get an inch thick for all I care right now. I need to save myself. He's out now taking a long walk with Brian and Hassan, and Aisha and I are enjoying the peace and quiet.

I feel as if there's something more I need to tell you, but I can't think of it right now. I'll send a note if it comes to me. Oh, one thing you've been mentioning is the possibility of doing lunch at each other's houses. That's a good idea, but let's keep meeting as long as it's comfortable for all of us. That could very well end soon the way things are going. Take care, and keep me posted on the results of your tests. So long from your partner in the dementia world.

Vicky to Ann

Regarding *10,000 Joys & 10,000 Sorrows*...certain parts of it were right on and she had such a Zen way of stating things, but I was annoyed with her that she didn't allow her emotions to show. She didn't explain how she got caregivers to come into the house, or the worry of working at the same time, not the nitty-gritty...just a reference to it. So maybe we will have a niche somewhere. I was really interested about the spells her husband had that made him go unconscious!

Seems like he was never incontinent or made messes around the house...maybe because she always had a caregiver? Overall, I did like the book though. It could have been a little more concrete emotionally. Like you, I thought there were a lot of good passages...I underlined them.

Ann to Vicky

After Ralph got home from his walk we had a big fight and he said he's really hurt. I don't give him enough time to clean the clutter, I always have something planned for him like today with Brian, and that hurt him. I told him I spend most of my time thinking of ways to help him, like getting out with Brian so needless to say, we had a big argument and things are very quiet. I can't point out to him that he has endless time to do things; that I'm handling everything and he can't seem to sort through the smallest pile of papers. He won't let me help him so I always feel backed into a corner. I have heard many times regarding dementia caregiving that I have to change, because he can't. I feel so teary right now and resentful. I almost feel like a little kid when they say, "maybe I'll die and then they'll be sorry." I must approach this in a more grown-up way. Bottom line is: maybe we should wait 'til next week for lunch so Ralph can get his work of the last 20 years caught up. Sorry, but I need to vent to someone, and the lucky winner is you.

Back to the book: Guess we should just call it Life in a Straight Jacket because there's nothing funny about it. I've also been thinking that with most of the books I've read, there's always help of some kind for the caregiver. I always think when I'm reading: "You think you've got it tough? Let me tell you how it is for 2 people on a limited budget with no outside help to speak of." Is that just me or do you feel that way? I think our book, if it ever gets written, will speak to many more people. Thanks for listening to me vent. Call me if you want to meet sooner, because I'm sure Ralph will feel differently tomorrow and will look forward to getting out and away from his 'many tasks.'

PS. Did I tell you we were accepted by EPIC NY Drug care, have our cards already, and will be paying much less for our drugs from now on? My little ray of sunshine.

Vicky to Ann

Congratulations on being members of EPIC! At least something is going right. The week after is fine with me…just put your arms around yourself and pretend that it is me.

Life in a Straight Jacket sounds good to me…I really do think our truths as to how bad we really feel would be helpful for other people because they must think that they are the only ones that are really bothered by all these things. I loved your line "maybe I'll die and then they'll be sorry." I know exactly where you are! Even though it has to get done sometime… I just think our guys aren't able to 'sort through' things anymore so it's probably a hopeless practice. Is there any chance he wouldn't know if some of it just disappeared? See, Jim wouldn't know, but Ralph has different capabilities than Jim.

This morning we went to breakfast at the Coal Tower. On the way out Jim got distracted by someone sitting at the entrance waiting to be brought to a table, and Jim must have thought he spoke to him, so Jim bent down and introduced himself with a smile on his face and then just stood there. Then I called to him because I was closer to the exit, and Jim turned the opposite way and started following someone else. I swear he doesn't know what I look like at all anymore. I had to call again and physically grab his jacket and pull him out of the restaurant. All the waitresses know he has Alzheimer's, but jeeze! He also keeps trying to get in the driver's side of the car, or he'll open the back door like I'm his chauffer. Basically I am, he just sits in the front!

If I didn't have the time after Jim goes to bed, I wouldn't accomplish anything other than meals!

Yap, yap, yap…I've got to get to bed. Know you are in my thoughts…Hugs.

Ann to Vicky

Things are going better this morning. As much as I would like to change dates and see you, I keep remembering that we can't really talk with the guys there, so we might as well leave it as is. I laughed out loud when reading your account of the Coal Tower happening. I wish I could draw or do cartooning because I have a perfect picture in my head. You're digging your heals in and grimacing as you pull on Jim's jacket while he is salivating and trying to run after a cute blonde that could have been you 30 years ago. Can you see it? We'll keep it in mind if we want to illustrate the phantom (at this point) book.

Ralph would notice if I threw out a postcard for a gallery opening 10 years ago. The next day he would say, "I had a card on my dresser with a picture of a canyon in New Mexico. Now it's gone. Have you seen it?" Or, if in the basement: "I had a foozlebob in an old Kleenex box and I wanted to repair it someday. Now it's gone. Somebody has been down here going through my stuff." I will say, "Who do you think took it?" and he'll say, "I don't know but it was here and now it's gone." Picture this multiplied by hundreds of postcards, clippings, and foozlebobs and you'll see what I'm dealing with. Meanwhile, last night I read a while in *10,000 Joys & 10,000 Sorrows* and went to sleep counting all my blessings: friends, family, my little ones; and the fact that Ralph's still gentle and can say he loves me; and I'm still healthy and possibly sane.

I still feel we're living parallel lives, because Ralph is constantly trying to get in the driver's seat, looks puzzled and annoyed when I tell him to go around, and yes, sometimes starts to climb in the back. I feel I relate to you much more than any author I've read so far, and I think there are probably thousands, if not millions going through the exact same thing.

Must get busy. Paying all the bills today, sorting and throwing out old clothes, and then...Nancy called and invited us for dinner. I asked Ralph because he was so mad at me yesterday for planning too many outings, and he said he'd be ready to go in 5 minutes. We'll 'talk' again soon, and hang in there because I'm always beside you in spirit.

11/10/2010
Vicky to Ann
Never Ending Stuff

I feel like life has slowed down to a crawl!

I mowed leaves yesterday in the morning drizzle. I put Jim to work blowing the deck and driveway (which he did), but of course left all the walkways covered with leaves and the bottom step of the deck...just didn't see it. Anyway, then I saw him wiping down the driveway with the new window mop that has a very soft nylon cottony mop head on one side (quite soft) and a squeegee on the other side, and the pole extends so I don't have to get a ladder. Well, he succeeded in making the cottony mop all muddy on the driveway. Luckily, I caught him before he destroyed the squeegee side. His thinking never ceases to amaze me. I washed the mop out and it isn't too bad but had to pick stones and leaf debris out of it.

Tomorrow, after my neurology appt., I am going to try to do the windows on the outside so I can then bring in the last hose.

It's getting so when we go anywhere I practically have to pull him by his jacket, because he moves so slowly. I know Ralph is not good on his feet and has fallen, but Jim seems good on his feet and has never fallen or tripped, but just walks so slowly! He is really sleeping a lot now. He can get up from a nap, and then say he's going to go in and take a nap. The time change has really thrown him for a loop, too. Even though he can't tell time, the change in the light fools him. It feels late to him and it will only be 3:30 or 4 PM. He wants to go to bed before dinner. Maybe I'll have to think about making lunch a bigger meal and perhaps making it at 2 PM...and dinner a lighter one. Even though sometimes he is not hungry at lunch, I am trying to feed him soup or something with vegetables then.

That's what's happening here. It will be good to see you next week.

I have my Christmas list made out...now just have to find the money to buy the stuff...and the time to do it when Jim is not with me. Shopping with him is like pulling a lead weight around.

11/11/2010
Ann to Vicky

Not getting easier, is it? I thought I was feeling better about things when I wrote Sunday, but then when we were at Nancy's, Ralph suddenly got upset for no reason and had a bit of a meltdown. Nancy calmed him down and he fell asleep, and then as she and Lou were telling me they understood how hard it all is on me, I had a meltdown too. Guess it's been coming on for a while and all it took was somebody feeling sorry for me. All was well in a short while and we had a good dinner and even enjoyed ourselves. I find the best thing for Ralph is for him to go to sleep for a while, and when he wakes he's usually calm and oriented. Nancy and I talked the next day about getting more respite for me. I guess I feel I'm going to need more help down the road and hate to ask for it now. However, I found myself feeling jealous of you Tuesday when I knew Jim was with Brian M. Ralph and I have been joined at the hip since Sat. afternoon when he came home from the market with Brian. You and I need together time!

Today we took a ride to Mumford, and then took the Oatka Trail to Leroy. We stopped at an orchard for apples and had a late lunch at a restaurant in Leroy. We had a good time and I've decided that 3 hours is about enough for Ralph to handle. After that, the confusion starts. We managed to get through the whole trip without any interruption from 'She.' Hooray...tomorrow Brian will stay here while I go to dance class and out to lunch.

We're both looking forward to meeting you Monday. Is Jines at 1:30 OK with you and Jim? Will you both be going to support group Tuesday?

I'm still working on *10,000 Joys & 10,000 Sorrows*. I find that sometimes the author is reading my mind but other times she loses me. I do understand how Hob's new reality sometimes becomes her reality too. I feel that way at times and it can be scary. Hence, the need for more respite. Too much togetherness. Also, the discussions of death made me think of some of our conversations.

Guess that's it for now. 11:30 and it still takes me forever to fall asleep. Even with the magic pill. My inner clock would rather have me sleep 'til noon and stay up 'til 4:00. That's 8 hours, right?

11/13/2010
Vicky to Ann

I know how you feel about being joined at the hip, but I have been living a bit dangerously, going out and leaving Jim. I went out with 2 gal friends to celebrate one of their birthdays yesterday, and I felt really guilty leaving Jim home alone. He was tired and went to bed with a sleeping pill so he probably would not wake up, but if he did and got scared, he would have been very upset. I did stress to him where I was going before he went to bed, but I bet the memory would have been erased if he woke up and found me gone. I know I am living on borrowed time...it's as if I'm leaving a child and if child protective service finds out, I'll be put in jail. My friends say to call if I need them, but I don't feel right calling them just so I can go shopping alone or, say, go have lunch with you...it feels like I am using them to have fun with someone else! So, I also have to get more help in. I have no qualms leaving Jim with Brian M., I've gotten used to that, but I do need someone when I need to go out, or take some time for myself. I have been putting it off. I can always ask the homecare agency for more time, but I don't really want to pay $19.50 an hour and I don't know what Brian M. will do with Jim to pass the time. I feel like Brian M. is his 'go out and have fun' friend. I need someone else just to stay in with him while I'm gone.

Also, it turns out I will not be going to support group after all. The Alz. Assoc. called today and wants me to fill a spot on a panel (someone cancelled last minute) at a meeting for caregivers at a Fairport church...about, of all things, relieving stress and asking for help! She was in a bind and I told her I would do it, but I am sad that I'm going to miss support group. At least I will see you Monday at Jines and then Friday for our gals' lunch. I really want to go, but I couldn't turn the association down. Maybe it will make me ask our freshman in college neighbor to see if he wants to earn some extra money. You'll have to give my 'hello's' to the group.

Doesn't it make you feel like a tight coil of wire that's being held in a spool by the one end that's taped to the edge, and slowly the tape is coming unglued and the wire is just going to fly around and uncoil itself 'til there's no more on the spool?

Anyway, if the college student doesn't work out, then I'll probably call a woman I was referred to years ago when Jim was adamant that no one come in. If we didn't have to think of Jim and Ralph's feelings about being left home, it wouldn't be so bad. The other night Jim asked me if he could go with me to take the friend out on her birthday, and I said "No." I felt really bad.

I wish we had a connecting hallway where we could meet without really leaving our husbands. We would be able to really talk about what the four of us are experiencing. It would make a big difference because you understand the feelings. I know my other friends understand superficially, but they don't know the degree of intensity of our feelings from middle to low...not really any strong degree of elation. Would you agree that you are never really super happy????

11/13/2010
Vicky to Ann
Reaching Out

I don't know why doing this stuff called 'reaching out' is so difficult, but it is.

After accepting being on the panel for caregivers, I could not look at the questions without feeling like a big fake and hypocrite! I sat down with Jim today and had a talk with him. I told him that I needed someone to be with him when I left for 2-3 hours. I said that I want to keep him home for as long as I can, but I needed his help in allowing me to do this. He initially got mad and his jaw became very set...like he was going to say he'd commit suicide if I engaged someone...but he didn't say that. I told him I loved him, but that I really need to go out with other women to have some relief, or I couldn't do it! He kept asking for one more chance to prove to me that he can stay by himself, but I really didn't respond to that. I will leave him alone Friday because I don't have anyone to stay with him. Then I took a walk around the block.

I stopped at one of our neighbors whose son is the freshman in college. I asked if he would be willing to come and 'just be there' if I went out in the evening for 2-3 hours...prearranged of course, and he could bring his books or whatever. He doesn't have to keep Jim occupied, just be there if Jim needs anything. Jim can watch TV or sleep if he's tired. I offered him $13 per hour...which I knew would be more than what he makes at Tim Horton's, and he said, "Yes," he would do it. He also has a light course day on Thursdays so if I want to book lunch like from 12-2, I could do that...all with his prior confirmation. So I now have someone who will come over other than Brian M. Brian M. is wonderful, but he costs $19.50 an hour, and that doesn't include the bowling or ice cream, etc. that I also pay for the two of them.

I also mentioned day care down the road so Jim knows it will be coming sometime, but not right away. Andrew's (the college student) schedule will change after this semester is over. Then I will have to wait and see what kind of freedom he has, but for now it is more time for me as long as I have the guts to schedule something. I told Jim when I got home what I did, and he didn't get overtly angry. This young man is very nice and I know Jim won't take his anger or feelings out on him. You'd think I was asking my parents if I could leave home or something...but I did it and it's a positive step...at least so far. I don't know how Thursdays are for you as far as a Dec. lunch, but that's what I will have to shoot for.

Ann to Vicky

Good for you! I had just opened my computer to send you a note when yours popped up. You'd think we were dating or something because I'm always so glad to hear from you, but it's probably a 'misery loves company' thing.

I'm bummed that you're not going to support group but I'll take notes and report. I don't know what I'll talk about because it's always the same old...He's going down, he's still having delusions, his vision is bad, etc. etc." Most things that I share with you I'd just as soon not mention because, 1) they're too personal and/or nothing can be done about them or 2) sometimes the advice is too general or superficial. I think I will mention the EPIC program and print out a couple applications in case someone could qualify. I'm especially thinking of the new woman who seems like she needs some financial help.

When I went to dance Friday, I found out our group is doing a show for the association in January at the hospital. I don't know if it's their winter party or not because I haven't been receiving notices. How about you and Jim? Any fliers?

I've been on a roller coaster ride again the last couple of days. It was great getting away for a few hours, and I was able to dance without a lot of foot pain. But Ralph seemed angry last evening and refused my help getting ready for bed. He went to bed without saying good night, which never happens. Then, this morning he told me I 'wasn't helping him' because I picked up a pile of shoes and slippers he had parked in this tiny kitchen. That hurt and I got very quiet because there's no point in arguing, but I needed to be left alone. Of course, this makes him upset and he insists on making up, and telling me how much he loves me. This helps him, but I don't get a chance to work through my feelings. Anyway, this afternoon he went out and worked at cleaning up the garden and did a fairly decent job. Later I brought up the idea of taking a train to Toronto in the spring to see *Billy Elliot*, which I'm dying to see. Nancy and Lou are going to see it in NYC and I know that it wouldn't be a good trip for Ralph, but Toronto seems doable. He agreed that it would be fun. A short time later he asked me where Ann went, and when were we going home.

My heart sank and I don't think I want to go after all. It makes me nervous just to think about it. He changes back and forth so fast it's dizzying.

One minute I think I'm going to be able to handle it all with love and caring, and the next minute I think, "Let me out of here!" I'm not as brave and selfless as I think I am.

By the way, I can't remember the last time I felt super happy. I'm just glad to feel somewhat happy some of the time. I know that in the grand scheme of things, we're better off than the majority of folks in this world...and that just makes me sad.

11/14/2010
Vicky to Ann

The panel is on stressors of caregiving and how to deal with them, etc. That's why I said I was a hypocrite...because I'm not very good at dealing with all this either.

I imagine it was fun to think about going to Toronto...a nice wish or dream...I did that last spring thinking about us going to the Grand Canyon. Maybe it would work for you, but I wouldn't try it. Having to take care of Jim all that time, and if he gets confused, etc. Jim could easily turn around and follow some other blonde lady...even a brunette, and then I would be searching for him. Too many variables. Going to Kip's is all I will attempt now.

I think I know how you feel...you are so stressed out that it's easy to get angry, and when Ralph tries to 'make up' it rubs you the wrong way. At least that is how I am. Jim learned long ago that he has to let my anger 'blow over.' I'm not an immediate 'kiss and make-up' kind of person.

This morning we went out to breakfast (the menu is easier to handle than dinner) and ordered orange-cranberry French toast, but when Jim went to butter the French toast he ended up with it all over his hands! I mean big globs of it. I think next time I will ask them privately to butter his French toast before they serve it to him...and do mine that way too, so he won't see the difference.

Maybe because of the time change, and the fact that it's getting darker earlier, the days are as hard for me to handle as they are for Jim. I seem to be full of energy one minute, and the next I'd like to crawl into bed and pull the covers over my head, wishing everything would disappear. I don't let it get me down for too long, though. I just try to keep myself moving.

Love to you and Ralph. This sure is a stinking disease, but you are right. There are a lot of people worse off than we are.

Vicky to Ann

Today I came in from changing the oil on the snow blower to find the faucet turned around in the kitchen and water was all over the window sills. He turned the water off but didn't see that it was facing the wrong way when the water was running! Ugh.

You can share my month with the group if you want...I think the time change is getting me down...the shorter days.

11/15/2010
Ann to Vicky
Enjoyed Lunch Today

We had a good time at lunch with you and Jim today. I'm so happy to see the guys talking together and comparing notes. It's heartbreaking at the same time. Things with both of them are changing so fast. And yet, they are so concerned and compassionate with each other.

11/18/2010
Vicky to Ann
Just Another Day

Boy, today was active in the beginning... eye dr., rec. center, grocery store...and then we practically slept for the rest of the day! Tomorrow Jim goes out at 9 AM to get a Christmas present for me with a wonderful neighbor. Then I go out with you gals. I'm going to try to clean the living room while Jim is away and then work on getting some Xmas decorations out, or maybe a mix of pumpkins and Christmas? I really need to spice up our life but I don't know what to do. I did order tickets...the Rochester Philharmonic Orchestra called and offered 4 tickets for the price of two...so we are going to the Christmas Concert even though it is at 8 PM. The other 2 tickets can be used anytime for any concert 'til July.

Kip is going to try to visit on Tuesday and leave on Saturday. So at least we will see him for 3 whole days. There is trouble at his work again. It always arises at holiday time.

This morning we both got in the car and Jim said to me, "You really should start the car earlier so that when I get in the car it's nice and warm." I looked at him like he was crazy! I should go out 10 minutes earlier with all my running around and getting him ready, so he can be nice and warm! I just about strangled him right there.

Ann to Vicky

I was thinking of writing you when I found your note. Ralph has been really out of it tonight. We went to the grocery store today to shop for my dinner party Saturday. He was OK, but every time I would say "wait here, I'll just run down this aisle for a couple of things," he would follow with the cart and then he'd head somewhere else and by the time I'd chase him down, he would be searching for me with a panicky look. In the end, I have to travel twice as far, and my foot still bothers me quite a bit.

Tonight he kept asking me who all the people in the living room were. Later, he came in the living room and asked who the big guy was sitting on the couch. Then, when I was helping him into bed, he said he wanted to get out of here and go home. I said, "Don't you think you're home?" and he said no, but that we will all be 'going home' soon. That gave me chills. He slept for about a half hour and then wandered into the bathroom. I thought he just had to go, but he took his pajamas off and when I tried to put them back on he said, "What are you doing? It's time to get dressed." I had quite a time getting him into bed and convincing him it was 11:30 PM. He was sure it was morning. I feel so sorry for him that I ache. So here I am, hoping he's gone back to sleep, so I can go in and read until my stomach unclenches. Gee, I'm so glad I'm entertaining 11 people Saturday. I might get bored otherwise. See you tomorrow. We'll talk about getting together on the 9th. I have 3 shows that week but we'll work something out.

11/19/2010
Vicky to Ann
The Thing (Christmas Gift)

Every caregiver should have a neighbor/friend like the one I have. She took Jim shopping for my Christmas present yesterday. She has done this for a number of years running, and I always give her ideas from which she can choose. This year I really wanted a NOOK. I ordered one and made sure that my neighbor would be able to pick it up when it came in. She gave Jim the idea, and he loved it. Giving my friend ideas helps shorten the shopping trip because, it would be hard for Jim to narrow the choices down to an actual gift with his dementia. He was so excited when he came home. I thought he was going to tell me what they bought. It allows Jim to have such a happy Christmas this way.

11/21/2010
Ann to Vicky
Whew!

Well, so far I've survived the weekend. The dinner last night was a success. The kids helped so much. Once I sat down to eat, I didn't have to get up again until dessert and dishes were done. Most everyone left by 9:30 but my niece stayed and we talked until after midnight. I was so tired by then that I couldn't get to sleep yet again. I slept 'til after 10 this morning.

We picked Hassan and Aisha up at 1:30 and went to see the *Wizard of Oz* at the local college. It was a wonderful show. Hard to believe its Community Theater and not a national troupe. Hassan kept whispering questions to me and tried to figure out the technical why's and how's, but Aisha never moved or took her eyes off the stage. They really are fun kids, and after a pizza and some time here we took them home. Now I'm crashing.

I'm pooped, so I'm keeping this short. By the way, if you get one of those NOOK things, how are we going to share books? I ordered *Keeper* by Andrea Gillies because 2nd hand was so cheap.

Vicky to Ann

We will share my NOOK! After all, while I'm reading a real book I don't need the NOOK, and maybe it won't always be so cheap either. I'll have to see after Christmas. Jim is so excited over my present he can't stand it. I don't know whether he remembers what it is, but he is pleased. My neighbor is wrapping it for him.

I really do like *Keeper*. I have stuff underlined all over, and she has really let go in some exchanges with her mother-in-law. She lets her feelings show and I like that because it's so real. Not finished reading yet, but soon. It will be a book we'll refer to if we write a book.

Glad your get-together went well. I don't know how you do all that running around...Obviously you're pooped. If I do something for half a day, I have to rest the other half.

11/22/2010
Vicky to Ann
Dr. D.

Well, we saw Dr. D. and Jim scored an 8 on the mini-mental status exam. Previously he said Jim scored a 12, not the 15 that I believed. Although Jim could not answer many of the questions asked of him, he was unaware that he didn't do well. He was fairly confident that he did O.K. This is a new reaction. Previously he would be bothered by all the questions he couldn't answer, but now he was cheery and very proud of his performance. I asked Dr. D. if we should discontinue the memantine (Namenda) or Exelon patch. He advised not to discontinue the meds because they keep the neurons in better shape, especially since Jim is visibly more functional than the MMSE reveals. He said when you score in the lower range, the scores are not that accurate and assessment must be made visually...how they move, etc. He had Jim stand with his eyes closed and asked him to walk across the room. He didn't sway or anything. I told him Jim could not read anymore, and yet when his assistant wrote a small sentence for Jim to read, he read it correctly. Also the doctor gave Jim words printed in different colors and he sees green better than brown, the next best is black. So that's an interesting finding. He didn't think Jim's asking "Has everyone left?" is a hallucination. Dr. D. wasn't too worried about possible hallucinations, but if things change or get worse he wants me to call him. He also said, "No more bike riding." I guess we are on the big downhill slide.

Kip comes in by plane tomorrow at 1 PM. Can't wait to see him.

Off to Skating with the Stars and some new library books. Enjoy your Thanksgiving!

11/23/2010
Ann to Vicky
Thanksgiving

Just a quick note to wish you all a Happy Thanksgiving. Don't even think about answering. Just enjoy your family.

I was surprised by Jim's MMSE score. I can't imagine what Ralph's will be. I was able to change his appointment from 1 to 3 on Dec. 1st. That means I'll do a show at 1, then jump in the car and get to Rochester General by 2:45. Ralph will be in a tizzy by then, because it's getting so the least added stimulus throws him for a loop. Today, Brian took him for a walk while I went to rehearsal. They were hit by a pretty good gust of wind and Ralph's still talking about it. As soon as I got home I picked him up and headed to Spencerport for haircuts for both of us. He wanted to go home as soon as we got there, but I talked him into staying. No way was I going to re-book. Of course, all the time we were there he talked about 'she' and "Where did Ann go?" The visions are around on a daily basis now, too. All that and I'm still recovering from the weekend. Makes me tired just rereading this.

11/26/2010
Vicky to Ann

We had a really nice Thanksgiving. For most people, Thanksgiving is a busy affair filled with many family members all gathered together for the celebration. Since our family was always a great distance away, ours has always been a celebration of three. It was really nice having Kip home, and Jim was in 7th heaven with Kip. They got along well together and they spent some time together without me, which was good. The first night Kip was here, Jim didn't want to miss anything so he stayed up 'til 11:30 PM. He was like a zombie, but refused to go to bed until I did. After our Thanksgiving dinner, we talked a bit about the doctor's visit, then Jim went to rest for a bit, but came back a few minutes later, angry because he could hear us talking about him. Kip went in the bedroom to talk to Dad and tried to tell him that what he recalled was when he was part of the conversation, and that we hadn't said anything behind his back. They both lay on the bed and talked, and Kip was skillful in redirecting Jim's thoughts to Kip's growing up and the many funny memories that they shared. The conversation went so well, I decided to stay out of it in case I said something that would derail Jim's mood. He went to bed at his normal 8:30 PM bedtime knowing he would see Kip the next day. It was great having him home.

We went to a nearby fish hatchery to feed the fish, and took a quick drive to Lake Ontario. Seeing the lake always amazes us. This time, the weather was much quieter there than inland, and we could see the small scallops of the waves at the horizon. That's not usually possible.

While here, Kip noted that if Jim is talking and has trouble, I interrupt him either to finish or add something to the story. He feels demoralized when I do that, and I really have to listen to myself. I have to make a concerted effort to let him finish and not add my 2 cents unless he asks for it. That is so hard for me because I want to rescue him!

Today I found him banging his blade razor IN HIS HAND with the blades oriented towards his skin. He already had a few paper cuts from it, but insisted that he does it all the time and that I was crazy. I showed him how to hold it if he wanted to 'dry it', but I don't really think he can see how I held it. I get so frustrated. I really have to practice taking an alternate tack so that he goes along with whatever whacky story I tell him. We'll see how it goes.

Jim seems to be more difficult lately. For instance, he lost his two winter hats, and we went looking for a replacement. He must have tried on 30 but none 'felt right.' We ended up buying an ugly blue and gold hat with a pompom. I cut the pompom off when we got home.

The next time we had to go out in the cold, Jim said he would not wear it because he didn't like the way it felt. I brought it anyway and after Jim felt the cold, he put it on gladly, not remembering the comments he made previously. It's just so trying! He is also sleepier and quieter, not active, perhaps bored. I guess it's reflective of his MMSE score, and we will just have to accept it and move on. The 'new norm' strikes again.

Hope your meeting with Dr. D. goes well. I summarized Jim's changes at the bottom of the meds sheet I brought in and I don't think he or his assistant read it! Why do I write these things?

11/27/2010
Ann to Vicky
The Rabbit Hole

It's going to take me all day to write this. I'm jotting things down as I think of them. Lately I feel as if I'm falling down the rabbit hole along with Alice and Ralph. When you're in the asylum 24/7 how long does it take before you become one of the inmates too? The past few days I've felt I'm really losing it: sad, depressed, wondering what's the use, wondering if I have any future, and then I got your note about holiday sadness and I know I'm not alone. Gotta go. Ralph is talking to 'someone' in the living room. More later.

11 PM. Another not so good day. Ralph has been declining, or I should say plummeting since Thanksgiving. He slept most of the day Friday, did a little better Saturday, but yesterday he started talking about his early life and an old girlfriend and why hasn't he heard from her. Then he talked about his parents, our wedding, his brother, and on and on. When I would say, "I know", he wanted to know how I could possibly know all those things. It's getting so I don't pay any attention when he talks about 'her' and where did 'she' go and "When are they coming to pick us up and take us home?" He talks to me about Ann too, so I wonder if he really thinks I'm someone else.

Yesterday we went to Barnes & Noble to get us both out of the house. He had been napping on and off all day, so I felt it would do him good. I had a 30% off coupon and Hassan's birthday is next week. We went to the 2nd floor where they have such neat games and puzzles. Ralph went into the side room where they have art shows and promptly fell asleep. When I woke him and asked if he wanted to go downstairs and look at more kid stuff, he said, "No, just wake me up when you're ready to go." Now, how in God's name am I going to get any Christmas shopping done?

I have an early morning rehearsal tomorrow, and then we have a lunch date with some friends. On Wednesday, I have a show and Ralph will go with me because we see Dr. D. after the show. I can't imagine what kind of shape he'll be in by Thursday. He's already worrying that Dr. D. will be angry with him if he scores low. He just doesn't get it, and it's getting more and more difficult to make him understand even simple concepts.

Guess I've kvetched enough for now. Took one of those cute little pink pills an hour ago and I'm ready to try reading a little, and hopefully sleep. Forgot to mention that I've been sleeping 'til 9:30 or 10, when I don't have an early appointment. I'm turning into a lazy old lady.

Vicky to Ann

You are NOT ALONE. Going through the same thing with Jim...I take him to a store and buy something for Kip's girlfriend, and then he thinks it's for our neighbor and how we should get something for her since she took him shopping for me. He says that at least 6 times a day and I tell him we have 4 weeks 'til Christmas. Yesterday I told him if he didn't stop asking about my neighbor I'm going to hate her by the time Christmas arrives (not really.)

I think I read something about 'going home' in *Keepers*, where it doesn't mean going to heaven, or necessarily going to the home he remembered when he was young, but going home to the place in himself that was once comfortable. He hasn't felt like 'himself' in a long, long time. Perhaps that's it.

I too feel sad and was not going to get a Christmas tree this year for the deck, but a friend convinced me to go next Sunday, so I gave in. It should raise our spirits. I also put some simple strings of lights on the entertainment center to plug in after dark...just set around the picture frames and the candles...and it makes it somewhat festive in here.

12/01/2010
Vicky to Ann
Are You OK?

I am worried about you because you haven't e-mailed at any length in a while...not that you have to e-mail me all the time. I just want you to know I am here if you need me...I would call but I don't want to wake up Ralph if he has gone to bed.

I really see a difference in Jim almost daily. He is no longer aware of himself. The other day, I went out and shoveled the driveway. Jim came out at the end and picked up two shovels full of snow off the lawn and then walked down the driveway wondering where to deposit it. I put lights on a wreath outside while he was futzing (about 5 minutes) and then called him to come in and take a nap. He actually thought he shoveled the whole driveway and wanted praise, so I told him it looked good and thanked him. Why is that SO HARD for me to do? I don't know, but it is. I guess I really work hard at taking care of things, and I don't get any kudos so I don't want to give them to him when he didn't do it...isn't that petty? You'd think I would be happy to make him feel good because I love him, but...that kind of thing is my really weak point!

Ann to Vicky

I'm fine and I'm sorry you haven't heard from me...just super busy, I guess. And by the way, I wouldn't call that your weak point. I'd call it 'being human.' We both need to give ourselves some slack.

I just got home at 11:30 from my annual shopping trip and supper with Nancy. Ralph stayed with Lou who made a great supper with fresh salmon, veggies, and salad. Ralph said it was the best meal he ever had! What? When did I become chopped liver? Ralph was sleeping when Nancy and I got home. Lou said Ralph kept asking who those two women were that were there and then left. Lou said he asked at least 12 times. I woke him up and we drove home. Guess what he wanted when we got here? I couldn't freakin' believe it! He's getting himself ready for bed now, and I guess I'll try to stay awake and away from him until he falls asleep.

Good news: I did get some shopping done.

Your dementia friend

12/03/2010
Vicky to Ann
Response

Wow! I guess I should count myself lucky!

Looks like snow is coming next week. We are supposed to go get our Christmas tree for the deck Sunday afternoon with some friends ... Monday night is Scuba ladies ... Tuesday, Voices ... and Thursday, a tête-a-tête with you. I hope the snow doesn't bungle things up. Remember, you are the one who has to drive the farthest, so if it looks terrible on Thursday, we can cancel. We'll wait and see.

Have a good weekend, and remember to get your old chastity belt out and dust it off! Good Luck!

Your friend in need...your friend indeed.

Ann to Vicky

We just got back from the Gay Men's Chorus Christmas Concert. Very good as usual. I don't think Ralph's in the mood tonight, but the kicker is, this morning he told me I should talk to the doctor about my libido problem...and 'libido' came out as clear as a bell. No stutter or stammer. I was speechless and that's not like me. Oh well, I guess I should be glad he still has an interest in life. I can't tell him how difficult it is to switch from caregiver to lover, never mind the fact that the sheer exhaustion from caring saps all my energy. I love him dearly and don't want to hurt him.

I know it's supposed to snow all next week but besides the 'Voices' and Memorial Art Gallery on Tuesday, we have performances on Wednesday, Thursday, and Friday. Let's play it a day at a time.

Brian is going to try and get tickets to Messiah on Thursday night and wants to take Ralph. If that happens, could we maybe meet half-way between your house and mine? What do you think?

Gotta go help Ralph get ready for bed.

12/05/2010
Ann to Vicky
Christmas

You guys!!! How cute is that? Just opened the e-card. It's adorable. I haven't tried to show it to Ralph yet. Not sure if he will be able to see it. We got your card yesterday and this one today. You're so efficient.

I'm off today to take Brittany and Marissa to Geva Theatre to see A Christmas Carol. Trying to do some decorating but things haven't been running too smoothly lately in spite of what Dr. D. says. I haven't even thought about buying cards yet. Maybe next week. Thanks again and I'll see you Tuesday.

I may not stay while Ralph is in 'Voices.' I already have to return something to Macy's, and I could do that in an hour. We'll probably grab some lunch at the hospital before heading to MAG (Memorial Art Gallery).

Love to you both.

Vicky to Ann

I only sent a few cards this year...only to my special friends/family. Others I sent e-cards. It's just too expensive and time consuming to do it the old way. I just have two to send to England now. I used to do a letter of what happened this past year, but to heck with that. It's too depressing!

Went for a Christmas tree today with a friend. When we got there Jim asked; "What are we doing here?" It's not obvious with a million Christmas trees around. At least he could help by carrying my friend's larger tree. He wanted to cut ours down but started sawing at the ground so I gave up and did it myself. Dropped off the tree to my friend and put it in her stand, then home to do ours, and left Jim shoveling the driveway while I went and washed the car. It was covered in mud balls because the parking area was muddy and we had to be pushed out of the area where we parked.

Supper is done and my hair is washed and Jim is in bed. Don't mind you running off while Ralph is in "Voices"...I'll peruse the library and bring a book of my own.

Anxiously looking forward to my scuba ladies' dinner tomorrow. Cross your fingers that the sitter is well received.

Vicky's Journal

Jim and I had a confrontation this morning. He is becoming less aware of his disease now and all of a sudden he wants to do things that he hasn't done in a long time, or has needed help with for a while but doesn't remember that he needs the help. He keeps telling me, "Let me do it myself" and then he tries and can't...but gets mad at me for helping because I get tired of waiting for him to do whatever it is.

He is starting not to remember parts of the house. If I say, "Your coat is on the coat rack in the hallway," he is rooted in one spot not knowing which direction to go. If he says his gloves don't fit, it's because he is putting them on the wrong hands or has the palm on the back of the hand, etc. Ditto his shoes.

But the good news is, after a while he doesn't remember what happened.

12/06/2010
Vicky to Ann
Senior Sitter

Things went well today with the new sitter for Jim. When I got home at 9:15 PM (from 5:45) Jim was still up with Andrew. Jim said that because he was company, he didn't think it was polite to go to bed while Andrew was here. I told him that in the future it would be fine. He was so 'worried' before Andrew came over, trying to repeat the name to himself so he would remember it.

At least it worked out for me, and Jim liked him so I can use him again. Jim doesn't agree with the idea that he needs someone in the house when I go out at night. I said; "Just humor me." I feel better knowing that there is someone there who knows where I am if Jim should ask. So far, he is going along with it.

I know I'm really bad at helping too much and not letting Jim do more...but I get so frustrated watching that I can't help it! I think that we should just hang in there and forgive ourselves...we all have a tolerance that even though it gets greater with the disease as it goes forward, that doesn't mean that we don't reach our threshold every now and again.

12/07/2010
Vicky to Ann
Dinner Thursday

About getting together Thursday: So you want to be near a mall so you can shop before we meet? Andrew will come here about 4:30 or maybe a bit earlier, so you have to allow me travel time to wherever we agree on. I was thinking that Marketplace Mall would be half way between both of us? I assume we want a place that serves wine??? But it's not necessary?

Let me know what you want to do.

Ann to Vicky

I was thinking about UNO's next to Borders' and across from Marketplace. That's probably equal distance and I probably will shop a bit before. Brian will probably be here most of the day, because I have a show in the morning. I can most likely go anytime.

Yes, wine is necessary. Ralph has been driving me crazy today. He keeps asking me where Ann went, and when is she coming back. Then, he asked me if I ever had a husband. Tonight he wanted to know where we are and how long are we going to stay. He said he thought we were somewhere near the eastern seaboard and pointed to the bathroom floor and asked if that was the spot. I said, "You know we're in NY State, don't you?" and he said he had no idea. I can't believe Dr. D. thinks he's doing so well. He's either talking nonsense or sleeping all day, and winter is just starting. A little while ago he asked what time we're going tomorrow. I assumed he meant to the show I was doing. I said about 1:00 and he said, "How can I pack all this stuff into the car by then?" I don't know what to do or how to answer anymore. I feel as if I already live alone. He just isn't there, and I'm disappearing in his mind. Any answers?

Don't know what I'd do without your shoulder.

Vicky to Ann

UNO's is fine.

I feel bad you are going through that! Jim isn't much better...he knows me but he's been sort of like a zombie. He woke up at 10 PM thinking it was tomorrow and ate some ice cream. He's still up, but I imagine he will go to bed when I do. I don't like him spoiling my quiet time! I totally expect him to pee in the closet sometime soon, not really recognizing any room anymore.

Take care and hope that tomorrow is better ... I wouldn't know how to answer him either...Do you keep saying, "I'm Ann"?

Ann to Vicky

You made me laugh at the closet visual. Yes, I tell him all the time that I'm Ann. I think he understands and then he'll say, "Did Ann get back yet?" Arrrrrrgh.

Did Jim go back to bed yet? I'm going to sneak into bed with a book and hope Ralph doesn't wake up.

12/09/2010
Vicky to Ann
Thanks

Getting together does help ease things a bit. Thanks for being there for me.

I got home and Jim was still up, but announced that he was tired. He didn't want to go to bed again because Andrew was here, and he thought it would be impolite. I told him it was OK and that Andrew knows he can go to bed, but I, of course, couldn't use the 'babysitter' word. I can't speak to Andrew separately right now but maybe sometime I will call him when Jim is out with Brian M. Jim still thinks it is ridiculous to be paying someone to stay with him.

Oh, well, I should thank my lucky stars that it's working out so far and that Jim has remained a gentleman.

Ann to Vicky

I agree. It does help ease things to get together. We'll try to do it on a regular basis.

I wandered around Borders' for a while, and then went back to Macy's. couldn't find anything I wanted. I munched that delicious peanut brittle all the way home. Can I have the recipe?

Ralph was like a new person when he got home from the concert. They all enjoyed it and the kids only got tired near the end. The complete Messiah is a long haul for anyone. I'm back sitting on my heating pad (Note: hurt my back again) before I take some Tylenol and go to bed. I think maybe the secret to dealing with Ralph is to be as laid back as Brian and not worry about who he thinks I am or where we are. No more questions that really don't amount to much. It's worth a try.

12/10/2010
Ann to Vicky
Doctor

Thanks so much for the recipe. Ralph loves it and he doesn't even like peanut brittle. I'll try it soon.

I went to the doctor today and I'm not very happy. First, he said it was probably just the same old degenerative back problem from before and that the only thing to do was conservative treatment, physical therapy (which he says works as well as anything on back pain,) acupuncture, etc., etc. Then, I told him how last night when I was walking, I noticed that my right foot stepped normally but my left foot seemed to flap instead of step. I said I thought it might be from favoring that side. He had me walk away from him on my toes which I did with no problem. Then he said to walk toward him on my heels. I couldn't do it. I couldn't raise my foot no matter how hard I tried. What a strange feeling that was. Almost as if it were paralyzed. At that point the doctor put me through a bunch of neuro tests. Then he told me he was starting me on large doses of prednisone and would see me in a week. He said it's another disc problem and was concerned about the nerve that goes to the left foot. Meanwhile, no heavy lifting, reaching, twisting, bending, and, get this, NO ALCOHOL. I said, "Thanks a lot, that's what keeps me sane these days." I'm sure he wrote 'raging alcoholic' on my record. If there's no improvement I need to see a surgeon. He seemed quite serious about it. So, that was my day. Ralph understands but doesn't at the same time.

Vicky to Ann

I'm sorry to hear that your problem is relatively severe, but then again, you didn't want to try and find the time for more physical therapy if it didn't work. I guess tap dancing is out too. The fact that you couldn't raise your toes is serious...it means the nerves are getting pressure. But, no alcohol, well, you don't want interference with drugs and technically we are not supposed to be drinking with antidepressants anyway. I'll just have to drink your share then. Thank goodness you told him about the way you are walking!

Please let me know if you need me to do anything...and at least if you have to have surgery maybe Brian can take Ralph over to his house for a bit. And we can take him too.

I'm gearing up for tomorrow's birthday dinner for a friend of ours. I've made the lemon cheesecake and the broccoli cheese lasagna and am going to make some more cranberry chutney for gifts...managed to take Jim bowling this morning. He beat me two games out of three. Go figure!

Hope your spirits lift so the bottle doesn't have to!

12/11/2010
Ann to Vicky
A Wee Bit O' Good News

My grandson, Alan, called me last night and said they had decided to do the Christmas Eve party and wanted to do a dinner. I wasn't in a very good mood and was a little miffed that they had decided to go ahead with it and had it planned, and then decided to call me and tell me about it. After I thought about it, though, I decided it was the best thing that could have happened. I'm off the hook!! I was only doing it 2 years in a row because they didn't think they could manage it with work and all. This way, we'll go there for dinner and gifts, get home in time for candles, kids hanging stockings, snacks, and that's it. Then I won't be too exhausted when the kids come back over Christmas morning. So I called Alan back this morning and said we'd be there and what could I bring. I don't sound very Christmasy, do I?

I didn't sleep much last night. Tylenol alone just doesn't cut the pain and my doctor doesn't want me to take anything else with the prednisone. My foot is still dropped, but I'm hoping that it will turn around (no pun intended) before my appointment Friday.

Hope your dinner went well. It sounded delicious.

My computer isn't plugged in and it's running out, so...take care, hugs all around.

Vicky to Ann

Hi there, glad you don't have to do Christmas Eve! Yes, my dinner went well, but I don't think I'll do that again. The entire time I was getting things ready in late afternoon Jim was napping and getting up every 5-10 minutes and just lurking at the kitchen/living room doorway. I had to keep telling him the company wasn't coming for 3 hours, then 2¾ hours, then 2 hours, etc. A couple of those times he showed up with his coat on and said; "I'm ready to go" like we were going out! It went much better once everyone arrived and I got the dishes in sync, and had a couple of glasses of wine. Jim was beat by the time they left at 10:30 PM. So, I put him to bed, and 10 minutes later he was up and asking if there was anything he could do, and wouldn't go to bed 'til I did. I finally gave up on my quiet time and just went to bed.

Ann to Vicky

FYI: My back pain is greatly reduced but my foot is still dropped. I keep trying to raise it, but it just won't work. Ralph has been miserable lately. He keeps telling me not to do too much, that he's here to help, but then he doesn't do anything. It's not because he won't, it's because he can't. And that's frustrating for him and heartbreaking for me.

At dinner tonight he asked if 'she' was going to eat and I said pleasantly, "There's just me". He said; "Are you Ann?" I said, "Yes" and then he said, "Thank goodness, I have to be so careful or I'll be crucified again." I asked if he thought I was crucifying him and he said, "There you go. I can't say anything!" Then he stopped speaking to me or answering me.

I really think he resents my having anything wrong with me. Nancy and Lou stopped over for a short while this afternoon before going to a party in the area, and Ralph was so friendly and talkative. It all hurts that he turns so quickly but I can't let it get me. I know he's confused and scared and is no longer himself, and knows it. I'm not sure how to handle this behavior.

We're going to a Christmas get-together with one of the Alzheimer's groups tomorrow. I think that may help bring his mood back to whatever normal is these days.

We'll be in touch,

Ann or 'She,' whichever you prefer.

12/13/2010
Vicky to Ann
Lunch Today

It was good we brought lunch over to Jim's friend…he's been having physical problems getting around and has been isolated for a while. He is such a good, sweet man.

How is your pain level? If your foot flop is still persisting you must be getting a little scared, huh?

Brian M. comes tomorrow if it's not cancelled due to snow. I have to go to the mall and buy Jim some new jeans, and get some new door knobs at Home Depot. I need to take the lock off the bathroom door and the other doors. I'm afraid Jim will lock himself in by mistake, and I want to put a lock on the den door where all our finances are.

Ann to Vicky

What good friends you are to Karl. He's lucky to know you. It wasn't a very good day to travel, either.

We went to the Just for Coffee party and as I looked around at all the folks we've met from the Alzheimer's Assoc. group, it seems as if Ralph has slipped the furthest. He just sat and did nothing the first half hour, and ate very little. Then he seemed to perk up a bit and helped himself to a second plate, but he kept asking me why Ann didn't want to come with us. I kept telling him it was me, and then he would ask how I got there, and where did I get the car. Funny thing is, we had stopped at a store on the way and picked out a gift for Marissa and he was oriented and looking at things. It's so hard to understand. Brian and Shino brought the kids over for Hassan's birthday tonight and he was OK. After they left he took an hour to get a bath and get his night clothes on, but he wouldn't let me help him. I put his pills and Miralax on the counter and he couldn't figure out what to do with them. I had to insist that he take them. Nancy called tonight to see how I was doing, and commented on how good Ralph was when they stopped yesterday. I filled her in a little and she can't believe how he acts when no one is here but me. I told her that's what's so frustrating to me, because I'm sure everyone thinks I'm exaggerating or just plain lying. And, by the way, I'm no longer 'crucifying' him; he says the woman who lives here is always 'chewing him out.' I'm afraid I'll be accused of abusing him before long. I'm feeling more and more alone when I'm with him. Oh, he also asked me this morning: "Where is that woman who does all the cleaning and cooking around here?" I just said, "She's right here" and walked away. I'm beginning to wonder if I'm doing this all wrong, or is it just the way the disease is presenting. Do you think he is good at hiding his delusions in front of everyone else but me?

Re: my disc problem: It doesn't pain me as much. I slept last night 'til about 6 AM and then it was too uncomfortable. It eases when I'm up a while. My toes can move a little when I'm sitting, but not when I'm standing. The foot is still dropped and I tend to stumble if I'm not careful about lifting my foot. My appointment is on Friday. I'll let you know how it goes.

I can't seem to stop writing this. Must be the prednisone high kicking in. I suppose I should try to get some sleep. I have a bunch of stuff to do tomorrow, but maybe the 'cleaning, cooking lady' will rescue me. Seriously, I must keep telling myself, "It's not him." He's disappearing from me just like I seem to be disappearing from his mind. I know you and Jim are going through so much too, but at least Jim still knows you're his Vicky.

12/15/2010
Vicky to Ann
Nothing

I really have to find something for Jim to do...like sorting screws and nails or something. He keeps asking if there is something he can do when I am cooking or doing something, and I know he needs to feel productive. He just sits around or walks from room to room. If the TV is on he can't tell a commercial from the regular program, and turns the channel because he doesn't like it!

Hope you are recouping a bit, and that your back feels better. I think all this snow is making us all feel nuts. Tomorrow night we take our friend out to dinner for shopping for me (Christmas present from Jim), that is if weather permits.

12/15/2010
Ann to Dr. D.
Update

Ralph has not improved since you changed his Seroquel med. from 25 mg. at night to 12.5 at night and 12.5 in the morning. He seems to be declining even faster. We saw you on 12/1. He's more confused and often doesn't seem to know who I am. He often asks if Ann went somewhere. There is this other woman around us constantly. He goes from totally oriented to completely out of it in a flash. I know the weather is not helping, but late this afternoon he became very agitated and was trying to get all the people out of the house so he could have dinner. He kept saying, "If you're not going to answer me, get out!" He told me he had a Howitzer in the back yard and wondered if they all knew that. His speech was crystal clear. I gave him 25 mg. Seroquel and he has finally calmed down. He ate and is now just sitting. It's getting difficult to communicate with him, because I have to be so careful of everything I say. He tells me (when I'm not Ann) that Ann chews him out and yells at him all the time. I have to let it slide and that's not easy. This is not the way I thought our marriage would end. I seem to be disappearing in his mind. The hardest thing is that when a friend calls or our kids are over, he acts more normal. I feel as if folks must think I'm either exaggerating or outright lying. I guess it doesn't matter but I'd hate to be accused of elder abuse. Brian (our son that lives close) is able to see more and more of this behavior. I hate putting him through all this when he's trying to raise a young family, but he's devoted to helping his Dad and me.

As for me, you'll be glad to know that my primary doctor has increased my antidepressant. I'm also on 40 mg. prednisone daily. I was dancing in a show last week (my sanity restorer) and I hurt my back again. My left foot has dropped and after 5 days on prednisone, I still can't raise my toes. It looks like another disc has ruptured and is pressing on that particular nerve. The pain has decreased except early morning so I'm getting up earlier. I'll be seeing the doctor again on Friday and he said that if there's no improvement, he'll send me back to the surgeon. I'll deal with what that means when I must.

If you have any ideas about Ralph's care, let me know. Just wanted to share and vent.

Dr. D. to Ann

I am very sorry for all that you are going through. No one thinks you are doing anything but a great job working with your husband. I cannot imagine how painful this must be, but you should take some comfort in knowing that you have done everything for him that anyone could ask. In that context, I can think of no nobler product of a marriage.

I think it is time that we increase the Seroquel again. If the hallucinations are making him upset, we should do whatever we can to suppress them. Let's try the 25 mg. afternoon and night.

I am sorry to hear about your back. It sounds like bed rest might be worth trying, at least for 72 hours. Can you arrange that? Do you have a respite care option?

I am taking the liberty of notifying our social worker. She is exceptionally nice and tremendously resourceful. She might have some ideas about respite care, day programs, etc.

Let me know how things are going.

Brian to Mom

Well, that's getting somewhere.

I can't imagine respite right now...whether it's taking Dad out of the house or putting someone in it. That's all he needs...more people around, or a strange place to visit. I can't see the logistics of that.

Meanwhile, you go ahead and lay in bed for 72, and I'll wake you up Sunday.

Does upping the Seroquel make him sleep more, or is that the Namenda?

Mom to Brian

Upping the Seroquel will make him sleepy, but if it stops the ranting and raving I don't care. I asked Dr. D. when he should take the extra med. and he said 25mg at lunch and then a nap and then 25 at night. He was quiet for a while tonight but then started in on all these people and why don't they come out and tell him what they want, and where have they been all these years. He's walking on tiptoes all the time and something about Fred's cabin and building another room, and why didn't he say how the hell have you been, and his old girlfriend is back in the picture, and where has she been and on and on and on.

I don't think he has any idea I have a problem, which is so unlike him. He's losing his ability to empathize but I suppose his world is so dark and scary, he can't think of anything else.

Brian to Mom

I think he needs as many diversions as we can give him. Being in the house all day with not a lot to do probably is what's letting his mind wander off and dwell on the negatives. I wonder if he feels abandoned by some of his living friends, and he's taking it out on the ghosts of his past friends.

Let's try for the one post-lunch nap and then keep him up 'til dark (this used to work well for Aisha). A combination of you taking him places, me Dad-sitting and getting him out for exercise should do the trick. After the 1st, I'll have some time freed up, but I'm trying to catch up on all the pre-holiday rush of files before the post-holiday slow-down hits. Hang in there.

When I was fixing the toilet, I suggested to somebody... can't remember if it was you or Dad or one of his ghost people, that maybe he needs to lay off the dairy for a while and see how things go. The milk, cheese, and ice cream combo might be contributing, although if that was a significant factor, the docs would have mentioned it. The apple a day bedtime snack wouldn't hurt.

Ann to Dr. D.

Thanks so much for your prompt reply. I don't know if they do bed rest anymore. It's much more uncomfortable lying down. As to respite care, nothing is sharply defined with the Alzheimer's Association. It all depends on what kind of grant money is being handed out. I'll double check but I'm pretty sure our health insurance won't help. There are lots of good agencies in this area, but a bit expensive for us right now.

I had a micro-discectomy 2 years ago and at that time, when the pain returned the surgeon said he could repeat the same surgery for the rest of the disc, but then it improved. This is the first time I've experienced the dropped foot. I'll let you know how things go. My son and daughter and their spouses are a great support team, along with our friends. I feel lucky to have them all, including you, in my life. I haven't given up yet. I think we have a few good days left with Ralph. He's always a surprise, just not always a welcome one.

12/15/2010
Ann to Vicky
My Life has Pits Inside of Pits

I can't even explain all that's going on. I'll try to call you tomorrow. I've talked with Dr. D. today. Ralph is so out of it. Babbling and ranting and hollering at all the people here to get out or he'd get the Howitzer out of the back yard. Oh, Vicky, this disease is so much worse than I ever imagined.

Yesterday, he had another impaction and I can't even begin to talk about the hell that was. And no matter what I do to help him and care for him, he just keeps getting mad at me, and tells me I have an attitude. Of course, we've both been stuck here in the house a couple of days so that isn't helping. I haven't felt good, but tomorrow I've got to get out or go mad. Brian says he'll be over at 9 to free me up. He's going to take him somewhere, anywhere, and I can finish up my shopping. I sure wish you lived closer so we could grab a cup of coffee.

Anyway, I'd still like to meet Monday if it's still good for you and Jim. Let me know.

I'll probably take Ralph with me to my doctor's appointment. Brian's going to take him to the theater on Saturday, and I can't ask him to do Friday too.

Oh, Dr. D. wants me to double the Seroquel and see if that helps at all, and my foot's still dropped.

That's it,
Your pooped friend

Vicky to Ann

Call me any time after 8:30 or 9:00...Jim will be asleep. I am so sorry!

12/16/2010
Ann to Vicky
Tonight

Ralph's still up (11:30) and decided he wants to shave. Doesn't want to wait 'til morning, takes too long. It's been a long week and I'm exhausted, but don't worry. The kids have been great and understanding. I don't know how they can understand, because he's so nice when they're around.

I'm thinking about calling a local senior care the first of the year. I'd like to see him go at least one day a week. Have you thought anymore about sending Jim? I'm going to try and go to support group Tuesday and see what days some of the other men go. I've got to stop being a martyr and start thinking about me a little bit more. Sometimes I think all the books I've read about dementia have been a waste of time.

Let me know about Monday. Hopefully things will have turned around a bit by then. We're supposed to go to a family party at my nephew's Sunday. Right now, I don't want to go. It's too exhausting to keep pretending. We'll see. Maybe the extra Seroquel will have kicked in by then. The pain is back, but I got out for 3 hours today. It felt so good!

Vicky to Ann

I didn't call because I figured Ralph was still going.

I can bring up the senior care place and see what Jim thinks about it if Ralph and the two other men are there...but I don't think he will go for it. It's worth looking into, though.

Don't worry about Monday. We are very flexible and so far I haven't heard from Kip about when we will be traveling. We'll just 'fly by the seat of our pants' like we do everything else. You can let me know that morning if you will go or not depending on Ralph's behavior. When you say Ralph yells at the people to go home, does he do it in the house, or is he opening the door and yelling? Either way, you have had two large assaults, emotionally and physically. How quickly things can get out of control, huh?

12/19/2010
Vicky to Ann
Our Plans

We talked today and we are going to Kip's after Christmas on the 29th, a Wednesday, and will come back here the 3rd or 4th of January. We were hoping to go for Christmas, but I'll try to get some necessary things done here, like cleaning (ugh). Hopefully, the weather will be as forgiving the week after next as it is supposed to be this coming week.

So, we will be here all this next week if you need us (besides Tuesday, of course, when I will bring some dessert over to eat while gift wrapping.)

Ann to Vicky

The MRI went well and I wasn't in a lot of pain so it was very relaxing. I almost fell asleep. Nancy picked us up and brought us back home, along with a kettle of chicken soup so I didn't have to cook. I also didn't have a lot of pain when I first woke up this morning, which I hope is a good sign. The biggest problem seems to be the numbness in my foot and now part of my leg. I keep the heating pad on my foot instead of my butt because it's so cold. They covered my legs with good warm blankets during the procedure so I was really quite comfortable.

I'm looking forward to tomorrow. (Note: Vicky helped me wrap gifts) I'll have everything ready to go and we should breeze through it. I don't know what to tell you about Ralph. He's been a bit miserable towards me, but I have to think a lot of it is fear. He also has trouble knowing that it's me with the problem. Probably also denial. Who knows? I hope we can make support group tomorrow. I'm going to bed right after I finish this, which is very early for me. I don't know when I've felt this tired.

12/22/2010
Ann to Vicky
MRI

When we got home last night there was a message that my MRI results were in. That was quick. I called back this morning and there is another ruptured disc which is no surprise. The Dr. said to be very careful between now and when I see the surgeon on Jan. 3rd. No sudden or strenuous moving, lifting, etc. I'm wondering if I should try and get in before the 3rd, but I suppose that's the earliest with the holidays and all. Dr. D.'s social worker, Susan, called me this afternoon and we chatted about day programs and how we're doing and such. She sounds very nice. I told her everything is on hold until the first of the year, but that I'm going to call the senior care place. She thought that was a good idea.

Meanwhile, I guess Ralph did a lot of talking last night at group, but today he's not sure who I am again. Apparently I haven't made much of an impression in 60 years.

Vicky to Ann

Try the picture idea...of showing him that recent picture of you and explaining that you are his wife. Try it for a few mornings and see if it helps any.

I got the NOOK Color at 11:30 and then went out to initialize it at B & N because I couldn't sign in properly but they just deleted the initial sign in and it started to work. It has crossword puzzles on it too, which I will love. It gives hints and I'm pleased as punch.

Has your sleep been any better? If there is anything more I can do for you, please holler. We have nothing planned in the next few days, except meeting with you on Monday.

12/23/2010
Ann to Vicky
This, That, and Merry Christmas

Not much new here. Would you believe I just finished wrapping everything this afternoon? Thank God you were here to take some of the load. I feel OK but very tired. I'm sleeping better, but my foot is so numb my walk is compromised and that's exhausting. Anyway, Ralph has done pretty well today. He tells me he always thinks there are at least 3 women here, and that's what's so odd. He's very aware of the fact that he doesn't know what's going on half the time.

Brian came over late today to take his Dad shopping. When he came in he said, "I've got good news and bad news. The good news is Aisha loves unicorn pillow pets. (I was giving her one.) The bad news is a friend of Shino's gave her one yesterday." I was crestfallen. I had just wrapped it and now I had to think of something else for her 'big' present. Off they went in one direction and I headed off in another. I really needed to be out shopping at 5 PM 2 days before Christmas. I ended up with something I think she'll like. It's a musical jewelry box with a twirling ballerina, and a girl's watch to go in it.

Brian called me from Barnes and Noble and wanted to know what I'd like. I almost said "a NOOK Color," but I didn't. I'm anxious to see yours. Bring it with you Monday if you think of it. And Monday is fine at this point. It will help make the time go a little faster 'til the 3rd. I hate waiting around to see if its surgery, PT, wait and see if it heals, or what. Just want to move on.

I'll be kind of busy tomorrow. This place needs cleaning, and I have to make a dish for Alan's party. So, I'll wish you both a Merry Christmas, and we'll talk soon.

Vicky to Ann

I almost called you tonight but didn't want Ralph to think I was a pain. I am glad he was better today. You must be praying for Christmas to be over. It's pretty quiet here because we have no family around...but maybe we have the better end of the deal. I called my aunt (my father's sister) who lives in NJ just to say "Hello." I also called my mother's sister outside of LA to make sure their home hadn't washed away. She is fine...too high up for mudslides and all her family was there. Nice to touch bases. I will call my sister tomorrow.

We are just going to have a nice breakfast and do I don't know what. I do love the NOOK, although they lead you to believe, or make the assumption from the booklet, that you get a great number of free books, but you don't really. But you can get parts of books to see if you like them and if you do, then download them. I am reading *U is for Undertow* by Sue Grafton. I have read most of hers. It also has crossword puzzles and Sudoku (which I don't know how to do yet) ... I can read it in a completely dark room with just the light of the NOOK, and the light is on very low.

Have a good Christmas and I am wishing and hoping your foot improves.

12/24/2010
Vicky to Ann
Just Me

How the hell did we ever end up in this position?

You, hopefully, are with family tonight. I am home and Jim went to bed at 8 PM. I just finished watching The Holiday and feeling sorry for myself! I suppose somebody has to do it, but why does it have to be 17 plus years? I wish I could be 21 again just for one night.

Oh, well...I'm going to take my NOOK and read for a while. My neighbors gave me brie and bread and champagne and chocolate. I had a little brie, and bread, and wine.

Hope your foot and back are feeling better.

Ann to Vicky

I agree...it really does stink, doesn't it? I wish I could have shared your evening. I hate to think you've been alone since 8. We went to Alan and Christine's and they put on a great dinner, very nice, but I was only going through the paces. Ralph was in and out. Nancy talked to him for a while and then she told me she couldn't believe the change in the past few weeks. I think the holidays make it worse and if it helps, just think, come January and February, everybody will be miserable, not just us. That's what's so hard about Christmas. The rough times look so much rougher. Take heart and know the holidays will soon be over. And we'll see you on Monday, come hell or high water.

Brian was over this morning with the kids' stocking stuffers. They'll have Christmas morning here with us. Stockings, breakfast, and gifts. Anyway, we got to talking and somehow I was talking about how we haven't made any funeral plans. I was telling him what I wanted and such, half joking but serious too. Then, when he came back this afternoon to pick us up, I said; "Cancel the funeral! I've been taking care of people since I was 18 years old and I'm going to have some 'me' time, not taking care of anyone before I shuffle off this earth." We both laughed but I meant it, God willing.

We usually light a lot of candles and have snacks on Christmas Eve, but not tonight. Hassan was sick this afternoon so he and Shino didn't go to Alan's with us. We got home at 11 and it's just another evening except I've got a Christmas service on TV. I didn't even bother to light the tree.

Hang tough...it's just another day and know I'm thinking of you with love and understanding.

12/28/2010
Vicky to Ann
We Leave Tomorrow

It was fun having lunch!

I think I just about have everything we need packed, minus the shavers and the toothbrushes. Last night, we picked up a night stand from Craig's list for $60 and have that squished in the car, too, with the giant framed fan and at least 6 bottles of wine. Of course, I had to take the miter saw that we bought Kip out of the box to get everything in. Now, I just hope that Jim doesn't get a headache the minute we are out of the driveway. Last night when we picked up the chest he got a headache from the seams in the pavement going calunk, calunk. God only knows what 7 hours of riding will do!

Probably will be back Monday night. Stay out of trouble 'til I get back, OK?

Ann to Vicky

Just found your note. You may have left by the time this reaches you. We enjoyed lunch too. Always do. Ralph seemed almost normal when we were with you, but when we left the house he wanted to know where the lady went that had been helping him all morning. Said she went upstairs and didn't come down. Then he swore there was a girl in the back seat on the way. Notice that all the apparitions are female?

Tonight, he has been very loving, but I don't know if it's me or someone else he wants to make out with. So weird. He seemed to know me, but then started telling me that he had relatives in Rome, N.Y. and proceeded to tell me where Rome is. Now, I have to get in bed with him and I'm going to insist on reading awhile, and hope he falls asleep fast. It breaks my heart to see what we've been reduced to. We've always had a good love life, and now we're sometimes like strangers. I have to keep hanging on and find joy in his good days when I am still the love of his life.

Have a good and safe trip. I'll miss you.

Chapter Three

2011

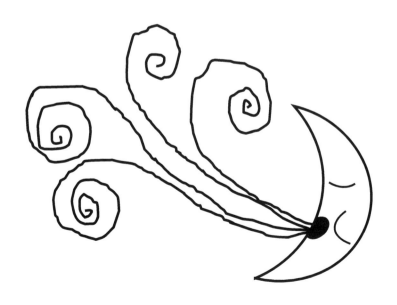

01/03/2011
Vicky to Ann
We're Back

We had a good time and good driving there and back. I painted Kip's bathroom, 3 coats plus the ceiling and closet, so now he can put things away. It was quiet, and for 3 hours Kip took Jim shopping for all sorts of things and really got a dose of what it is like. He is so much better at answering and speaking to Jim than I am...good psychologist and can direct him by what he says without telling him what to do.

While at Kip's, we refinished the table I bought from Craig's List with polyurethane (had some glass rings on it) and it looks great, especially with new knobs...so that is all done and only cost $60.00. Will make a good end table for him.

We are unpacked and glad to be home...and back in a normal routine with normal meals, etc.

01/05/2011
Ann to Dr. D.
Appointment

Would it be possible for you to see Ralph before his scheduled April date? He wants very much to speak with you about some things that are bothering him about his memory. I want him to be able to express himself to you before he loses that ability. At this point it's difficult to tell whether or not the extra Seroquel is working. The holidays have been exhausting for him, and I'm hoping to see a little more energy now that they're behind us. However, he spends a lot of time trying to figure out just where he is and who I am. He doesn't seem to know we're married and/or I'm his wife. I'm not sure who he's looking for, and I've run out of ideas on how to cope.

Anyway, let me know if an appointment in the next few weeks is possible and, as always, thanks for your help.

01/09/2011
Ann to Vicky

I was going to write this morning, but it takes forever to get ready to go anywhere these days. We went to the Support Group Winter Party. It was nice, but we missed you. The regulars were all there, but the problem was; most of us were there by 11:30AM, but the food didn't arrive 'til almost 12:30. That's when the Tappers were supposed to start their show. I felt bad for them, trying to perform while people were either eating or just getting their plates. Anyway, they did a great job, and Tara was glad I had suggested them.

I guess we haven't written because things are same old, same old, with some new same olds. Ralph is more confused and has been insisting on talking to Dr. D. because he can't figure out what the 'deal' is. Why is he living here, how long does he have to stay, and so on. He also insists he's never been married. At that, I told him if we're not married, I'm not going to work my tail off taking care of him anymore. That stopped him, but I don't think I'll tell our group facilitator about that. Sometimes, you just have to react or go nuts. I wrote to Dr. D. and we'll be seeing him in February instead of April. I want Ralph to express his feelings to him while he still can. Other than that, he's been pretty good. This past week we went to MAG (art gallery), Geva (theater), the planetarium, and the event today.

My foot is still dropped and numb. The back pain is better, but my right hip hurts for a couple of hours in the morning 'til the Advil kicks in. I think it's from walking funny. I had to take the brace back, because I discovered I needed authorization from the insurance company or they wouldn't pay for it. Haven't heard if it went through or not.

I'm glad you have a project to do (pillows for Kip) to keep you busy on these dreary winter days. I feel bad for Ralph and Jim. There's so little for them to do. I've decided not to try day care just yet. Brian said he'll plan on spending more time with his dad so I can get out. Speaking of which, I can't wait until lunch on Friday.

01/10/2011
Vicky to Ann
Resistance

While you have someone who is living someplace where he shouldn't be, and you're not married, it seems we are all living in a boarding house or some such place. Although it's not hallucinations, Jim wants me to shut the door when he's getting dressed in the bedroom so that no one else sees. He's always asking if all the people left, or are the other people up yet. He also doesn't want me to shave his neck...he doesn't want to look nice when he goes out. He wants to wear the same clothes until they rot off him, I guess. He says he doesn't give a damn what he looks like, and I say; "Well, I do!" He fights me every step of the way. I told him; "Fine, I'll hire someone else to take care of you." Then, he said he doesn't need anybody, so I said, "Fine...I'm moving out!" Not really.

I must admit I was being a bit childish. We were supposed to meet our neighbor at the end of our driveway...we were going out to lunch...and I made him go out too early. It was cold (suck it up...I'm out here, aren't I?) Our neighbor was a little late so Jim said; "I'm going inside." "Fine," I said, knowing he wouldn't be able to remember the code to the garage door opener...and he couldn't...so he came back down the driveway and said; "So, you've won." He was mad for a little while but it quickly disappeared.

The other day I went out with the scuba ladies, and Jim went out with one of the husbands. They went to a local restaurant, and as his friend was being seated, he looked around and Jim was nowhere to be seen. He looked and finally found Jim sitting with some old guy at another table, because Jim couldn't remember who he was with, even though he's one of our closest friends!

Then, we went to the rec. center and I burned off all the emotions because I walked really fast. Now, I'm level headed again.

Why can't I be civil and clever with my responses like Kip?

Well, that's my take on the week.

Ann to Vicky

I guess we're going through very similar scenarios, aren't we? I was talking to Beth from support group, and she said her husband doesn't think he's married either. She said, "It hurts, doesn't it?" I replied, "Maybe its wishful thinking, but who knows?" And Diane said her husband sits right across from her at the table, talks about 'Diane' and says he wants to go home, too. I feel so much more normal when I'm with our group.

The reason Kip handles it all so well is because he's not with Jim 24/7 like you are. (I mistakenly wrote 224/7 and when I noticed it, I thought that's what it feels like.) Anyway, Ralph is much better with Brian and Nancy too; so much so that I almost get jealous of them. I can talk and talk with Ralph and it doesn't reassure him, but he believes Brian when he tells him that his brain sometimes plays tricks on him.

01/19/2011
Ann to Vicky
Support Group

I thought it was a good discussion last night, but do you think I went too far in my segment? It was so nice to have just women for a change, and I didn't mean it to be funny. I'm just so frustrated with this identity thing. I'm beginning to understand how it must feel when Alzheimer's patients cease to recognize their spouses or children. I'm trying so hard to think of this caregiving as my purpose for being, but where is the real me? Have I lost my identity to myself as much as to Ralph? Can you make any sense of this?

Ann (I think)

01/20/2011
Vicky to Ann
Support Group, Husbands' Girlfriends, and the Blahs

Even though Jim recognizes me, I feel as if I've been 'swimming' around the house, just attending to Jim's needs and not doing much else. I attribute it to having a cold, but maybe it's just another low that we have to deal with. I don't feel like I used to, and if I think back over the words I would have used to define myself a few years ago, I am none of those things now. I am just a thing that provides comfort and needs (and not doing a spectacular job of that, I might add.) It's as if all we are doing is waiting for the other shoe to drop and trying to put up a good outward appearance so no one figures it out...that we can't or don't want to do it anymore.

I don't think you went too far. We need to hear what most of us will go through, and it gives you validation that your feelings are real and terribly crushing. You can say, "Well, he doesn't know what he's saying or thinking," but it doesn't make you hurt any less.

You are correct in feeling that Ralph never would have cheated on you in your marriage, just like I feel that way about Jim. Do remember that the constraints that gave them morals and ethics aren't functioning very well now, so the girlfriends break through. It doesn't mean he would have acted that way before the disease. I hope that helps you.

Group was good. I just wish we all had more time.

01/22/2011
Vicky to Ann
Hi

Well, Jim's stitches are healing well, although he doesn't like showering. (Note: Jim had a pre-cancerous lesion removed from his forehead.) He wants to get into the bath tub, but I won't let him do that for another few days. Today, he appeared without his bandage an hour after I put a new one on. He has a Herpes cold sore on his lip and I don't want him to pass that to the incision, so I told him he had to leave the bandage on. Also, his eye is getting more swollen from all the fluid falling downward on his face. Hopefully, that will disappear soon.

I figured out why all the toilet paper is disappearing. Jim's been stuffing his jockeys, in case he dribbles later I guess! No evidence of that, but whatever. He's going through toilet paper like there's no tomorrow.

Not accomplishing much here except the bare minimum.

I have your anniversary card but forgot to mail it today. I'll take it to the post office tomorrow. I know anniversaries are really kind of tragic now. It's not an easy day to celebrate. Good luck on your Dr.'s appointment Monday.

Ann to Vicky

I didn't realize Jim's surgery was that invasive? I thought it was one of those zap/cauterize deals. Little problems are so much bigger when Alzheimer's is in the picture. Hopefully, it will heal in spite of Jim.

By the way, about the toilet paper problem. Before we all invest in Kimberly-Clark, why don't you try those new pads for men? They're large pads with all the absorption in the front (not adult diapers, just pads.) We used them a few times when Ralph stopped taking Flomax. Needless to say, he went back on it and things have been OK for now, anyway.

Don't worry about our anniversary. I can't remember when yours is, and I hope I didn't miss it. I'll have to check last year's calendar. I'm not sure how I feel about ours. This morning, Ralph's friend, Dan, (who we've both known for 40 or more years) took him out for coffee. When they came back, Ralph said he wanted to tell Dan about us. Then he stopped and said, "Never mind." After Dan left, I asked him what he wanted to tell him. He said that he didn't know how to introduce him to me. He said that on the way home, he told Dan he wanted him to come in so he could introduce him to his new wife. Funny thing was, when Dan picked him up, Ralph told him we were celebrating our anniversary this weekend.

So, ♫Happy Anniversary to me♫. My life feels really bleak lately, but as Beth said the other night, there are a lot of folks who are much worse off. I try to think in a positive way, but it doesn't always work.

Take care for now and don't worry about doing the barest minimum. I may have you beat.

Ann's Note

This year's anniversary turned out to be the sweetest (although bittersweet) in a long time. This morning, Ralph said he wanted to go out and walk around the block. I gave him the usual rules (take your cane, be careful, don't go on the main roads, don't be gone too long, etc. etc.) He agreed to all of the above, left, and returned almost an hour later as I was starting to worry and look for him. He handed me a bag, and in it was a lovely anniversary card signed by him. I was stunned! The closest store is almost a mile away and on a very busy street. He said that he took his time, was careful, and that the clerk in the store helped him find just what he wanted. My heart melted and broke. I can't say any more except that I love this dear, sweet, gentle man, and will do everything I can to make this awful journey bearable.

02/02/2011
Vicky to Ann
The Latest

Jim told me the other day while we were riding in the car that he wants to enroll in driving classes again so he can drive next summer. I said, "Absolutely not!"

I reminded him that he hasn't driven in over 5 years and had given up his license. He would have to take the test all over again and he can't even read! Hopefully, he forgot that he said it. He told me that with practice he would do fine...that he can still learn...isn't it sad??

He has been driving me crazy lately, because clothes that he has worn a million times suddenly 'don't feel right' and he won't wear them. I feel like strangling him. Now, he doesn't like any shirt if it comes up too high on his chest and comes close to his neck. I have ordered new long winter underwear for him since the old ones are shrinking, and some new shirts that go over the head and zip at the top so he can adjust the neck closure. Hopefully, that will help.

I assume your days have been going slowly...as mine have.

I finished the pillows yesterday and they turned out well. Now, I'm enjoying the latest book you loaned me.

Ann to Vicky

I was going to turn off the computer, found your note, and here I am.

My days are going slowly, but also fast enough that I'm not accomplishing anything. Today I was going to completely clean my desk, papers, junk, etc. Then, I opened today's mail and found a bill for a procedure for Ralph. We had already paid the co-pay but they were charging a 'facility fee.' The procedure took 5 minutes, was in the regular exam room in the doctor's office. I won't go into detail, but 3 calls to the billing rep. and 3 calls to the insurance company got me nowhere. I was venting it all to Ralph and he seemed to understand. Funny thing is, tonight he started telling me all about it and how Ann had to make all these phone calls, and he felt bad about how much work it was. Go figure.

When I read your note, it made me think about how Ralph and Jim are both going down-hill, and yet in such different ways. Ralph doesn't have any illusions about his driving and he's pretty mellow about what clothes he wears. On the other hand, Jim seems to know you (as long as you're not in Wegmans.) Ralph asks me over and over where everybody went, or "Where is our boarder" or, "Is Nancy home yet?" and my personal favorite; "Where's Ann?"

02/12/2011
Vicky to Ann
New Developments

I was approached today by the director of recreation at the rec. center, and they are concerned about Jim's safety while working out on the machines in the weight room. They don't want to discourage him from coming, but I agreed that he should be supervised from now on, and that he would not use the large bar bell pulley weight system.

That means no more walking around the track for me because Jim doesn't like to do that. I guess I will have to go with him and watch him work out. He's not going to take that well, but that's the way it is. At least, if we can keep our lunches to Tuesdays, I can get out then.

Hope things are going relatively OK with you.

Ann to Vicky

Boy, 'relatively' is certainly the operative word here, isn't it? Relative to what?

I'm sorry that your one good exercise is being taken away. Just what you don't need. I still haven't been able to take Ralph back to Silver Sneakers, and one of the reasons is that they told me they couldn't deal with his 'dizzy' spells. I think he gets a little light-headed and makes more of it than what it is. Maybe you can start weight lifting along with Jim, and someday join a ladies' wrestling team.

I feel bad that Ralph isn't able to get out and walk, and I haven't taken him to the Silver Sneakers track either. It seems as if it's one thing after another with all the appointments. We've both been sleeping longer, so by the time he's dressed and had breakfast and fiddled with his shaver for an hour, its noon.

I was sorry I went back home after lunch Tuesday. Ralph had another impaction and the rest of that day and night was hell.

I won't go into detail. Suffice it to say that when he wondered who I was the next day I could have throttled him. I asked him who took care of him the night before and he sheepishly said he guessed I did. He still wanted to know if I was going to stay overnight and where I was going to sleep. Yesterday he said there were still gaps in his life. He remembered our first house very well but says he wasn't married, even then. I asked him if he remembered having 3 kids there, and he said, "Yes." I asked him who took care of the children when he was working, and he thought about it and then said he really had no idea. Makes me feel as if I wasted my life caring for my family. I certainly won't be remembered for it. I sometimes think of Jack and wonder how he handled Ginny's not knowing him. I guess what bothers me is that Ralph remembers everyone else.

On top of all that, Ralph re-injured his arm again. It was just starting to heal. When I try to find out just what happened, he goes into such detail I really don't understand what he's saying. I'll probably have to take him back to the doctor if it doesn't appear to be healing. He already has an appointment with his GI doc. to see what more we can do about the impactions, and he sees Dr. D. Monday. I'm going to write a detailed note for his assistant to give him before he meets with us. It should save some time and I can think about what I want to say.

My friend, Anne, returned from Florida Wed. and we met for coffee this morning. We sat and talked for 2 hours and it was heaven. Thank goodness Brian was able to take Ralph out for breakfast so I didn't have to worry. I thought I might leave him alone for just an hour, but he was so mixed up last night I didn't dare. He thought he was out in Penfield and didn't know who was going to drive him home. He was amazed at how similar the Penfield folks' house was to his own. He said even the furniture looked the same as his. He was floored when he went into the bedroom and that looked the same too. No matter how I explained it all to him he just couldn't understand that he was home.

I probably should think about calling it a day. I have Aisha overnight and she wakes up pretty early now that's she's in school. People must think I'm crazy for keeping the kids overnight so much, but the truth is, they keep me grounded in reality. I'm much more content when one of them is here for the weekend. It's too easy to get depressed otherwise. Tomorrow, we're going to Alan's to celebrate Nancy's birthday. I'm looking forward to it and hope Ralph is a little clearer and will enjoy it as best he can.

02/13/2011
Vicky to Ann

You sound worn out and I empathize with you about, "What has my life meant?" but think of the love you have extended to your children and their friends all your life, and what a wonderful Mom you were. Yes, a major part of that is missing due to a terrible disease, but it doesn't mean it was done for naught. Look at what great kids you have, and the good memories of your life with Ralph. You are a special person and have accomplished a lot in your life.

We may have to go see Dr. D. too. I'll wait and see. I tried to tell Jim delicately about being accompanied at the rec. center, and he got very angry and says he wants to dispute what they told me. He wants to talk to them. I told him, "No, they were right in being worried." I told him either he agrees to their stipulations, or we won't go at all. I'm going to have Kip talk to him later today, too. Jim keeps insisting that there is nothing wrong with him, and I said, "Oh, yeah? Well, look at your underpants and your long winter underwear and the tissues all over the bathroom floor. Why is that all there?" I gave him his underwear and said, "Let's put this on," and he said he would do it himself and closed the bedroom door. A few minutes later he asked for my help and said, "OK ...you've won."

It's a sad life we're living, isn't it?

Ann to Vicky

You always know the right thing to say to help me out of a dark mood. You are such a dear friend, and I appreciate you more and more.

We went to Alan's for dinner and I still have Aisha with me. She's staying another night because Shino and Hassan both have a bug and so far Aisha's OK, so it seemed logical to keep her. Shino had to fly to

Boston this afternoon to interpret a court session tomorrow, and she's feeling better. Brian jokes that they won't allow Muslims to bring bombs onto planes, so they have to bring viruses instead.

Coming home, I turned the wrong way onto the expressway at a ramp I'm not used to, and went miles out of my way. By the time I got home, I was exhausted. Now, Aisha's not able to fall asleep. She keeps getting up to check on the Valentines she's taking to school tomorrow. I'm going to lay down the law as soon as I finish this. I have to roll her out at 7:30 and try not to go back to bed. It may be tough.

Thanks again for all your support. We certainly are on similar journeys, you and I. Something tells me we'll both survive it.

02/14/2011
Ann to Dr. D.
Note Before Appointment

IN A NUTSHELL:
Physical: In January, Ralph had a laser procedure done on his right eye, improving his visual acuity from 20/80 to 20/50. This is helping his vision somewhat, but his perceptual vision is declining.

He continues to have problems with impactions (from meds??) He will be seeing his GI doctor later this month to see if we can improve that situation. The problem usually ends in a nightmarish day for both of us.

Three weeks ago, Ralph tore a bicep muscle. His doctor is hoping it heals itself as surgery at this point is not feasible. He doesn't think Ralph would do well with physical therapy either. If I don't protect it with a sling when he's up and about, he keeps re-injuring it.

Mental: Ralph had some melt downs in December and January, and wanted very much to talk to you. I think you're the one person he trusts completely. He tells me he has gaps that are disturbing to him. For instance: he doesn't always realize he's in his own home and wants to know how he got here, and when he can leave. The main problem is he thinks there are at least three (I wish!) women taking care of him. He doesn't always realize I'm his wife and insists he's never been married. He remembers his children, but has no idea who cared for them. I'm sure this is a typical scenario for you, but I'm hoping you can reassure him a bit and make his world more comfortable. I'm never sure if I should gently remind him of 'who, what, and where', or if I should go along with his unreality. He continues to need more and more help dressing, undressing, and all that goes with everyday tasks. He doesn't have a problem with swallowing yet, (Thank God,) and is able to eat without assistance. His speech is declining, but I'm amazed he's doing as well as he is. He makes up words if he can't find the right one, but that's pretty much the new normal. I worry about the future when he can no longer express himself.

As for me, my back continues to be a problem. I have a herniated disc that is pressing against a nerve, and has left me with a dropped left foot. It has remained dropped since early December, but the surgeon is taking a 'wait and see' position. He doesn't want to do surgery as long as I'm now pain free, but my gait is a bit unsteady, and I can't dance (my therapy) for the time being.

02/16/2011
Vicky to Dr. D.
Jim

This morning, Jim is insistent that he wants to learn how to drive this summer if someone teaches him. He won't accept that he can't or won't be able to do it. He says either I bring him to someone who will teach him or he will kill himself. He is tired of being trapped.

Dr. D. to Vicky

If he drives, he will not be covered by insurance, no matter how much you pay the insurer. Read the fine print; the driver is 100% responsible for giving up driving if he has Alzheimer's disease, and Jim does. If he gets in an accident, you could lose everything you own.

If you have guns in the home, dispose of them now. Give them to a trusted relative, or take them in a box to the local police. Call them and tell them you are coming. Don't walk in carrying a gun.

If you feel he will hurt himself or others, you need to take him to an Emergency Room. The two largest hospitals have psychiatric ERs. If he won't go, and you feel there is immediate danger, call 911.

We might need to consider a residential dementia care option. We can adjust the meds, stopping Ritalin and doubling the Mirtazapine, but they may be insufficient. Keep me informed.

Vicky to Dr. D.

I think things are in control for now. I wasn't considering telling Jim he could take the driving test. I was trying to tell him in no uncertain terms that he will NOT drive. He doesn't want to hear that Alzheimer's has made it impossible for him pass the driver's test or get insurance, etc. His problem is he wants to believe that he can still learn. Maybe if I give him the chance to try, he will realize that he can't.

What I am going to do is to pretend I called a driving school and tell him that before anyone can teach him to drive, that he has to learn the DMV driving manual and take a test (which is true.) I have to go to the DMV anyway, and so I am going to get a manual and work with him. Then, he will think he is making progress. I'll keep you posted.

I don't want him to be placed in a residential setting if I can avoid it. He has been gentle and not harmful to himself or others so far. I just think that he is so frustrated with no independence.

I'll keep you updated on how it goes and thanks for the suggestions.

Dr. D. to Vicky

That is a reasonable and realistic plan. I hope it works. Good luck.

<u>**02/24/2011**</u>
<u>**Ann to Vicky**</u>
<u>**Don't Feel Sorry For Me**</u>

Guess what? I called the Alzheimer's Association and I can have 40 hours a year of respite care at home. It's basically for Ralph, but I'll be able to rest. I've requested 5 hours on Mon., Tues., Wed., and Thurs. of the week after surgery. Someone will come and help Ralph with breakfast and lunch, pick up, light housekeeping, and even LAUNDRY!

<u>**Vicky to Ann**</u>

That's wonderful. Wow! What a blessing!

<u>**02/26/2011**</u>
<u>**Ann to Vicky**</u>
<u>**In Touch**</u>

I'm doing next to nothing today so I thought it would be a good time to catch up with you.

I think I've picked up a bug of some kind and I'm afraid it may interfere with my pre-op. I've been coughing and just feeling lousy. I had a fever Wed. night, but felt fine Thurs. Yesterday I had to go out in the storm and finally got my blood work done. Then we went out to breakfast and I picked up groceries. I felt OK, but tired. Today, I can't get out of my own way. I tend to get bronchitis easily because of my life long asthma history, so I'm hoping my doctor will give me an antibiotic when I see him Tues. He doesn't prescribe them easily, but knows how susceptible my lungs are. I won't be happy if I have to reschedule the OR after all the planning with the Alz. Assoc., so I'm staying in for the weekend. We cancelled a memorial reception for this afternoon. I thought Ralph would give me a hard time, but he didn't. He thought I should take it easy, too. Surprise!

Brian M. worked for three hours Thursday. He cleaned and polished all the wood cabinets and scrubbed the stove and oven. Did a great job. After he finished, we sat in my gleaming kitchen eating cheese and crackers and drinking wine while swapping family horror stories. He didn't leave until after 6:30. I guess we've connected. He's coming back next Thursday to scrub the tile and grout in the kitchen and bathroom. Yay!

Hope you're both coping with this latest weather issue. It makes the whole dementia thing a lot harder, doesn't it?

Hassan is visiting today. Brian dropped him off when he picked up Ralph for the market. He's no problem (we have TV and they don't) and Brian is bringing a pizza later. No sense using my nice clean stove.

Vicky to Ann

Glad you had a good time with Brian M.

Jim has been complaining about his right arm and I thought it was due to his snow shoveling, but tonight he figured out that when he drops his head, his arm hurts. I vaguely remember the arm from before, but he hasn't complained lately, so I forgot all about it. Probably has a bone spur in the neck that puts pressure on the nerve in certain positions. I explained that if it is a spur, there is either surgery or 'don't do that' and I said surgery would not be good for his brain. Anyway, what I'm trying to say is that we laid low today. I was fixing a friend's Roman shade (doing a lot of fine sewing), so we just watched golf. For some reason, Jim has been up since about 3 AM, not being able to sleep even with Trazodone, so we napped this afternoon.

Finished the Roman shade, so now I can attend to my boring stuff. Just got in from shoveling the driveway. Yesterday, we got about 10 inches and it looks like we have at least another inch, and it's still snowing. Also, I've been trying to take some pictures of the birds at the feeder with my telescopic tripod...1 good one for 20 bad ones.

Jim, because of lack of sleep, was very dopey this morning. When I came up from the cellar this AM, he had a bunch of short sleeved shirts that he says are too tight in the neck (a new development with his clothes), so I had to refold and put them all away. Every week it's a new complaint about some type of clothing. He needs help today finding the bathroom, but so far, no accidents. He walks around like a zombie. Then he says, "So, what are we going to do today?" like I'm a cruise director or something! I guess I should be grateful for the snow because who knows where he would be if it was nice weather. I'm going to have to install an invisible fence this spring. (Sorry)

02/28/2011
Ann to Vicky
When it rains, etc., etc.

I need to share and I don't want to talk about this with my family. I went to my pre-op today and was coughing much more. I explained to the surgeon's NP about the long standing asthma/lung problem and how easily I get bronchitis. She said she would order a Z-pac and if I felt my primary might object I could wait and pick it up after I see him. That was fine, they finished the pre-op and gave me a copy of the EKG to give to my regular doctor. Nobody said anything. While we were waiting for Ralph's appt. (GI doc), I casually looked at the EKG printout. It said, among other things...abnormal EKG, probable inferior infarct, age indeterminate. So now I'm wondering if I'll have an angiogram instead of the discectomy. I've been searching the web and there are a number of similar cases. EKG abnormal, infarct, etc. and they all had to cancel their surgeries. I know I shouldn't worry until I've had Dr. P. see and explain it, but I've had an EKG every year and he tells me they're normal. Meanwhile, after we got home, I couldn't stop coughing so I went and picked up the Rx. I wolfed two of those babies down and my temp just went over 100.

Sorry I dumped on you but I needed to, and you're always there for me. Oh, I tried to explain it to Ralph and I think he 'got' it. He's been awfully nice to me. Not so last night. We had a row and, of course, it was all my fault, the way I treated him, and so on. He stomped off to bed and I sat watching those boring Oscars and crying. I was feeling very sorry for myself, when a tribute to Lena Horne came on. It ended with a quote of hers: "It's not the load that breaks you down. It's the way you carry it." I decided it was meant just for me, and I gave myself a good talking to.

I'll let you know how things are as soon as I get home.

03/01/2011
Ann to Vicky
To My Favorite Shoulder

All is well. It is as we thought. Dr. P. said my EKG has stayed the same forever. The one taken yesterday is read instantly by a computer and he said most of them come back abnormal. He also said it's a good thing I started the Z-Pac. He doesn't want me to still be coughing come surgery time March 11th. I asked him if he thought the surgery was worth a shot. He said the only other option is to live with it. The surgeon has been in contact with him and said this is very unusual, and that with all the nerve damage I should be in a lot of pain. They both want to make sure I realize that it may not improve at all, and if it does, it may take 6 months to heal the nerve. I'm sure surgeons worry about patients wanting to sue because they didn't improve, but I know the odds and I'm willing to take them. I have a feeling it will get better, and I may even dance again.

Everything else checked out fine, but Ralph and I decided not to go to the art gallery this afternoon because I'm coughing my head off. Guess I'll take a nap. Take care.

03/09/2011
Ann to Vicky
Surgery

I called the surgeon's office today because I'm still coughing. She says as long as I don't have a fever they'll go ahead with the surgery.

Ralph is having a lot of trouble understanding it all. He keeps asking when my surgery is, and when is that other lady going to have her back surgery. He tries hard to grasp it and gets so confused. I feel sorry for him, but he'll be with Nancy and they get along so well together. Do you want me to let you know when I'm scheduled?

Vicky to Ann

Yes, I would like to know when you're having your surgery, just so that I can think about you when it's that time. I will call later in the day to find out from Nancy how you are doing. Do you need me to stay with Ralph while Nancy takes you to surgery? I don't mind doing that if you want me to come to your house, or do you think he'll be fine with Nancy in the waiting room?

I'm thinking good thoughts for you and I am hopeful that your foot drop will resolve after surgery. It may take some time because the nerve has been compressed for so long, so don't be discouraged if it isn't miraculously all better after the surgery. But I bet things will slowly go back to normal.

I am glad you feel comfortable sharing your true feelings with me. When you said that sometimes you don't really like your husband anymore, I totally know what you mean, because I feel that way too. And, of course, it probably makes you feel guilty, but what's said is the truth. I, too, sometimes don't like the person I am with. There are so many demands and complaints; it's like...so what's next? What will it be tomorrow? But their lives are so narrow now...there is nothing to fill the void.

Today I gave Jim a Sloppy Joe open-faced sandwich and by the end of the meal his left hand had dried BBQ sauce all over it. I felt like I was dealing with a 1 year old, having to get a wet washcloth and wash his hands after eating. This prospect is so sad, and I wonder if I will be able to slog through it to the end like I want to. How do we bathe them and diaper them when they get that bad...and yet I don't want to institutionalize him if I can help it.

On a happier note, by the time you are ten days out from your surgery, the weather will be that much better. Love and hugs.

03/12/2011
Ann's Note

My back surgery was uneventful, but it will take months (perhaps years) before I know if the nerves to my foot will regenerate. Ralph is still having trouble understanding what's happening.

Vicky to Ann
A Bit of a Row

Hi there...hope you are progressing well.

In the last couple of weeks there has been a significant change in Jim's personality. He has started showing a reawakening of his striving for independence. It has been a very significant change for him. All of a sudden, he wants to start driving again. This time, he has no awareness of having Alzheimer's. When he talked of it last summer, he knew he would need a lot of training. Now, he acts as if he is perfectly normal. He even mentioned that he didn't know why he gave up driving in the first place! I want him to forget about this, but I don't think he will.

Presently Jim and I are having a bit of a row. I don't want to speak to him. Just one of his imagined problems. It will blow over soon.

Ann to Vicky

I was just going to write and you beat me to it. I feel much better today than yesterday. Yesterday, I had a lot more pain and I've had ongoing fever since Friday. The temp finally went down this afternoon, and I think it's going to stay down. I'm having a lot of trouble staying awake though. I think I could sleep 'round the clock.' I'm so glad I found respite care through the Alzheimer's Association. Our aide is very nice.Very comfortable to be with, like Brian M. She fixed Ralph's breakfast, cleaned up the kitchen and bedroom, and went for a long walk with Ralph while I took the first of many naps. I'm beginning to realize that I really did need some help.

Nancy told me yesterday that she didn't realize how hard it is just trying to keep him on an even keel. Also, Ralph has been quite miserable to me. I don't know if he is afraid or just trying to cope with everything. He's doing better, but that's probably because I told him I was going to send him to Nancy's while I healed.

I don't think I'm going to support group tomorrow. I'm most comfortable when I'm either standing or sitting with my legs up. Sitting is uncomfortable after a few minutes. Say 'Hi' to everyone and tell them I'll be back next month. I want to take advantage of all the great help and just relax. Trouble is, I might not want to go back to how things usually are.

Last but not least, your dinner was delicious. I'm not eating much at a time, so we'll be having it again tomorrow or Wed. Thanks again. I don't know how I would manage without all the great support. I appreciate it so much and I'll pay it forward whenever I can.

Hope you and Jim have resolved your quarrel. It's not getting any easier, is it?

Let me know how support group goes.

03/15/2011
Vicky to Ann
What's Up

Yesterday Jim was more withdrawn...almost like his mind was busy, and he was very slow to answer questions, if he answered them at all. Sometimes he would say "Wait", like he needed the time in order to think about his answer. I didn't understand what was going on, and that evening he was verbally resistive. I can't even remember what we were talking about, but I just said, "I can't stand this anymore" and began to cry. I went into another room and shut the door. Crying didn't accomplish a thing. It didn't change his mood, or scare him, so I figured being upset wouldn't do either of us any good. Jim then took a bath to stave off the symptoms of dry eye, and so I laid out his clothes, but I wasn't willing to talk to him much. When I put the clothes on the counter he said, "Don't come in!" He also had complained about his arm hurting when he moved his head in certain positions, complained about pot holes, complained about his mouth being dry despite drinks with ice cubes, and the humidifier going non-stop. Then, after a nap, he woke up pinching his nose and squinting, saying he had a nose bleed. There was no blood. I actually got out a flash light and looked carefully...he has a few pink blotches in his throat, but no real blood. He was also sticking his finger way up his nose, so if he didn't have an injury before, he would now. I told him it looks irritated, and that I would give him some medicine that would make him feel better in the morning (cough syrup)...my attempt at 'going where he is.' He didn't fall asleep that night and kept asking me questions 'til about 2 AM. That entire day, my heart was palpitating and I wondered if all the days in the future were going to be like this. I noticed as I was trying to fall asleep that Jim's breathing was much faster than mine. Was he scared or upset?

The next morning when we both got out of bed, he said we had better tell Vicky about this because she would think that we were having sex. He didn't want to get in trouble. He didn't recognize me as his wife. Who would want to go to sleep with a stranger next to them in bed? I told him I was his wife, but I asked him if he would feel more comfortable if I slept in the other room, and he said yes. So I guess I am relegated to being just a caregiver. I am now a stranger. Today, so far, he has called me Annie, and a neighbor's name. We'll see if it's permanent. I am trying to take it all in stride. I am now walking in your shoes!

Vicky to Ann
Tonight's Meeting

We had 8 people there, but two people were new and came in late. The facilitator was also an hour late. You know, we can practically run the group ourselves anyway, because so many of us have been there for years.

Some people talked about incontinence issues and sleeplessness in regards to going on a trip. Everyone gave the same advice...take the trip now while you still can! A new lady talked about her father with infarct dementia, but she has no diagnosis from a neurologist, so the group suggested she take him to the Memory Care Clinic for a proper diagnosis. It's amazing the people that come with a diagnosis from their GP! Another person who has been taking care of his mother without help from family, is completely worn out, and is looking for placement. He says he wants to place her so he can love her again. That sounds familiar doesn't it?

I spoke about the problems I related to you earlier. Jim recognizes me tonight, so I guess I will take a chance and sleep in our bedroom rather than the guest room. Brian M. came and sat with Jim while I went to support group.

Take care and continue to get lots of rest. That anesthesia really does knock it out of you.

03/17/2011
Ann's Note

This was the last day of respite care from the Alzheimer's Association. All went well until the aide offered to walk with Ralph. He adamantly refused and insisted he could go alone. (He likes to walk at his own pace.) A half hour later, a postal delivery truck pulled up in our driveway. I was hoping maybe it was a get-well gift for me, but no such luck. The driver helped Ralph out and half carried him into the house. It seems he was walking down a slight hill and fell on an icy patch. The aide and I thought he was OK, but he complained of his wrist hurting. Since it's becoming increasingly difficult for him and/or me to gauge his pain levels, we decided to take him for x-rays. The doctor said it was just a sprain (no breaks) and put him in a soft cast.

So, that was the end of my post-surgical recovery. Back to 'normal', like it or not.

03/17/2011
Ann to Dr. D.
One More Thing

Again, thanks so much for your concern. I meant to tell you and forgot (tell me it's not anesthetic dementia,) but Ralph has had 3 episodes in the last month where he went blank and stared for perhaps 20 seconds. It's almost like a petit mal seizure. Sometimes he gets weepy afterward. Dr. P. said it could very well be part of the picture, but wanted you to know about it.

It's not always easy to talk when Ralph is right there, but here's how I feel about walking:

- Ralph absolutely needs to walk. He has fewer and fewer joys these days.

- Someone should always be with him.

- If that's not possible, I should take a deep breath, make it as safe as I can with rules, canes, etc., and let him go. How sad if he had to give up his exercise and then fall in the house and break a bone.

I don't think we came to a decision about the Seroquel. Let me know.

By the way, your social worker, Susan is great! Having a good support team makes this almost bearable.

Dr. D. to Ann

I know how difficult it is to be inactive when there is so much you could be doing, but you need to take it easy. I think your husband's spells are best viewed as pauses in the coherence of the usually continuous relationship between ongoing experience and what we call spontaneous behavior. I do not think they are worrisome. Of course, other things can happen, but I do not know that we should be doing anything about these events. His illness is progressing; we cannot stop that. We are doing all that can be done. Keep resting, and keep in touch.

03/23/2011
Vicky to Ann
The Doctor's Office & More

Yesterday, Jim woke me up at 4 AM to tell me there was a man in our bedroom, and he stole a lot of our stuff. I got up and checked a number of places to make sure it was a hallucination, and then told Jim that everything was all right. Shortly after, he called me and insisted that I touch the roof of his mouth. He said it was so dry, he would be dead shortly. It is dry because Jim is a mouth breather at night. I have been running the humidifier non-stop. There's not much more I can do. I got him a drink of water, but he didn't hold it in his mouth at all; he swallowed it quickly and told me his mouth was still dry. "I want to go to the doctor's office NOW!" I told him at 4 in the morning no one is there. They are all home sleeping. He replied that I didn't know everything; that we should ride over and see if anyone is there. I said, "No," but got him OJ with ice, and he drank it. He chewed the ice and swallowed it, and then told me his mouth was still dry. This went on and on and he got more agitated and angry with me, but I didn't think he would hit me. Jim took a bath at 6 AM, then we ate breakfast, and I waited for the doctor's office to open. They reluctantly agreed to see Jim during their 'walk-in' hours for simple things like dry mouth.

When Jim entered the office, the staff and our doctor were 'blown away' by his appearance and the change in him from his last visit. While she was asking Jim questions about what was bothering him, Jim yelled, "I want to see a doctor NOW!" She responded by telling Jim she is a doctor and that she was trying to help him. Jim said, "Feel my mouth. I want to see a male doctor." She recommended Biotene mouth spray and mouth wash. At the end of the appointment and in a quiet voice, she stressed to me that I should get in touch with Dr. D. immediately. She later called me to make sure I was physically OK staying with Jim. She wanted to make sure I wasn't in any danger. I didn't think I was, but?? She thinks all the obsessions with the body are part of the disease, and that perhaps he needs Seroquel.

That afternoon, I went over to the day center where many of the support group dementia people go, and filled out paperwork so Jim could possibly attend. I said that I wouldn't start Jim until his medications were straightened out. After the director took all the pertinent information, all I had to do was complete a medical history sheet and bring in a change of clothes. I was hoping that Dr. D. could tweak Jim's meds so that he wouldn't be 'on the edge'. Maybe then, a day center (for a day or two a week) might be an option.

Early today, after going to the eye doctor to make sure Jim's punctile plugs were still in place, we received a call that Dr. D. would see him at 1:20 PM. When we arrived, they gave him the MMSE and he did very, very poorly. Even though I explained to the staff what was happening, Dr. D. asked me to tell him what was going on. Dr. D. wanted to watch Jim's expression and body language as he listened to me tell the story. I told of the obsession with his body, wanting to go to the doctor's at 4 AM, the outbursts in the doctor's office, the fact that he doesn't know who I am most of the time, and that Jim wanted to leave home and move back to N.J. with family, not with me. Jim added that our marriage was not working, and that we should call it quits. He showed his 'attitude' with Dr. D. when he was asking Jim questions. Dr. D. explained to Jim that at his stage of the disease, he wanted to add Seroquel because it was more appropriate, and that he would try to simplify Jim's pills over the next few weeks. That should make Jim feel better, and hopefully bring down his agitation level, allowing both of us more sleep.

I know Dr. D. would prefer that I institutionalize Jim now, but I just want to see if we can quiet this phase and I can keep Jim home a while longer. Perhaps we can get through these obsessions and it will be better.

Tonight, I noticed that Jim has forgotten how to dry himself off after bathing. He was trying to scrape the water off his body with his hands...until I gave him a towel and showed him how to dry himself, and then he got it.

Hoping for a better day.

03/26/2011
Ann to Vicky
Bits of Trivia

We didn't mention Monday yesterday, so I thought I'd better confirm it. 1:30 at Jines, right? As I write this, I'm remembering you mentioned calling ahead for a booth so I guess we did talk about it. Anyway, I hope Jim is staying stable and will remain so for a long while.

I drove to Webster and back today with Ralph and Aisha. Marissa has a piece in an art show in the high school, and I told her we would come see it. Long way, but she was happy to see us. It's good to have my wheels again, but I wish I had enjoyed my time off more. I'm back to the old grind and doing everything, and Ralph doesn't see anything that he could be doing to help. Just assumes I'm completely back to 'normal'. At least his mood is better, so I guess I should be thankful. He went to breakfast and shopping with Brian this morning and Webster this afternoon, so he's even more confused than usual tonight. Told me I should be glad I didn't have to go to the high school like he did, because 'there were mobs of people.' He must be thinking that Aisha, the five year old, drove.

Guess I'll get back to my book. Another in a series of *The Mistress of the Art of Death* by Ariana Franklin. Aren't Saturday nights exciting? Love ya.

Vicky to Ann

Hi Ann, yes, we will be there at 1:30 PM at Jines.

I tried to get Jim interested in the golf tournament because Tiger Woods was playing, but after a while he couldn't distinguish which one was Tiger. You could say he is liberated and not prejudiced, but really, he is just blind! After a bit, he changed the channel because he was bored. But that didn't help.

I scraped down the back hall ceiling because it's that really spiky stuff (Jim textured it when we first moved in) and I wish we had never done it. It looks better and then I repainted it because I have to paint the skylight walls, the regular walls, and the closet doors...not all at once, a little at a time. It was too cold for Jim to go out to walk, so he just snoozed in the sun the entire afternoon. The Seroquel isn't giving Jim any side effects at least, but he still wakes up in the middle of the night ... more like 5 AM. I give him some mouth moisturizer and tell him he has to sleep until it is light out.

He didn't recognize me at all today, I don't think. He asked my name a couple of times so I put on a name tag.

Tomorrow is another day ... this is getting old fast!

Ann to Vicky

Things are going OK, but Ralph is still trying to figure out his 'stuff.' I can't tell you how sick I am about all that. I started to write a really scathing letter to you about his obsession, but ended up telling him just how I feel. And, strangely enough, he seems to understand where I am coming from, and the hurt feelings dissolved as I realized I just have to back away from those issues. I have enough to deal with without assuring him that no one is taking his 'collections.' Speaking of which, he wants to know if you'd be interested in any wine making materials since you do make wine at home. He has a large jug of some kind and a hose, and I don't know what all. If you think you could use any of it, let me know and I'll throw it in the car.

Managed to take a walk and spend time on the exercise bike. See you tomorrow.

Vicky to Ann

See you tomorrow. Today was a better day for Jim. I was trying to update our book file, which now should be called Life in a Straight Jacket instead of Laughter in a Straight Jacket. It's amazing to look back over the past year and see the progression.

Another thing Jim won't eat besides dense meat (pork, steak, gristle.) I prepared Greek turkey burgers, French fries, and corn. He won't eat

French fries at home because they are too crispy...he was afraid that they could slice open his insides! I ate all of mine. I guess my stomach is made of steel.

Ann to Vicky

It's odd, and we must be on the same page, but just this morning Ralph was being difficult. I thought that we should change Laughter to Life in the book title, because there's nothing about it that's funny anymore. He's so darn unhappy, and I'm tired of thinking I can help his always somber mood. If I thought he would be happier with someone else caring for him, I'd do a search and then trade my house for my freedom. Then I'd turn my back on the whole sorry mess and try to find some joy. It probably wouldn't work, and I'd be miserable, but it's fun to think about.

PS. You tell me my experience with the identity issue has made it easier for you and I love the idea of the name tag. I'd try it but I think it would make Ralph angry. However, I wish I could take it more in stride like you do and not feel hurt every time he asks where Ann is. I know he can't help it, but I still feel bad and lost and alone. Oh well, it is what it is.

03/28/2011
Vicky to Dr. D.
Jim Ruppert on Seroquel

Jim seems calmer on Seroquel. He also was diagnosed with thrush and is taking fluconazole for his dry mouth. The dry mouth isn't going away fast enough. I've also been giving him Flonase for post nasal drip...he still has it, and insists that it is blood dripping down the back of his throat, and that he is slowly dying from this. No amount of conversation will convince him otherwise, but he is not agitated or angry... just frustrated and resigned.

I will write you this Thursday when he has been on the Seroquel a week. Then we will discontinue the Lexapro and add the Seroquel morning dose.

Thanks so much for seeing us so spur of the moment like that.

Dr. D. to Vicky

I am glad it is helping. These are dynamic issues; he may need more or less in the future.

03/28/2011
Vicky to Ann
Lunch

I really looked forward to lunch and I had fun. If I hadn't had a stone sitting next to me it would have gone a bit better, but I still had fun. Did you notice how unemotional Jim was? It was like he was in suspended animation, just staring straight ahead.

After we had a nap, we got up and had a simple dinner. Jim was very stoical the entire time. Finally, right in the middle of the national news, he said he wanted to talk to me. We had to go into the bedroom to talk, because he didn't want 'the others' listening in. Anyway, he told me that he was going away with his sister, that the family was moving, and that I couldn't go. He asked if I would be all right. He couldn't give me specifics, but he has been pressing me lately to visit his sister and Kip. I told him his sister would be arriving next Thursday. That didn't seem to please him. I asked if he would see his mother and father (who are dead,) but he didn't know. He just felt really bad that I couldn't come with them. We'll see what develops as the week goes on.

Thanks so much for the chocolates. I will enjoy one a night with my wine.

I'm glad that today was a good day for Ralph, and therefore, a good day for you.

03/30/2011
Vicky to Dr. D.
Update on Jim Ruppert

Jim has done well on the Seroquel at night. Should I drop both Lexapro now (morning and night,) and should I give him Seroquel in the mid-morning or half the Seroquel mid-morning?

I have not noticed any hallucinations since on the Seroquel at night; he wakes at 5 or 6 but allows me to guide him back to bed. He is insisting that he is going to go stay with his family and live there permanently, and I can't come. I assume he is thinking of his childhood when all his aunts, uncles, and cousins were all around. They are now spread all over the country. He says he wants to see them all every day, and he will talk to them about not going to work.

I told him we will go after his sister comes to visit next week. Hopefully he will forget about it.

Dr. D. to Vicky

I am glad things are going well. His early AM problems suggest to me that we should double the nighttime Seroquel to 50 mg. and leave the AM Lexapro in place for now.

These changes may be too much for Jim. The only way to know is to try it. Please keep me in the loop.

03/30/2011
Vicky To Ann
Topsy Turvy

Things are a bit better...Jim is still waking me up too early, but with a drink, an ice cube, and a gentle push, he will go back to bed 'til almost seven. Doesn't it sound like I have a new baby?

Lately, Jim has been very serious about leaving and going to his 'family' as if he is traveling back to his childhood. He says he has to go to them and wants to live there permanently, so he can see all his aunts and uncles and cousins. He said Mom and Dad too, but I told him they were dead. He didn't deny it, but just said he would see the others that are alive. I asked what he would do if they had to go to work...and he said they wouldn't, he would talk to them about that, as if they would agree to stay home and 'play' with him...he didn't use the word 'play.' I asked who would take care of him, and he said he could take care of himself. Up to now, I have left the other set of car keys hanging on the kitchen hook. I don't think he would even know how to start the car if he sat in the driver's seat. I said, "You have Alzheimer's," and he responded, "I do not!" He wants to 'hang out with the guys'. He's tired of hanging out with women. I could just see them all together at age 10-12, doing what boys do. I mentioned that some might not live there anymore, but he wanted to go and find out. It was as if he wanted to hop in the car right then and drive...no planning or bill paying, or packing, etc. The more he talked about this idea, the more he said something that rocked my world. He said that our marriage wasn't working, and he didn't want to be married anymore... after 42 years and 18 of those with Alzheimer's. He didn't want my help. From wife, to caregiver, to 'the enemy' or 'warden.' That is how he saw me. "I can do it myself," he would say. Just like a two year old.

I notified Dr. D. of the present problems, and he said to double the dose of Seroquel at night and take away his Lexapro in the evening. He will change other meds after we see how this affects Jim. It's all about getting just the right dose without too much. I sure hope Jim forgets about moving back to his family. I suggested that we could go to New Jersey in a couple of weeks, after I pay bills and pack and all. I was hoping that would buy me enough time for Jim to forget about it. I don't think my ploy worked. He didn't look convinced. I feel like I should throw him a big family reunion, but I don't think he would recognize his relatives if he saw them. He's thinking of when he was younger, I'm sure.

Also, I can't make our lunch on the 12th. I have to meet with my lawyer about what funds I should withdraw money from if I should need more help, or heaven forbid, a nursing home.

The week following is bad because my lawyer is going away and she has things booked for next week. I have to do it when Brian M. is here with Jim, so I can speak freely with the lawyer. If you could make it Thursday, I could ask Brian M. to sit on Thursday if he has availability (14th). Let me know, otherwise I'll just see you both for group next week.

Glad I ordered 4 boxes of wine from Bully Hill for the spring and summer. I'm afraid I'm going to need them. I'll keep you updated.

03/31/2011
Vicky to Ann
Stupid Me

Stupid me. I had a dermatology apt. this AM at 8. Jim said he would not go outside. HE PROMISED HE WOULDN'T. When I got home, he was across the street with no coat on, asking my neighbor if she'd seen Jim's Uncle Bill because Jim was sure he was coming to visit. So if I had any doubt, I know I can't leave him one second. He even had my spare set of keys on the coffee table, so they are hidden now.

Ann to Vicky
My Week So Far

It sounds as if Jim has entered an entirely new phase. I noticed a difference Monday. I don't think he really recognized Ralph and me. It's all so sad. Perhaps he'll be a bit more oriented when his sister visits. Also, it looks as if we won't try any more quick lunches, just you and me. They'd haul you off to the slammer for sure.

I wanted to tell you about the highs (few) and lows (many) this week, but I'm finding it hard to put my feelings into words. It's all about Brian trying to help Ralph deal with his 'stuff'. Both of them had found a young man who is interested in buying whatever Ralph wants to sell. He came over Tuesday, seems like a really nice guy, owns a bike shop, and is getting into a little antiquing on the side. Wrong, wrong move. After hours of hemming and hawing, Ralph finally agreed on what he wanted to sell. Most of it was junk, but even so, he ended up with $420 more than he had that morning. Since then, he has obsessed and griped and talked about all the things that 'they' want to get their hands on. He even is thinking this guy snuck things out that he wanted to keep. He talks constantly about things that he treasures, and now they're gone. I started to blow up tonight but then I looked into his vacant eyes, and realized I just couldn't. This has been a bone of contention with us for most of our married life, and I couldn't solve it then, and I damn well can't solve it now. I have to turn my back on it all, and concentrate on cleaning out what I can. Am I bitter or resentful? You bet. But I have to focus on all his good points and how he's always been a loving husband and father. A truly good man.

A friend from support group and her husband wanted to come visit us on Wednesday. I was a little uncertain about it because Ralph couldn't understand exactly who was coming. He kept thinking I was going to be entertaining two or three women friends. Finally, I got through to him who was coming, and we ended up enjoying the evening. We had some cheese, crackers, and grapes, and of course, some nice white wine. When they got ready to leave, Ralph started getting ready too. When questioned, he said he wasn't quite sure where he lived. It has to feel like a nightmare to him. Time for bed. I took a sleeping pill, so hopefully it will work. I need to refocus and remind myself that I'm the best caregiver ever. Then, I'll go to sleep and grind my teeth. Thanks for listening.

04/01/2011
Vicky to Ann

Wow, do you know that what you just wrote off the cuff could be part of a book? It is so full of emotion and caring. You are the best caregiver ever! Congratulations on the $420.00.

This morning I played like an ostrich, and put my head in the sand. After breakfast, I took a 1 hour nap until I figured I better get my butt up and moving. Once up and occupied, I was fine, but getting up feels like swimming through molasses. And I didn't even take a sleeping pill last night. Of course, between the snoring and being awakened to get Jim dressed at 5:30 AM after a bath, and the complaining 'my mouth is dry', my sleep was interrupted many times.

You are wonderful!

04/02/2011
Ann to Vicky
Book

I ordered that book last night as soon as I read your note about it (*Alzheimer's Diary, A Wife's Journal* by Michelle Montgomery). I need to find more people who think about this disease the way you and I do.

Things are going better. I have to put my money where my mouth is and do the same. It's just that my junk is cleaner (books, needlework that I'll never do, pictures, etc.) Ralph may be calling you today or tomorrow about bringing that jug out to you. We're going to an art reception at B & N tomorrow afternoon. It's from 2-5, and I'm sure he'll tire out quickly. Maybe we'll make a quick visit afterwards, if you're going to be home. Don't stay home on our account. It's no big deal.

About Jim: More baths are better than no baths, which I understand is often a problem in the later stages. Does he realize that too much water dries your skin faster? Best you don't tell him that. I'm sorry you're going through all these changes. They seem to be coming at you fast and furious.

I just threw out a ton of old stuff in my refrig./freezer. Going to do the big one tomorrow, then defrost. That will give me a little start on spring cleaning. Hang in there, talk to you soon.

Vicky to Ann
B & N (bookstore)

What was the occasion at B & N...a special book signing? I was there taking Jim to the card store to buy me a birthday card. There were cars and busses all over the place. Hope it was fun.

I can pick up the carboy if you can bring it to lunch on the 14th, or maybe I'll pick it up at your house next time we're over.

Jim seems to be doing better, but he still wants to leave and go to his 'family' after Nancy leaves. Boy, I can't wait. Think of all the time I will have to myself. I should call one of his cousins and tell him Jim is coming. What a shock that would be!

Back to my reading...500 NOOK pages but it is good!

04/03/2011
Ann to Vicky

I don't know what was going on at B & N yesterday. The art show reception is today. The work will probably be there a couple of weeks in the community room (2nd floor.) It's called the Artist Breakfast Group, and Ralph belonged to it for years. Just a glimpse of who he was.

Yesterday was a nightmare. Another impaction. 'Nuf said. I'll write more later or tomorrow.

04/03/2011
Vicky to Ann
New Normal I Guess

Jim is still waking me up at 4 or 5, but after I get him dressed again, he will go back to bed. He wakes me up by wandering around the house saying, "Hello, is anybody here?" Today he let me sleep 'til 8:30 AM.

He now treats me like 'that boring caregiver,' unwanted but necessary. We went to Mendon Ponds Park, and the nature worked its magic. Jim seemed happier and more relaxed. After we got back, Jim said he was worried about our neighbor who takes him gift shopping. He said, "I'm afraid she's dead." I said, "How do you know?" and he said, "Because I went there and saw her." I tried calling her so that Jim could speak to her and hear her voice, but she wasn't home. I left a message for her to call. She called an hour and a half later, and I put Jim on the phone. He was so relieved. For that entire hour and a half he was worrying. [There was an irrational fear in my head...how did he see her dead? Could he have been violent and done it himself?

But there was no time when he was away from me, and he wouldn't, would he? No! He is a gentle man.]

Tonight as I was getting Jim ready for bed, he said he needed to go to the bathroom. I said "OK, go." I went into the computer room to update the journal...with the door closed. I came out after a bit and asked if he was ready to go to bed. He said he couldn't go with all these women in the house! I said, "There's only you and me, and I have been here for 40 years!" (Why do I have to be so snotty? Because I'm frazzled.) I asked, "What do you want me to do, wait outside the house?" He said, "No." Anyway, after some trying, he gave up and and went to bed. Thank heaven.

I wish Jim were as 'with it' as Ralph. At least Ralph can take his own pills with a prompt. I put Jim's pills in a cup and he still doesn't take them, even if they are right by his tooth brush.

It occurred to me why you are more tired sometimes than I...I get 3½ hours of alone time that you don't get. I really value that time, and when Jim was going to stay up later tonight, I said, "Oh no! You have to go to bed. If you fall asleep on the couch I can't carry you to bed." So he went to bed. I can't wait to move into Kip's room after Nancy leaves. The snoring on Seroquel is really bad sometimes. Last night he was quiet and I don't know why.

Hang in there...ever think about painting the bathroom brown? Lately I have had to clean the toilet every time Jim has to poop. It was never like that before. And it's not like it's an emergency for him to get there. One more thing to do, I can do it...Sure! Just add it on. Sorry, I'm just being flip.

Hope things improve on your end. Love and hugs.

04/04/2011
Ann to Vicky

I think I'm more tired than you because I've got 14 years on you. I just got Ralph into bed and I'm not far behind. You think Ralph is more with it, but tonight he stood out in the kitchen for 20 minutes without taking his pills. I had put out his 3 pills and glass of Miralax, and then I was in the living room not paying attention. He finally came in with my pill box and said he needed to take those. I said, "No, the ones on the counter." He came back with his pill box and said he had to take those because they were all green???? Now, I'm thinking I should hide all the pills. He hasn't gone back to childhood like Jim, but he's still pretty out of it.

We went to the reception at B & N this afternoon. We had Aisha with us, but it wasn't much fun. I finally left him with a friend and took Pooky (Aisha) to the children's area. I bought her a craft kit; a little ceramic tea set with paints to decorate them. Then, back up to check on Ralph. He was enjoying himself, but one of the guys came up to me and said he wanted to go talk to Ralph, but was afraid Ralph wouldn't know him. I said, "Of course he'll know you. Go over and talk." I'm beginning to ramble, so I guess I should call it a day.

Uh, oh, Ralph just wandered out in a bit of a stupor. Gotta go.

Vicky to Ann

Well, I didn't want to mention age...

Ann to Vicky

That's OK. Sometimes it's a good excuse, as if we needed one. Is Jim still getting you up before dawn? Ralph goes to bed later and later, but he sleeps in the morning. When I can drag myself out of bed, I have breakfast and read the paper before the daily onslaught.

About the 14th: I'll see if Brian can help out. I'd like to save Brian M. for Easter week if possible. I'm thinking maybe both Brians can clean the porch before the holiday. I'm planning on an Easter breakfast. That way, the kids can have their baskets and their annual egg hunt, and I can keep things simple. I'm checking the net for easy breakfast casseroles. With a couple of kuchens, fruit, juice, and coffee, we're good to go. This is one of those times when no one really understands the challenges we're facing, but it's my fault for making Easter brunch an annual tradition.

What was Jesus thinking? Couldn't he have downplayed it all so it didn't become a national holiday? I'll be going straight to hell for that one. Oh, well…

Vicky to Ann

Oh, I loved that one…if you go to hell, I'll be right there with you! As a matter of fact, I think we are…in hell.

Jim has been getting me up at 5 or so to get him dressed after he takes a hot bath…to help his dry mouth??? Don't understand that one. But he went right back to sleep, so when I did get up, I was ready to tackle the day. Today is the most normal I have seen him. His old sweetness was back, and I was more me. His speech is becoming more halted, and I can't hear him well. He mutters, and he's always calling for help when he's at the other end of the house. I am also trying to convince him to pull down both his underwear and pants to go to the bathroom, instead of stripping nude. So far I have shown him at least 20 times. He keeps thinking the pee will soak his clothes.

You are such a good mother…having everyone over for brunch.

If Nancy came 3 days ago, my house would have been clean. By the time she gets here, everything will be dusty again…except the bathroom. I just didn't want to wait to do everything in the last day and a half. I'm too busy with Jim for that. I know she will understand, but it bothers me anyway.

Kip's job may be on the line again. They are restructuring to save money. Don't know what will happen. They asked him for copies of all the training sessions he gives. He's hourly and works about 60 hours a week. They wanted him to convert to being salaried previously, but they would pay him for a 40 hour week. He said "No." Don't know what they will do this time, but if they let him go, they will be losing a big asset. He doesn't need all that stress on top of worrying about his dad. It is not easy for him, being a family member some distance away. Lots of guilt not being here more often, but he needs to live his own life. It's got to be tough. He sees the drastic changes, while I only see a little at a time.

04/06/2011
Vicky to Dr. D.
Jim Ruppert Update

Jim has been doing fairly well with the 2 Seroquel at bedtime with his mirtazapine, and his Pulmacort. He goes right to sleep, but still wakes at 4-5 AM and sneaks in the bathroom for a bath (presumably to ease his dry throat which is very severe.) I know by reading the pharmacy side effect sheets, that all Jim's medications can cause dry mouth. Jim is a mouth breather, especially at night, so that exacerbates the problem. I am giving him mouth liquid, mouth spray, and mints that help him salivate. Nevertheless, he is still uncomfortable, which increases his orneriness. He doesn't have the wherewithal to use these things on his own, unless directed.

After the bath, he still wakes me up to help with his dressing, but I can usually get him back to bed for at least another hour.

I have not noticed excessive sleepiness. Before he was on the Seroquel, he took 2 naps (one in the morning and one in the late afternoon,) and he still is just about comatose by 7:30 PM when he goes to bed.

Jim continues to 'see people'. One day this week, he told me our neighbor was dead, and he was worried about her. He said he went to her house and saw her, that's how he knew she was dead. I had to call her in order to satisfy Jim that she was all right. Jim was very relieved. However, he remains irritated with me because he says I am a big 'know it all'. I know his failing ability to do the simple ADL's (activities of daily living) embarrasses him and he takes it out on me because I am there. He still sees me mostly as a caregiver, not as his wife... typical, I think.

His other obsession, other than dry mouth, is his post nasal drip that started when the snow melted. He thought it was blood dripping down the back of his throat, and that he is slowly dying. I had him spit some in a cup, and it looks like healthy saliva/nose fluid, not yellow or green. I told him it was probably due to the spores, etc. that are outside now. He doesn't believe me, but I give him nasal saline to sniff each night, and Flonase once a day. Jim still has some post nasal drip.

He has the idea that he must spit it out every time. I said to swallow it... women do it all the time, they don't spit. He thinks if he swallows it, he will be peeing a lot more. He also restricts his fluid intake during the day, which is bad, but of course he doesn't understand that. Sometimes, I go into the bathroom and he is standing over the sink and spitting for a long time. Anyway, he has these weird ideas/obsessions and frequently gets mad at me, saying that I just don't understand. He implies that I'll be sorry when he's dead! In his eyes I am the 'wicked witch of the west.'

What to do about dry mouth?

Should I drop the morning Lexapro?

Do I begin ½ Seroquel mid-morning?

I forgot to mention at night Jim gets the Exelon patch. Is there any reason to continue the Exelon patch and Memantine now? I don't think he cares for his life to be extended at this point, but if it just makes the time he has easier to manage, then I'm game. I just can't see the point of prolonging the illness.

Dr. D. to Vicky

I think it would be reasonable to stop the Exelon patch now. If there is no substantial adverse effect in a week or so we could stop the Memantine as well.

Please let me know how this goes. You are doing a wonderful job in a very hard situation.

04/06/2011
Vicky to Ann
Changes for This Week & My Birthday

I wrote Dr. D. of Jim's progress (if you'd call it that.) I also asked him about whether we should stop the Exelon patch and Memantine (Namenda.) He called and said that we could stop the Exelon patch, and if there is no adverse effect we could stop the Memantine. Wow. I meant it when I asked him, but I guess we should be afraid of what we ask for! It was as if I got kicked in the gut. The end has begun. I really wasn't expecting him to say that...

I'm looking forward to Jim's sister, Nancy, being here if just for the distraction. I do have wonderful friends and relatives. Everyone called me or sent me cards today to wish me Happy Birthday. I am blessed. And that means you, too. Hope things are going OK at your end.

04/07/2011
Ann to Vicky

I'm not sure when Jim's sister is arriving but I'm going to try and call you tonight. Let me know if 11 is too late. I'd rather talk after Ralph goes to bed. I'm late getting started today because I slept 'til after 9. Now, I still have papers to get ready for my lawyer appointment at 3:30. I tend to forget how long it takes to get Ralph ready for the day. At least, he's very cooperative lately and thanks me for everything I do for him.

I, too, felt a little sick when I read your e-mail. Is Memantine the same as Namenda? Ralph has never been on any of the other drugs you mentioned. Just Namenda and Seroquel. Dr. D. says none of the others would work on his dementia. But, still, you must be thinking this is the beginning of the end, and I'm feeling so badly for you. We spend years planning, caregiving, searching out nursing homes, and reading all the books, and yet it really doesn't sink in until something simple like stopping drugs happens. Then we really see what this is all about. I have tears in my eyes and a knot in my stomach just writing this. My heart aches for you and I know Ralph and I are next.

I'll call you tonight, and my arms will be around you all day.

04/07/2011
Ann's Note

We met with our elder-law attorney and had a long discussion about our options. These included keeping or selling our house.

Pro: Selling and moving to a senior living apartment would give me more time and ease caring for Ralph without the constant maintenance a house requires. Depending on what senior complex we go to, it could be easier to place him when necessary.

Con: Senior apartments are expensive and we can't live any cheaper than in our own home.

We also went over all our finances, and what we can and cannot do now and in the future. She also told us about a program that provides day care at home. I'll be setting up an appointment with them.

She talked about the necessity of applying for Medicaid now, even though we have funds and home equity. Many nursing homes require that step because private assets are used up quickly after placement. Currently, the average cost is $110,000 to $125,000 a year. Mind boggling!! We must find ways of protecting as much of our hard earned money as possible.

We will be seeing her again. She is a great elder advocate to have!

04/08/2011
Vicky to Ann
Jim

Nancy arrived yesterday. Jim didn't recognize her at the airport, but felt comfortable with her ministrations. We had a nice dinner after she arrived, and she is settling in.

Jim has been without much outward emotion this past week, and yet has worried about everyone dying. We went to our GP this morning and Jim thought our doctor was dead, that's why they weren't calling us in right then. Jim was awful while in the exam room. He was there for a review of general meds. She was assessing his joint pain by pressing in various joint areas. She was hurting him and he got up to leave the room. I blocked his way and asked him to sit down. He said he had dry mouth. What I think he meant to say was that he had to urinate. I took him to the bathroom, but since he doesn't see me as his wife, he didn't want me in there. All I can say is that he was nasty, agitated, and paranoid, even with the Seroquel on board. Such a sad thing for his sister to witness. Jim has always been the gentlest soul, and his doctor was his idol. Neither his mom nor his dad was like this towards the end. The long and the short of it is that his dry eye, dry mouth, and post-nasal drip are being addressed with meds. Dr. D. is taking care of the behavioral issues.

I called Dr. D. and he is adding a Seroquel at 3 PM, but doesn't want to give a dose any earlier in the day because of its sedative effects. I suspect this will lead to putting Jim in a nursing home. I am getting out the applications of the top three we visited, and getting them ready for submission. Thank heaven we looked at them early and know which ones we want. I had no idea that needing a nursing home would develop this fast. I thought we would have time to submit an application, and when they had an opening we would decide if the timing was right or not. I will schedule a PRI and go from there. If I have to place him it will be a relief. Hopefully he will be able to go out with Brian M., because I have some really important things to do without Jim's presence.

I doubt if support group will be possible this time. I can't bring Jim unless he radically improves, and I wouldn't leave him in the care of anyone else.

So far this is the worst day ever!

Ann to Vicky

So many things are going through my mind. I know it's been a long haul for you two, but things seem to be going downhill too fast. Maybe that's how it usually is. I'm thinking of others in the support group where placement was needed unexpectedly. Do you think it would help to get home care for Jim on a regular basis? It would free you up, and keep Jim at home at the same time. I know that's just prolonging the inevitable, but it's still hard to picture Jim in a nursing home just yet. Are you getting the PRI done soon?

I explained yesterday's elder-law meeting to Ralph, and he seems to understand, but now today he's saying he wants to start a simple wood working class in one of the day care centers. When I said we had to go through some other steps first, he accused me of being negative to all his ideas. So, I guess we won't talk about it until I get all our financial ducks in a row.

Hang in there, and please let me know if there's anything I can do.

Vicky to Ann

Have to see if the meds straighten Jim out, then it will be day care or home care next (or nursing home)...depends on what happens in the next few days.

Ann to Vicky

We must be on the same page. I was just wondering if Jim would be in some kind of care very soon. Opened the computer and there was your note. I think for your sake, it's definitely time for more care.

Ralph is in and out the last few days. One minute he understands what's going on, and the next minute he has no idea what he's doing. I'm going to ask Dr. D. if I can increase the Seroquel at night. He's beginning to wander around the house at all hours. Never seems to know why he's up. Brian took him to Springwater this morning, and we're going to Nancy's for dinner. I hope he can cope with that much activity.

The attorney suggested calling Oak Ridge at Home, a long term health care program. They will come out and do an assessment and go from there. She said the medical community is beginning to realize that dementia folks don't usually need full scale nursing homes. In-home care or day care is the wave of the future. You probably have your your plans in order, but I just thought I'd share.

Looks like monthly lunches are coming to an end, but you never know. Jim has rallied before. Let's hope that if you get more help, he will do better.

Vicky to Ann

Today was much better than yesterday. He only gave me trouble once. I asked him to put in his eye meds and he said, "No way am I taking that stuff," and looked at me with no recognition. I said, "OK," and sat down and waited 10 minutes. Then I told him the ophthalmologist ordered these drops for him, and he took them without thinking. If I stand over him, I'm too much like a warden. He went with Nancy and me to the Bird House to get a bird bath, but other than that, he slept. Perhaps our talking together was too much for him. Tomorrow will be better.

I am going to update Jim's companion, Brian M., and call the day care to ask if they will consider Jim. Then I'll call Dr. D.'s social worker, Susan, and update her on my scheduling a PRI and handing in paperwork to the nursing homes. I'll also ask Brian M. if he wants more hours. That's my plan.

Today, every time he went to the bathroom, he took his clothes off and got in the tub. By 1 PM I had redressed him four times. Nothing thereafter. Now, he gets 1 Seroquel at 3 PM and 2 at 7:30 PM with a Mirtazapine.

04/11/2011
Vicky to Ann
Home Care

I am having the interviewer from the home care agency come out Wednesday. The agency is funded through Medicaid, so it wouldn't fit our needs, but the interviewer could steer me in the right direction. The first meeting is gratis. She also suggested an alternative day placement possibility.

I also talked to the head of the first day care center. She said they couldn't take someone who might wander, nor could they take someone who is belligerent, for the sake of the other clients. She will, however, wait to see if Jim stabilizes on his present meds.

Ann to Vicky

Wow! Things are happening fast in our lives. I'm surprised about the Oak Ridge program. On the flyer the attorney gave us, it says, 'Services are covered by Medicare, Medicaid, some retirement plans, and long-term care insurance.' I'm sure the representative will explain all that.

We had our taxes done today, which is another task off my back. I also went on-line and finally figured out how to cancel Ralph's Sales Tax Account. The tax guy helped me fill out the final form I must send to the state. Ralph had a small business after he retired, never made a ton of money, but we had some vacation money from it. Anyway, I've had to file a return for it every year. That's done.

Then we went to the gym that offers the Silver Sneakers program. Ralph will go tomorrow at noon for an assessment of what he needs in the way of exercise. I want to be with him because the woman in charge seemed to disregard his dementia, talking about having him lift weights so he doesn't stoop so much. Anyway, it's good to get him back to a regular exercise routine.

You'll be pleased to hear my black mood lifted along with the bug I had. I felt so lousy I thought I wasn't going to be able to deal with all this, but after a good night's sleep I'm back to "I am woman, hear me roar." I'm re-energized to get the infamous 'ducks in a row'. Thank God.

Funny thing happened last night. I don't know if I sounded a bit groggy or not, but I took half a Trazodone about 9:30 to help me sleep. I didn't consider that I hadn't had any food since Sat. night, just a little ginger ale. Anyway, I was getting pretty sleepy when we talked. I tried reading in bed, but the pages looked as if someone had sprinkled brown sugar over them. I kept blinking and cleaned my glasses, but all the pages were 'dirty.' I gave up reading, but when I closed my eyes I saw lots of colorful spirals whirling around. I dozed off and when I awoke, they were gone. I thought, "Man, that's like a little dose of Alzheimer's." When I woke up this morning, I checked the book and the pages were white as snow again. Guess I took a little trip.

Let me know how things are going. Hoping Jim is behaving. I do so want you to keep him home a while longer.

04/12/2011
Vicky to Ann
Seeing the Lawyer

Had a good day yesterday with little incident, except for Jim wandering out of the house to our neighbors across the street while I was gardening. The neighbor brought him back to our house.

Today, Brian M. came to sit with Jim while I went to an appointment with my lawyer. Jim decided just as I was about to leave, to take a bath. He already had 4 baths today. There was no dissuading him or things would escalate, so I talked to Brian M. while Jim bathed. Then I had to quickly get him dressed and leave.

I warned the lawyer that placement might be imminent; at least payment for more aides in our home was in the offing. I will need money from our funds to pay for that. I gave her a full accounting of all our monies. Then the lawyer gave me the 2011 guidelines for Medicaid. In order to meet the guidelines, I'll have to spend down our money to the allowable levels. The guidelines won't leave me with much, especially since I am 63 and probably will live for 20 more years. If I spend down so Jim is eligible for Medicaid (meaning Medicaid will pay for his nursing home care,) I will be a pauper scrimping by on Social Security, which in this day and age won't cover my costs of living in this modest 1000 square foot house. I am going to get all the necessary paperwork together just in case I have to apply for Medicaid for Jim's care. The list of documents is quite extensive, and quite time consuming to accumulate, so I am going to start now. If for some reason we don't need to apply, so be it. We also went through all our legal papers to make sure everything was in order from our prior visits: wills, health care proxies, living wills, life insurance ownership and beneficiaries, and bank account ownership. Long ago, Jim's share of the house was sold to me for $1, and we put our car in my name only. We will continue to meet with the lawyer as Jim's case evolves.

04/13/2011
Vicky to Ann
Look Mommy Look! See What I Can Do

I tried to prepare Jim for the nurse that would come today to talk about Oak Ridge at Home. It is an agency that helps the elderly to stay at home longer. We do not qualify age-wise yet, but she took down some history so that she could advise us of possible avenues, and also have the information on file in case we did become eligible. She started by asking Jim the questions about what he could do and what he found hard or impossible, but he didn't like her being here and so he refused to answer. Since he refused to answer, I began giving her the information she needed. While we were talking, Jim got up and started balancing on each foot, one at a time, waving the raised foot around in circles. While he was doing that and showing off doing push-ups, he told her not to ask questions until he was finished. It was just like a small child saying, "Look Mommy look, see what I can do."

04/19/2011
Ann to Vicky
What's Happening?

Haven't heard from you since our lunch. I figured things are either very good and there's nothing to write about, or bad enough that there's no time. Then I remembered that Kip was coming home on the weekend. How did the visit go? Mainly, I just want to know if you're going to support group tonight. You can fill me in then. Hope you can make it.

Vicky to Ann

[Note: We went to support group but didn't stay too long. A new substitute facilitator for the dementia group came to our door, and asked me to take Jim home.]

I didn't hear what Jim was really doing to disrupt the group...can Ralph tell you? All I heard from Jim was that he was frustrated with the group because no one was sharing what it's like to have Alzheimer's. I tried to reason with Jim that even though he is a family therapist, he is not the facilitator for the group anymore (and hasn't been for a while,) and it was the facilitator's first time with his group. He needs to cut him some slack. It's not helpful to be disruptive. There was no time to find out what Jim was doing exactly to disrupt the group, so we just went home. That means no more group sessions for Jim. If I want to go, I will have to get him a sitter.

Jim also lost his glasses today. I don't know what number of replacements we are on now!

Ann to Vicky

So, do you want me to call you at 11? Otherwise I'll write what I know, which isn't a whole lot. Also, I'll touch on the rest of the time.

Vicky to Ann

Sure...call me before you go to bed...if it's not too late. I know it's now 10:30. Had to call my sister, because we haven't spoken in a while.

04/20/2011
Ann to Vicky
Catching Up

I just found your e-mail. I wouldn't have called you so late if I saw it last night. I'm sorry. I know I run off at the mouth at times. Enjoyed the chat though. Ralph is just now getting up. I think yesterday was overwhelming with our financial meeting, Silver Sneakers, and then support group. As I listened to everyone else, I decided Ralph's doing pretty well.

Ralph is eating breakfast and is still talking about last night. It sounds as if they did a lot of sharing about what it's like to have Alzheimer's. What set Jim off? We both want to know how Jim is doing today. Ralph said he thought I should have called you last night and when I told him that I did, he was pleased. Guess our next call can be earlier.

Gotta do a pick-up sweep through the house and porch so Brian M. can clean. Then, sort through the pile of paperwork that's backed up. We'll talk soon.

Vicky to Ann

Maybe I'll call you later. At about noon, Jim decided he wanted to go home to see his friends in New Jersey, and he wanted me to take him there to live. Nothing worked to change his mind. He left the house about 4 times, but always came back to make threats. He finally left with one shoe and one slipper, and started walking down the street. I got in the car and pulled alongside, telling him we'd go for a drive. He assumed I meant N.J., but I took him to some friends of ours. The wife tried talking to Jim and reassuring him, but that didn't work. Finally, he agreed to talk to Dr. D., and so I called his secretary asking if Dr. D. would call me. Still waiting, but did e-mail him of what happened. Gave 2 Seroquel at 2 PM when we got home. My friend's husband and another close male friend came over to talk old times with Jim as a diversion. (No mention of what he was planning to do or anything.) They just now left and the Seroquel seems to have done its job, but Jim is not dopey yet. I also called an assisted living place near us to schedule a meeting Tuesday to submit my application...they may have an opening. I will see what Dr. D. says. If adding another Seroquel will keep him in control, I'll still try. Otherwise, in he goes.

Ann to Vicky

Please call if you can. Ralph has been very concerned about his friend. He wanted me to call, but I said you're waiting to hear from Dr. D. Then he wanted to come over, which was fine with me, but I told him you had friends over who had just left. He's afraid Jim's going to have to be hospitalized. Is there anything I can do to help?

04/20/2011
Vicky to Dr. D.
Re: Jim

I called your secretary today to get in touch with you. Jim was 'in another world' and wanted to go home to live where all his old friends were, in New Jersey. He left the house a number of times but always came back. Finally he left and started walking down the street. I picked him up in the car and told him we'd take a drive...and he assumed to N.J. I brought him to a female friend's house, and she talked with him for a while. He finally agreed that we should call you. I brought him home and managed to give him 2 Seroquel at 2 PM (This all started about 12:30.) My friend had called her husband and another male to meet us at the house. They talked a while about a lot of fun memories they all experienced in their times together. They left at 4:21 PM and Jim seems O.K.

Should I start giving him Seroquel in the morning, or maybe around 11 AM, one at 3 PM, and then his usual 2 at bedtime? What would you recommend? I have an application for an assisted living facility that is locked and has a dementia floor, but I don't know if they have openings. Should I pursue that, or do you think the Seroquel might keep him at home?

Sorry to be such a bother.

Dr. D. to Vicky

I think that an extra dose of Seroquel should be fine as a temporary measure. I think your rather frightening day is a strong indication that he needs residential care on a locked dementia unit. The long-term effectiveness and safety of dementia care is far better than that of chronic high dose Seroquel. The dementia care unit is better for all involved.

This is a hard decision to make. But I am 100% confident that it is the right one. I hope things settle down. Good luck.

04/21/2011
Ann to Vicky
Courage

COURAGE DOESN'T ALWAYS ROAR. SOMETIMES COURAGE IS THE QUIET VOICE AT THE END OF THE DAY, SAYING, 'I WILL TRY AGAIN TOMORROW.'

by Mary Anne Radmacher

Did you ever hear back from Dr. D.? Hope things are better and I wish Kip could come home again this weekend. You need him even if Jim doesn't seem to. Brian M. and my Brian were here today. It was great. Porch is clean, porch windows washed, screens up, living room vacuumed, and garage swept. Poor Brian M. My Brian came complete with kids, and Hassan wanted to help but never stopped talking. Aisha never started. The wine and cheese were welcomed by both at the end of the time (Brian M. and me, not the kids.) He loves to share his family stories with us.

Vicky to Ann

Dr. D. called at 9:45 last night, and OK'd 1 Seroquel at 10 AM, 1 at 3 PM, and 2 at 7:30 PM. This is a temporary measure only to be used until he can be placed. He doesn't want Jim on it long term just so I can keep him at home. He said that Jim needs placement, and that's all there is to it.

Today was a busy morning for me...getting all the applications complete and preparing a cover letter of sorts as well as copies of my car loan, financial holdings, meds sheet, POA (Power of Attorney,) and health care proxy/living will. I tried to make sure they were complete, and put each in a folder with the nursing home name and person in charge of admissions. While doing this, Jim was in the living room and would call out every few minutes to see where I was.

When I finished, I called all three places to see if they had openings. The first two did not, and I couldn't get through to the third. I decided that I needed to hand these things in, and so I told Jim we were going for a ride to drop off some tax stuff, and afterward we would go for ice cream. Jim waited in the car while I went to all three and handed in the forms. It's Thursday, so I know it may not get looked at 'til next week, but at least they are in. The cover letters explains it all.

We stopped for ice cream cones, and then went home for a nap.

By the time we got home, there was a message from the third NH. The admissions director said she would look over the information and we would talk tomorrow afternoon. We will have breakfast with the couple that rescued me yesterday, and then I have to get new tires on the car. It's weird to throw in something that is so mundane, but I have to do it sooner or later, so might as well get it done.

This whole time my adrenalin was pumping, and when the papers were in I felt a big sigh of relief. After the nap, I felt oh sooo guilty! I kept thinking of all the things Jim won't be able to experience anymore. Tonight Jim told me he thought I was trying to kill him with all the pills, mouth sprays, and eye drops. That made me realize I was doing the right thing. He was also getting more and more scared listening to the news. How can one's emotions do such a flip flop from one moment to the next?

When this is resolved, I will be free of the imminent happenings that make the adrenaline rush, but I will be faced with years of payments, not the ups and downs as life is now, just a heavy weight hanging over my head. We never escape...things just change. That 'new normal,' I guess.

Ann to Vicky

I just don't know what to say. Even though we all knew this day would come, it's still a shock. I wanted to call you, but Ralph just went to bed, and I don't want him to know yet. This will devastate him, both for Jim's sake and for his own. I'm afraid the reality will hit him hard.

I'm a little surprised that Dr. D. didn't consider help at home, unless he feels it would be too much for an aide to handle. I wonder if he will be that matter of fact with us, even if it means a sub-standard nursing home. Thank God you can afford at least the first year.

I wish I could just put my arms around you. Would it help if we stopped by Sat. or Sun. or don't you want Jim to know anything's up? How are you going to break it to him? Do you think Kip should be there with you? I feel so helpless. I'll tell Ralph we're cancelling lunch Monday, but not why. All I can wish for you is as easy a transition as possible. You're a very strong lady, and I admire how well you're handling it all. It's been a long journey, and you need to rest and think a little about your own 'new normal' as well as Jim's.

We're with you with love.

Vicky to Ann

Placement might not happen right away. An acquaintance of mine is a social worker at St. John's. I called her to see if she could help in any way. She would like to have Jim there, so maybe she will push for us...depending on the PRI, and of course, we have Dr. D.'s consent. I called Kip last night and he will come down for placement, whenever that will be.

We really cannot consider help at home because of Jim's agitation and anger. And we can't continue the present meds regimen indefinitely. When we went out to breakfast this morning, Jim could only take a half hour of the noise and confusion. He made the excuse that some of his old friends were coming to visit. So that means definitely no Monday lunch. Now Jim is tired in the morning, even before the Seroquel.

The PRI (the patient review instrument that is necessary for placement) is Monday morning. If there is an opening at St. John's, I will take it. Otherwise, I'll try to opt for an assisted living that is locked. That's assuming Jim will pass the PRI. I think he will now because of the 'escaping.'

04/24/2011
Vicky's Journal
The Day of No Return

Today was the day of no return. We were on our way back from the restaurant that we had breakfast in the day before. We thought Jim had left his cap there, but he hadn't. All of a sudden, Jim said that he was tired of the way we were living, and he wanted out. At that moment he opened the car door to leave. The car was moving at about 25 miles per hour, and I think that surprised him, so he shut the door momentarily. Before he could try it again, I pushed the 'lock' button. He was not 'with it' enough to hit the 'unlock' button. Jim didn't try to get out again until we were safely in our driveway. As soon as we stopped, he was out of the car in a flash and ran down the driveway and into the street. He kept moving, but looked back as he was heading down the street. That moment stuck in my mind...he looked like a scared child...and in a way, he was. I hopped back in the car and went after him. When I reached him, I pulled the car in front of him to stop his progress. He never thought to walk around the car and over the neighbor's lawn to avoid me. I pleaded with him to get in the car and come home so we could talk more about his plans. When we arrived home, I gave Jim 2 Seroquel, and called our very good friend who had been over for the previous incident. He came to talk to Jim, but no matter how hard either one of us tried, we could not convince Jim to relinquish his idea to go to New Jersey. I had to execute a mental health arrest.

I called 911 and explained what I wanted. They asked if they needed an ambulance, and I said, "Yes." Jim needed to be transported to the hospital. Our friend met the sheriff and the ambulance to explain what had transpired in the last hour. The sheriff knew what to do, thank heaven! He asked Jim what the problem was, and Jim responded that he wanted to walk to New Jersey. He said that he didn't love me anymore, that he was sorry. The officer told Jim that his eyes looked funny, and asked if he felt alright. He asked Jim to lie down on the couch, and also asked if he could have a paramedic check him over, because Jim did not look well. Jim believed him, and did what the officer requested. After a bit of quiet monitoring, they told Jim that he needed to be checked out at the hospital because he looked very ill. They convinced Jim to walk with them to the ambulance, and off they went.

Upon arrival, they put him in a semi-private stall, and eventually did a work-up. Unfortunately, as with any hospital where a 'not so sick' individual is brought in, he was put in a queue for care. It took forever to get results. Jim could not understand why he needed to be there, and wanted to leave. After his roommate was discharged, Jim became agitated, went to the door, and screamed at the top of his lungs for a doctor to come discharge him. They tried closing the folding door to the room to lessen the noise, looking at me as if asking, are you alright with him...will he hurt you? I mouthed that I was OK. They still needed a urine sample, but Jim was in no mood to give them one. I explained to Jim that they needed the results of all the tests before they could release him. After waiting around most of the day and into the night, he was moved to a private bay in pediatrics. Then, they moved Jim to a semi-private room on the ortho floor. His bed was within view of the nurses' station. Jim seemed relatively quiet, so at 11 PM I went home to bed.

When I came the next morning, I found out he had hit his roommate...opened the bathroom door and was surprised by the roommate. It scared him and he swung. The roommate was not hurt, but from then on they ordered a 1:1 aide to sit with him all the time. That helped calm him.

I talked with the floor social worker, and gave her the names of the three nursing homes I like best. Days passed as we waited for the forms and PRI to be received and reviewed. Because of the hitting incident, accosting a patient, he was denied admission to all three. If it had been staff, I don't think it would have been as bad. Those nursing homes were the best, and if they denied him, I was certain the others would also. (The top three nursing homes were about $11,500 a month.) I didn't want him going to a poor quality place. I also knew that if they couldn't find some place that would take him, we would have to look at behavioral nursing homes. There are only 3 listed for New York State, and vacancies are slim. Sometimes they even have to place people out of state! (Behavioral nursing homes here at the time run about $20,000 a month, give or take some additions for special needs.) I called the support group facilitator to see if she could give me some advice, and she reminded me that some assisted living dementia facilities are locked. She said I might consider them. She knows Jim very well and also knows of a facility, so I gave them a try. I arranged for an interview with Jim by one of their nurses, and they were going to give Jim a try. They really think they can give him a better quality of life. Although it is a locked facility, inside there are two pods of rooms and recreation areas with TV's, movies, and activities, and areas to go outside without getting out of the facility. It's perfect.

Vicky to Dr. D.

Had to make a mental health arrest today because Jim tried to get out of a moving car and later tried to leave home for New Jersey again.

The Monroe County Sheriff was very good and understanding. The hospital social worker can place him. It is scary how fast this behavior developed. I was slowly getting the applications for nursing homes ready before all this 'fell into place.'

Will let you know where he ends up.

Dr. D. to Vicky

I am sorry that it came to this. I am glad that you managed to have him brought to the hospital before something bad happened. I will hope to see him tomorrow, but I will be very busy. I would be happy to have you tell the caregivers that I have been involved, and I am happy to play whatever role might be helpful.

04/27/2011
Ann to Vicky
Jim

We're on our way to the Atrium for the dance concert. I'll call you tonight when I get home. If you'd rather I didn't because you're probably exhausted, send a note. It sounds as if your cloud finally has a silver lining. He couldn't be in a better place for now.

Vicky's Journal
The Move, etc.

This assisted living place was confident that they could handle Jim. So arrangements were made to move Jim in the next day (at half the price of a nursing home.) Kip came home and helped me arrange Jim's room with familiar things. We put a list of likes and dislikes on Jim's bathroom door, called 'Getting to Know Jim'. We told him that because he didn't want to live with me anymore, we found him a room of his own. Kip rode with Jim in the van, and I drove separately. The night after the move, Kip and I couldn't sleep, but neither knew the other was awake until about 4 AM. I got up to go to the bathroom and heard Kip stir. We said we both had been lying there awake, waiting for the phone to ring! But it didn't, so then we slept soundly 'til morning. This move was the hardest thing that Kip and I have ever done.

Not only did Jim need his meds changed because of his 'wanting to leave home', but he also lost a lot of mental ground in those 5 days at the hospital. It didn't matter how many hours I spent with him, it was not a quiet and loving home environment.

Although the assisted living place was beautiful, well-staffed, and 5 minutes from my house, Jim just seemed like a fish out of water. He couldn't do much of anything except feed himself. That was the one thing he had to be able to do, because they can't feed you in assisted living by definition. As with some other residents, despite his picture outside his room, he always needed to be taken there, because he never knew where it was. After a while he seemed to be adjusting, but rarely talked to others. He did not like the staff dressing him, and so would wear the same clothes for a number of days. Who knows how long he went without a shower. I was always on edge, but at least he was in a good place with lovely surroundings and wonderful staff, and I could sleep at night.

Getting To Know Jim:

1. Jim usually sleeps in his clothes...belt, slippers, and all!
2. Jim usually sits down to pee.
3. Jim is almost always cold, so frequently he will wear his red winter jacket indoors.
4. If Jim displays agitation (pursed lips, jutting jaw, or folded arms,) one or more of the following may help:
   a. Give him space.
   b. Ask him to show you push-ups and count for him.
   c. Ask him to show you how he balances on one foot.
   d. Play soft music on his player and dance with him.
   e. Toss the ball with him and compliment him on his skill.
   f. Take him for a walk or sit in the courtyard in the sun.
   g. Ask him about his job working with children.
   h. Sing.
5. Jim does not like to be pulled, trying to coerce him to do things.
6. Jim is embarrassed to be undressed by a woman.

05/02/2011
Vicky To Ann
After Placement

Jim has withdrawn inside himself. He sits with his eyes closed most of the time. I feel like I have deserted him there. As if I've left him to die. Today, when I went to visit him, it seemed as if he didn't care that I was even there. When I took him back to his room so he could see some pictures I hung ... he didn't remember or could barely see any of it. To the picture I put over the toilet, he said that it's just a room where you go to the bathroom, why do you need a picture. I want to bring him home so badly, although he'd probably just run away again. I don't know how I'll ever get used to this.

We have often talked of wanting to be free, but now I can't imagine having fun while he is in there. It's a nice facility from the view of a fully functioning person, but for him it's a lonely place. There is nothing crueler that this disease.

05/03/2011
Ann to Vicky
Jim and Ralph

I was explaining a little more about where Jim is, etc. and Ralph says he wants to see him. I explained that he had to get used to the new place first before having visitors. Then I thought, maybe it would do Jim good to see Ralph soon. He always seems to know him. Anyway, just a thought and you can let me know when it might be a good idea.

05/03/2011
Vicky to Dr. D.
Placement of Jim Ruppert

Last Friday, Jim was placed in an assisted living dementia care locked facility. I have changed Jim over to the medical group that covers this facility. They only see their patients once a month and that occurred the day before Jim got there, so Jim won't be assessed until the end of May.

Jim is still on the 25 mg. Seroquel mid-morning and mid-afternoon, then 2 at bedtime as well as the Lexapro at breakfast. If you would like to change his meds now that he is in a locked facility, feel free to do so. I have provided the nurse's name and phone number so you can speak directly with her.

I will still keep Jim's visits to you, since you are Jim's Alzheimer's specialist. Our next visit is June 22nd at 2 PM.

Jim's facility deals only with dementia patients. The three top nursing homes in our area refused him because of behavioral issues. In the hospital, he was even more confused because of the environmental change, and was disruptive and almost violent in the ER. He had an altercation with his roommate on the floor. The roommate was in the bathroom when Jim wanted to use it, and when Jim opened the door he was surprised to find someone inside. I think he hit the roommate. Jim mellowed as the week went on, partly due to the scheduling of 1:1 coverage by aides 24/7.

As far as I can understand, Jim is going to bed at 7 PM or so and waking in the early morning. He is then sleepy most of the morning. He is beginning to come out of his fog more now, his walk is more regular, and he's opening his eyes more frequently. He was always sitting with eyes closed, listening to what went on. It breaks my heart, but I know this was the right move.

If I can be of further assistance to you in adjusting Jim's meds, please don't hesitate to ask.

Dr. D. to Vicky

I think that there is no question that this was necessary. You did all that could be done, for as long as it could be done. I am happy to be involved as you and they see fit.

05/03/2011
Vicky to Dr. D.

Since Jim won't be seeing the facility doctor until the end of May for his first visit (and he won't prescribe anything before seeing the patient,) I would like you to make changes as you see fit for Jim, otherwise he will just be in a holding pattern for weeks. I think he is still on the Lexapro 10 mg. in the morning and the Seroquel morning and afternoon, and the 2 Seroquel before bed, as well as the Mirtazapine.

They told me that yesterday after dinner he was yelling for me. This morning at 9 AM, he was upset because he must have hallucinated that there were lots of children that were in danger, and no one would help him rescue them. He was scared for their safety. His hallucinations always involve people that are being hurt, and he feels so helpless. He is trying to protect them and that is why he gets angry.

If you feel his meds need adjusting, please talk to the nurse in charge. Anything you can do to make him feel less upset, and still have some quality of life is key. I know these things are delicate to handle.

Thanks so much for your help, and thanks for your kind words.

Dr. D. to Vicky

I talked to the nurse. He was agitated yesterday, but fine today. I asked for small changes, just a further reduction of the Lexapro for now to 5 mg. per day for 2 weeks, then stopping it. We will consider increasing the Seroquel further if he is persistently agitated.

05/03/2011
Vicky to Ann
Ta-Dah!

This morning Jim is still having his hallucinations. It continues to be about children being hurt, and no one will come to his aid (so sad for a school psychologist and family therapist.) I tried to talk him out of the funk. I shaved him, did his nails, and his neck, and signed him up for regular haircuts. I went back after dinner and he was walking normally and talking like his old self! I was so relieved. He went to bed because he was tired, but didn't mind that I was leaving.

They said that he has been sleeping through the night; he is just scared in the morning after he wakes. What a relief. I feel almost normal again.

Ann to Vicky

I'm really tired tonight and just found your note, so I'll keep this short. I'm so glad for both you and Jim. Thursday and Friday this week are really busy, so perhaps Monday or Tuesday will be good for visiting Jim. I'll talk to you later this week. I'll tell Ralph the good news in the morning. He'll be relieved too.

05/15/2011
Ann's Note

Today was Jim's birthday. Vicky wanted a small, quiet gathering with a few friends. Ralph and I, and a few folks were there to help them celebrate. We met in the private dining room at the assisted living home, and it all went very well considering the circumstances.

There was much laughter and reminiscing. Then, Ralph suddenly stood up and said he wanted to say something. Now, Ralph never enjoyed speaking to a group, even in the best of times, but he needed to be heard. He talked slowly but fluently about meeting Jim and Vicky, and what they meant to him. Then he told about the time, recently, when the four of us were at lunch and two former co-workers of Jim's came up to our table. They told us they missed Jim a great deal, praised his skills as a therapist, and talked about how he touched their lives. Ralph said it meant a great deal to him to glimpse Jim as he was before we knew him. Well!! The other guests were surprised, but Vicky and I were astounded. Another mystery of this disease. After we left, I told Ralph he couldn't have given Jim a greater gift.

05/15/2011
Vicky to Ann
Thanks for Helping Celebrate Jim's Birthday

Thanks to both of you for coming to celebrate Jim's birthday. I think all his long-time friends were there, and that made it nice for him. It was a decent sized group, but not too big that it confused him. It felt fairly normal, and that's what I wanted to achieve.

Ralph did such a fabulous job saying those kind words about Jim. I was flabbergasted he spoke so well, and with such composure. Wow.

05/21/2011
Vicky to Ann
Contented

It's amazing. Jim has never asked 'am I in a nursing home' or anything. He is more alert now, because he was quite traumatized by the hospital visit. I don't think he will ever regain what he has lost. He lost much of his affect the month of April, but he seems content where he is, and when I took him out to the eye doctor he didn't want to escape. He went right back with no problem. I was relieved.

05/24/2011
Vicky's Journal
Finding My Footing

Three weeks into life on my own, and I still don't know what to make of it all. I don't know what the rules are or how I am to structure my day. All of a sudden, my days aren't filled with caring for another person. Even though I know it is irrational, I feel guilty and a deep sadness that I had to start this whole process, and that it can't be undone. I know it's the disease that started the behaviors, and I know bringing Jim home to live with me again would be insane. Would he run away again, or is he so damaged by the week in the hospital that it doesn't occur to him now? In a perverse sense, he has his independence now. Independence from me. He has his own room and bathroom, he can get up when he chooses, wear what he wants, and go where he wants in the assisted living facility. He is distracted from his space by other residents around him, and the aides that help orchestrate the day. He is not subject to the wishes and needs of just one person. There is an order to each day that is the same, even though the specific activities are different. The order probably adds some measure of comfort unconsciously, even if the residents don't know what comes next.

When I come and go, my presence doesn't seem to leave a few moments of happiness behind. I really don't see much emotion anymore; they call it 'flat affect'. And yet, sometimes when others visit he says, "Well, we better check that out with Vicky," as if I still call all the shots. I didn't interpret my care of him as being a director or warden, but he obviously did. I tried so hard to engage him and take him places where he would find joy. It hurts me to think that my visits don't matter. It is the disease, after all, not a conscious decision to act the way he does. For months he has been looking at me and seeing a caregiver, not his wife, and now he doesn't even see that. I can sit right next to him, but if I don't announce, "Hi, I am your wife and I came for a visit," he doesn't respond. When I do make the announcement, he responds, "I know that," but it's just a cover-up to make us think they get it when they don't.

In the beginning, I visited him every day. I could not stay away. I wanted to see if he was getting used to the place, if his clothes were changed, was he shaved, was he engaging other people? Sometimes he wasn't shaved and his clothes weren't changed, but it wasn't for lack of trying. When an Alzheimer's person doesn't want to do something that you want them to do, you either: make them think it was their idea, try to distract them and try again later, or go with the flow. Trying to force them only makes them resistive, agitated, and ultimately angry. That needs to be avoided. So, if it doesn't hurt them to leave them the way they are, then that is what the aides do.

After a number of days, I started skipping a day here and there, to see if Jim would notice my absence. Nothing was said, so I guess he didn't notice. I go when I want to see him for me, and sometimes I don't want to go and don't, but I feel guilty the entire day. It's as if he's noticing and thinks that I don't love him anymore. I was told by some friends that I have to figure out what is right for me, and do that. No one can tell me how many days I should go. I see the sense in that, but I am not ready to commit to any particular pattern. When I do go, I don't always know what to do with Jim, because there is so little that causes any emotional response. Taking him out for ice cream doesn't always get a rise out of him. Some days he says he has had a busy day and just wants to sit. I have tried throwing a ball with him to get his blood moving, but he doesn't always like to do that. Sometimes I take him to the center courtyard, and sit in the sun under an umbrella and enjoy the breezes. He has never made any attempt to walk out the locked door either. His lack of emotion and tiredness is most likely from the medication that is used to help control his outbursts and hallucinations (Seroquel.) I have not seen him 'happy' in weeks.

When I visit, I try to learn the residents' names as well as the staff. They are very friendly, and are always willing to talk if I have questions or ask how Jim is doing. They have remarked that if they ask Jim to do something he doesn't want to do, he says, "Now we are having a disagreement about this, let's sit down and talk about it." The old psychologist comes out again! Some learned skills you just never lose because you've done it so often in your lifetime.

How do I go on with my life? I find it hard to be motivated to do anything. I have to force myself. I'm not lying in bed with the covers over my head, but my 'to do' lists aren't full, and it doesn't give me joy accomplishing them. I feel that I'm in limbo with Jim in a facility. I know I need time to grieve, and time to recoup my 6 months lack of sleep. My friends definitely are trying to keep me busy and well fed, and I am so lucky to have them. I am more and more aware that we all have life altering events we go through, that others don't know about.

Ann's Notes
Synopsis of May

Three years ago, after Ralph had been diagnosed for three years, we put our name on a waiting list for an apartment in a nearby independent senior facility. I didn't think much more about it as I didn't think it was an option we could afford. I didn't know at the time that the next three years were going to be so difficult for both of us. On May 19th, we received a call from the complex. Our name had come up, and there was an apartment available with our specifications. I asked how much time was needed to think about it and make our decision. We had a week and a half!

Long story short: we went to look at it, Ralph liked it (important), and with the advice of our attorney, Dr. D., and our family, we said we'd take it. After that came the whirlwind of listing our house, showing it, selling it, and cleaning it out before our move on July 22nd.

06/02/2011
Vicky to Ann
I Am Back

I am back and had a good respite at Kip's (New Hampshire.) I spent one entire day in 89 degree weather putting in a front garden of grasses and Hostas by his front walkway. I had to remove lawn, which was a pain with all the NH stones, but it's done now and filled with river rock around the plants.

The second day I sanded, primed, and painted his sliding glass door, touched up the ceiling in another room, and installed the shelving in his bathroom again, after the paint job I did last time.

Kip worked the entire time, but we went out to dinner twice, and I cooked for him once. Not that we were not close before Jim's transfer, but Kip and I are so much closer now having gone through that experience together. I really missed him and he missed me...and of course, we both are missing the old Jim terribly. It was fun to get away, accomplish something tangible, and think about something else for a change.

Ann to Vicky

Glad you're back. Reading about all the work you were doing this weekend reminded me of when Ralph and I helped Brian and his wife then, Barbara, get settled in Vermont. After they were settled in, we drove back two consecutive weekends and painted the outside. Old farm house, 2½ stories, 2 coats. We went out to dinner all the time. We were almost too tired to eat, much less cook. Now, what little energy I have is being used up fast cleaning out this mess.

I called The Meadows Tuesday and said we'd take the apartment, and today we listed the house. One minute I feel good about it, and the next I'm scared to death.

I'll try to call tonight before 10 or after 11. There's a British sit-com that Ralph likes, and he wants us to watch it together.

06/09/2011
Vicky's Journal
The Call

At 7 AM today I received a call from Jim's assisted living facility. He tried to strangle an aide. He took her to the ground and he had to be pried loose. I dressed very quickly and drove the 5 minutes there. When I arrived, they were waiting for an ambulance to take Jim to the hospital for assessment to see if there was something wrong medically that would make him react the way he did. Jim was out in a hallway and two aides came out of the laundry door behind him and let the door slam. Jim is bothered by loud noises and must have sprung into a 'fight or flight' response to defend himself. He took one aide by the throat and threw her to the floor using 'legs' (a wrestling move that has stayed with him.) Luckily, she was not hurt, but they sent her to urgent care anyway to make sure. She was definitely shaken up and was near tears.

The ambulance arrived and they took Jim off to the Emergency Room. I followed in my car. He was fine in the ER, unlike last time, and for the evening and the next day they had a 1:1 aide with him. He also had a nurse who had worked at a behavioral center previously, and he was wonderful with Jim and me. What a difference the training of a nurse can make.

I told Jim why he was back in the hospital, and he looked at me in shock, not believing that he would do something like that to someone! He must have thought I was lying.

06/10/2011
Vicky's Journal

There were no tests that showed any physical problems. The assisted living center agreed to take Jim back as long as there was a 1:1 aide with him during waking hours for 10 days to watch Jim's behavior. They feel that the incident was partly their fault because of the slamming door. They educated their staff to be mindful of door closings, etc. that might trigger incidents like this one.

I have to pay for the 1:1 aide, so I asked if I could take the 3-10 PM shift each day to reduce my costs. They agreed, and so I have started fulfilling my part of the bargain. They contracted for an aide from a local agency, so as soon as that is set up, Jim can return.

06/15/2011
Vicky's Journal

So far the days have been uneventful. Jim must feel odd having someone sit with him all day long, and me in the evenings. I take my dinner and eat with him in the dining room with the others, but for now he is at a separate table, so I join him there. This time has been good for me in one respect. I am learning all the staff names and what special people they are to do the jobs they do.

One of the special aides who monitors Jim is a golf instructor. He previously asked if we could take Jim out to a driving range to see how he would do. He thought since Jim loved playing golf, it would be good for him. I agreed to accompany them today. It was very disappointing. Jim had no clue what to do with the golf club, where the ball was, or anything. He was not capable of taking 'practice swings.' The aide and I hit the remainder of the bucket and we left.

Jim doesn't remember how to get into bed or lay on top of the covers so that his head is on the pillow. He is always cockeyed and his arms are out in mid-air. He also doesn't recognize a toilet or its use. He thought the hamper was the toilet. Pretty soon he will be peeing in the closets! I put Velcro on all his pants to make things easier, but he can't manage that either, so I will have to switch to stretch waist pants.

He does recognize me as someone who visits him, but he won't let me assist with his clothes, because he doesn't see me as his wife. I don't know whether he is getting bathed or not. He did let me help him shave, though.

I noticed two days ago that Jim's left ankle and foot are swollen, but not the right. I don't know why that would be, unless it is congestive heart failure. In that case, wouldn't both feet be swollen? Now, the right foot is swollen just on top of the foot. Inactivity? I have to get him compression stockings.

He is a lost soul. There is no emotion on his face. He just sits. He does listen to TV, though.

06/23/2011
Vicky to Ann
Hello

Went to see Dr. D. today. Slowly and methodically, he asked Jim a group of questions about: what he did when he worked, how he got his training, was he happy at the assisted living facility, does he eat well, etc. As he was listening to the answers, I could see the wheels turning. At one point, Jim said, "That doesn't seem relevant to my being here, so I'm not going to answer." Jim would never have said that before the disease.

He had Jim give a blood sample for baseline testing, and he prescribed Depakote to help stabilize his mood. It is normally used to smooth out the highs and lows of bipolar disorder, but can cause liver damage. He has to bring Jim up slowly to the therapeutic dose, taking more blood samples as we go. He wants to see Jim in 3 months to see if there is a positive change on the Depakote. That is in addition to the Seroquel Jim already takes.

Hope you are both slogging through the 'must dos', and fingers and toes are crossed for the sale of the house.

Ann to Vicky

It sounds as if Dr. D. is going to stick with you through thick and thin, doesn't it? Wouldn't it be great if Jim could come back home for a little while? Or would it? Probably not, but if he can be happier where he is, it would make you feel better.

We have the house sold to a point. The buyers wanted an inspection done, and they are paying for it. The engineer was here for almost 3 hours yesterday, and there are a couple of issues. When we put in the new furnace a year ago, somehow the venting system took away from the venting of the hot water tank. I don't pretend to understand it all, and Ralph has been really out of it lately. The inspector also questioned the root cellar Ralph dug almost 40 years ago. It is starting to cave in. The agent said not to lose sleep over it. Yeah, right.

I'll call you later about helping pack on Saturday. Whatever you want to do is fine. I think we'll try to pack the kitchen, wash and pack the good china, that sort of thing. You're more than welcome to join the fray. I'm feeling more and more overwhelmed. I'm hopefully going to finish sorting almost 60 years of pictures into a couple of boxes. I'm going to have to be ruthless about it. Then, a woman from The Meadows is coming over at 4:30 to give us tips on moving. Nancy is coming over after work to sit in on that.

06/27/2011
Vicky to Ann
Try to Stay Positive

I felt so bad for you on Sat. having to make all the spur of the moment decisions about things that you have collected your whole life. Just hang in there for three weeks more and the clouds will start to clear, and you will have the things that you hold most dear at your fingertips! Thanks for the 'lemon' pitcher. I really love it. Great for water or lemonade.

Please don't hesitate to call if I can be of more help.

Ann to Vicky

Thanks again for all your concern and hard work. I'll call you tonight with all the latest stuff. But at least it's good stuff.

06/29/2011
Vicky to Ann
We Are Back In The ER Again!

I had taken Jim to the dermatologist this AM for an 'all over' exam, as well as a look at his left eye brow where the cancer was removed. He was not cooperative in taking his clothes off because he was cold. We finally got him to comply, but barely! I noticed at the office that Jim had a large urine stain on his underwear. When we got back to the assisted living, I tried to get Jim to change clothes, but no amount of cajoling worked. I blew it and said, "Fine. I don't care if you smell and wear dirty clothes." That was really mean, and it didn't help the situation at all. Jim went down the hall and when I left I passed him. He was unphased by my words.

When I got home I went out to garden (to ease my soul,) and forgot to take my cell phone with me. At 2:30, when I went in the house, I found a message on the answering machine that assisted living sent him to the ER again. This time, they sent him to the hospital that is affiliated with the assisted living center, because he was throwing chairs in the dining room. They said he even picked up a table with very little trouble.

This hospital was terrible for a dementia patient. Because of his actions, they put him in a psychiatric part of the ER where the room had all white walls and ceiling. The only thing in the room was his bed. No tray, no bedside table, nothing. The doors were divided in two so that they could close the bottom like a horse stall that you couldn't open from the inside. There was a camera on the ceiling and a security person down the hallway monitoring him from a distance. I was crushed that he was all alone, and I was mad that they would isolate him this way. They treated him like a drug addict. He had no pillow, no food, or meds for the first 9 hours he was there! I had to ask for a chair so I could sit down. They were not very attentive because they were busy. The evening shift finally came through and they were helpful. He had to be accompanied everywhere, and they would only let him use the bathroom where the toilet and sink were aluminum and bolted down so they couldn't be moved. Do you know how cold it is to sit on a metal toilet? I finally got him a pillow and something to eat. Went home sometime after 11PM. I was bushed, and there was no place I could sleep. They said if Jim became agitated, they will give him a dose of Haldol to make him sleep. They removed the chair when I left. Will keep you posted.

07/03/2011
Vicky's Journal

Jim's next few days were not much better. They insisted he wear a hospital gown and underpants, and he was very cold. No blankets, just a sheet. Someone from psychiatry wanted a consult with the head guy, and we were waiting for that. In the meantime, none of Jim's regular meds had been given, but of course there were orders that if he became agitated they could give Haldol as needed (used to be given in the old days to control patients by keeping them sedated-flashback to *One Flew Over The Cuckoo's Nest*.) It took 'til 5:20 PM the second day before they became aware of the meds he was on, which they still didn't administer, and someone ordered 25 mg. Seroquel morning and 125 mg. Seroquel at night. He was on 50 mg. Seroquel at night previously, so the 125 mg. snowed him! He slept for an entire day, and when he was awake in the morning they gave him a Seroquel, and he zonked out for hours again!

The greatest disadvantage with this hospitalization is that this particular hospital has no affiliation with any of the neuro-behavioral care units (behavioral nursing homes) in New York State. There are three of them. If he had been sent back to the first hospital, he would have priority in the behavioral nursing home close by. Jim's present hospital has no ties with any of the three. Behavioral beds are scarce and these are reserved for the people in affiliated hospitals. Jim was not eligible for a regular nursing home because of his agitation/violence issues. So unknowingly, the assisted living did Jim a big disservice by sending him to this particular hospital.

At the end of Jim's fourth day in the ER, they finally found a private room for him, so he could be moved. Because of his over-sedation, they needed to stop everything until the Seroquel got out of his system. Because he was sleeping so much, he was not eating or drinking, or peeing. I was especially worried about that. I had asked for a 1:1 aide, and they hoped to have one tomorrow. Everything was slow because Jim was brought in 2 days before the 4th of July weekend. Another coincidence that led to poor treatment.

They have to verify that Jim's actions weren't due to some infection that made him act out. They also have to establish some sort of baseline before they can try new meds to control his behavior, if such a thing is possible. A nurse from the assisted living came by to assess whether they would take Jim back, but they could not do the assessment because he was too sedated to participate. I seriously doubt that they can take him back. I did question Jim about his actions that day, and in one of his more lucid moments, he told me he was protecting the children...his tragic hallucinations.

Vicky to Ann
Quick Update

Jim is finally on a floor! I asked the charge nurse for a 1:1 aide and it was approved, but they take someone from their already busy staff, not an agency or outside worker...crazy system...so they are short.

For the first time in days I left at 3:30 today, and Kip came home for the weekend at 7:30 PM. We are going out to dinner, and then back to see Jim in hopes that a 1:1 will be there.

Nothing regarding placement will be done until Tuesday, because of the holiday. At least he has a nice private room with a lounge chair and his own regular bathroom. And he will receive more regular treatment like a 'real patient', now that he is out of the ER.

Keeping family updated has been hard because my cell doesn't get good reception in the hospital. It keeps cutting out. Have to do family calls when I get home at night. I am also keeping our financial advisor and lawyer abreast of what's happening. Will write more when I know more.

Ann to Vicky

I was just going to call you and then I checked my e-mail. Thank God Jim was moved from his 'cell.' It sounds like something out of a Dickens novel. I still can't believe the horror of this whole stinking disease.

I took Ralph to see the apartment yesterday, and he was very confused. Still doesn't know who and how many are going to be living there. Hopefully, he'll come around when things settle down.

Today we went to Springwater to admire Brian's goats and turkeys. It was a long day, and we're both dead tired. We stopped at a restaurant on the way home, and I've decided eating out is fast becoming a thing of the past. I thought we were inconspicuous, but when I paid the check the owner said, "You certainly have your hands full, don't you?" I guess we stuck out like two sore thumbs.

I'm glad Kip is home. I'll talk to you very soon, or call me when you have news. Hang in there.

07/04/2011
Vicky's Journal
A Line for This and a Line for That

The last two days Jim had a 1:1 aide shared with the person across the hall. That worked out well. Jim was awake this morning for breakfast and ate well, but then they gave him his Seroquel and he zonked out again. His orders were bed rest, but I thought he should be up in a chair when he could. He's probably lost a lot of weight over the last few days, and bed rest isn't helping. I didn't want him to lose any more muscle mass. I finally managed to have him put in a chair late in the afternoon for a little while. Things are better in more 'normal' surroundings.

They told me today that Jim has developed pneumonia from trying to eat when he was so sedated. He aspirated his food and saliva that has bacteria in it and that leads to infection. They also had to catheterize him because he wasn't peeing.

His enlarged prostate made it difficult for them to get a line in, so they had to wait for a specialist to do it. So now he has a bag for pee and an IV line in for the Ceftriaxone for his pneumonia, he gets Seroquel 3 times a day. He also gets Depakote twice daily. Other than the Foley catheter and the antibiotics, that's what he had when he came in to the hospital 6 days ago! Is that aggravating or what!

Kip went back to New Hampshire late today. It was good to have him here.

07/05/2011-07/08/2011
Vicky's Journal
What Happens Now

Jim was seen by a speech therapist to evaluate his swallowing. She changed Jim's food to nectar consistency, because it elicits a stronger swallow response. She was adamant that he should not be fed unless he is really awake.

The assisted living facility told me they would not take Jim back. No surprise there. Luckily I have some very wonderful friends who provided a truck and manpower to move the heaviest things out of Jim's old room and into our garage while I was at the hospital. The remainder I emptied in one car load on the way home.

The first day after the long holiday weekend, I met with the social worker from ED again. She wanted to follow Jim's case through to placement rather than handing him off to the social worker on the floor. She ordered a state Level II review for Jim. Without the state's go-ahead Jim could not be placed in one of the three behavioral facilities, even if they had a bed. While we were waiting for the results, she suggested I physically visit all three places so that 'a face goes along with an application' in case Jim is approved for Level II care. She said it always helps. I met with a person from the closest behavioral facility located in Rochester, but they assured me that there were no openings. I never met with anyone at the facility in Penn Yan, N.Y. (1½ hours away.) They had no openings either. However, I did meet with a representative from the Newark facility on Thursday afternoon. It just so happens that a patient died the night before, so there was a bed available. Jim was in a group of 8 patients wanting admission for that 1 bed. I received word this morning that 1) Jim was approved for Level II care, and 2) the Newark behavioral unit accepted Jim!! What made the difference was that I had enough money to pay for one year of care for Jim. I may not have much after that, but I had MONEY. What a relief. The social worker told me that sometimes patients wait months in the hospital for a behavioral bed. Sometimes they are even placed out of the state where they live...which makes it impossible for family to visit very often. I think that is outrageous. While they are waiting for a bed in an appropriate facility, they are also not getting the care and attention they really need. Also, sometimes while waiting for a behavioral bed, the hospital/health care tries to force payment for room and board. The pièce de résistance...Newark costs $21,500 per month!

The biggest hurdle is over, and Jim's doctor from assisted living (still his primary) took Jim off the Seroquel and Depakote to bring him out of his fog. His antibiotic was also changed. He has not been allowed to walk because there is not enough staff on the floor. I was very worried about Jim's decline since hospitalization.

07/08/2011
Ann to Vicky
Just A Thought

It's probably just a shot in the dark, but do you think spousal refusal would work in a case like this, or are some of your assets still in Jim's name?

Vicky to Ann

I have a spousal refusal form that I signed ages ago at the lawyer's in case we needed to use it, but Jim has some money in a 401K that they would go after to pay for his stay. One of our support group men used the spousal refusal after his wife was in the nursing home 5 years. Right now, it would not be well received in helping him get a place. The longer he stays in the hospital, the quicker he will die being confined to bed...and I don't want him to die that way!

Good thought, though.

See Spousal Refusal in 'Caregivers 101, Things We Have Learned.'

07/11/2011
Vicky's Journal
Day Thirteen of Hospitalization

Jim's antibiotic was changed to a pill form, so he could continue by mouth after discharge to Newark. Jim was more awake and talkative than in prior days, and he was more understandable (previous days his speech made no sense.) They finally took his Foley catheter out yesterday and he has been able to pee. At 10:30 AM the transport team arrived and strapped him in, and off they went. I drove to Newark separately and arrived early enough to set up Jim's room before he arrived.

The people at the Newark facility were wonderful. They took a complete history of Jim's likes and dislikes as far as food, clothing, interests, and environment. They gave him a tour of all the community rooms ending up with his own room. They had a code of ethics to make sure each person was respected and treated with courtesy and dignity. An example of this follows: I was going to have Jim put on an undershirt underneath his shirt, because he was cold. I started to take his shirt off in the common TV area, and was told not to do that there, but to take Jim back to his room and do it. I just wasn't thinking...I'd been in 'hospital mode' too long.

07/14/2011
Vicky's Journal
Jim's Progress

Since Jim was admitted, the staff had him in a wheel chair for a few days, getting him up occasionally. As he seemed to get stronger, they let him walk. I don't know if he has had some incontinence, but now I noticed he is no longer wearing diapers, but is wearing regular underwear. He is back to eating normal foods now. The very day they let him get up and walk, he showed them he could do 23 push-ups and that was after the hell of the past 2 weeks! He is something else! Give him a chance to show off and he comes through. He has always been proud of his body.

He has alarms on and around his bed, so they know if he is out of bed or falls. The alarms keep ringing until silenced, so it is not something that can go unheeded. The staff are caring, good natured people who don't get flustered by much. They are also well trained in how to approach people when they are agitated. They make sure that each person is well dressed and groomed down to the jewelry and hair for the women.

But behavioral places take some getting used to. It's not like walking into a posh nursing home. The day I toured, the lighting was very low. It helps to calm those who are agitated, and some were that day. The walls were cream colored, and high up on the walls were numerous quilt pieces on display. There were no pictures or objects on the wall that could be used as projectiles, or if broken could cause harm. Each person had a shadow box by their room with their name in large letters and pictures of family on display. I made Jim's a story of his life with early pictures of him with his parents and sister, some of Jim wrestling and pole vaulting in high school, our wedding photo, and a description of his professional life so people would know his strong drive to help families and children make their lives better. There was one place in the room where pictures could be taped, but again, no pictures in frames or decorations that could cause harm to anyone.

Single use razors were used to shave the men (or electric razors which were kept at the nurses' station.) Tooth brushes were kept in their shared wardrobe with their clothes...that is also locked during the day. There was a much higher staff to patient ratio here. Besides needing 1-2 people to get each person dressed and cleaned up in the morning, they must monitor each person's behavior and take them out of the situation, if necessary. They had to document where each person was every 15 minutes. It was very well run, and Jim was receiving great care, but it was very stark and institutional looking. Just the week before, their TV was broken by someone, so they received a new flat screen TV mounted behind Plexiglas and wood. Every two rooms shared a bathroom, along with a sitting area enclosed with a low wall. This allowed those who didn't want to be in their own room, to sit on 'their front porch' and watch the world go by.

I brought up the idea with Kip...the next time Jim gets an infection, not to treat him, just give palliative care. Kip was worried about Jim experiencing pain with that kind of care, but I assured him that's what palliative care means: caring for a patient to relieve or prevent pain and suffering by reducing symptoms of the disease, rather than the focus of cure. He isn't too keen on the idea because it is his dad, and he's not ready to let him go yet.

With the 40 minute drive both ways, I am getting tired of staying the full day with Jim, but on the other hand, I want to be there to make sure he's not all by himself. I feel so bad for him, but there is nothing I can do to make it better. Whatever happens is meant to be. I have to learn to trust the staff, and take a day or two here and there to revive myself.

07/22/2011
Ann's Note
Moving Day

People ask me how I could manage sorting, cleaning out, packing, and unpacking with all the time I was devoting to caregiving. Simple answer. I couldn't, but I had a great support team. Brian, Nancy, and Lou worked their tails off helping me. We had 40 years of accumulation to deal with. Nancy has a gift where she can look at shelves of 'stuff' and instantly determine what to keep, throw, or sell. She and Lou's sister, Linda, and Vicky spent a Saturday cleaning out my kitchen, wrapping and packing everything I was taking with me. All I did was stand around like a zombie saying: "Keep, throw, garage sale, you can have it if you like it," and "I don't know."

Nancy and I made countless trips to the new apartment to settle the kitchen and closets, and measure where the furniture would go. Sometimes, we would take Ralph with us so that he could slowly become oriented to his new home, but most times, Brian would look after him so we could work without worrying. Brian contacted potential buyers for Ralph's woodworking tools and equipment. A huge part of the job was placating Ralph, who at that point was trusting no one. Everyone was extremely sensitive to the problem, and spent a lot of time talking with Ralph about the many aspects of his craft and gaining his trust. It was heartbreaking to all that this talented man was losing yet another huge part of himself.

At last July 22nd arrived, the moving van pulled up, loaded all that was left, and we were off. A chapter of our life together had closed. I think we both realized it was one of the best chapters.

07/23/2011
Vicky's Journal
The Days March On

When Jim came here he was not on any Seroquel or Depakote. They let him stay that way for about a week and a half. He is not sleeping well at night, especially if he doesn't go to bed by 7:30 PM. They think he gets overtired. This past week they X-rayed his lungs and there was one spot that wasn't clear, but he has no temperature and no increased white count so they are watching it and will repeat the tests later. He is also now on Seroquel again morning, afternoon, and evening. He gets tired in the afternoon as usual. They will continue to increase meds as necessary SLOWLY.

Four days ago I brought in our wedding album, and after looking at all the pictures he seemed to remember that I was his wife. He said how lucky he was to have married me. He was very loving. Today I am another Vicky. He didn't want the other Vicky to think he was two-timing her! Now I am 'the other Vicky who visits'. So quickly we are forgotten. Sigh.

It's so hard being alone. I get to thinking about Jim as a young man, and I feel so sorry for his life now. I want to see the old Jim, and I look for him, but he just doesn't come out of that body. It pains my heart so. Somehow, I have to continue my life. Right now I am just coasting.

07/29/2011
Ann to Vicky

No one could totally understand what we are going through. It's an awful disease to be saddled with, and all we can do is be there for each other. I like all the support group friends, but I really feel bonded to you.

I continue to struggle with my back issues. I had an MRI yesterday, and am waiting for the results. In the meantime, I'm not getting much unpacking done. For every 5 minutes I spend unpacking, I spend 15 minutes dealing with Ralph. Very frustrating, but it will get done eventually.

Take care of yourself and remember the Alzheimer rule: Put your own oxygen mask on before putting it on your child...in this case dementia loved one. We must try to stay healthy.

08/07/2011
Ann to Dr. D.
Update

Where to begin. We took the advice of family, friends, and support team, and moved to a senior apartment on July 22nd. It was a hectic six weeks of listing, selling, and cleaning out our home of 40 years. Ralph has had trouble adjusting to the move, but was starting to settle in. However, he was showing more anger about his life and criticizing my care. I expected that.

Last Wed., we were in an accident and Ralph was injured by his seat belt. He spent two days in the Emergency Room. The conditions there would send anyone into a frenzy, but to keep a dementia patient there for any length of time is like 'bringing coals to Newcastle'. He had a psychotic episode in the middle of the night. I won't describe it here, but I hope you can bring up the report on your computer. They had to use heavy anti-psychotic drugs to calm him. The rest of the time he was cooperative and his usual gentle self. To add to the situation, Ralph and I were told he was being discharged to home that next morning. At that point, he had a 1:1 aide/guard.

Anyway, we never left the hospital until 7 PM, and Ralph was starting to sundown again. If I had the time, I would start an advocacy group to insist there be at least one unit in one of the hospitals for dementia trauma patients. At the very least, I intend to warn all my support group and Alzheimer Association friends that no matter how trivial an illness or injury seems, "Do not, under any circumstances, leave a loved one alone in the hospital." No matter how much I explained his condition to staff, it became clear to me that no one had the experience needed to understand the dementia patient.

We saw Dr. P. yesterday, and he couldn't discuss anything beyond Ralph's injuries (car insurance protocol.) However, I expressed concern not only about his mental decline, but the fact that he's lost 12 pounds since March 1st. I can see that he is wasting. Dr. P. thinks he will go back to what his baseline was before the accident, but I'm not so sure. He's declining so fast, I think you might want to see him. I don't know if anything can be done. All I know is he is much worse today than he was a week ago.

Dr. D. to Ann

I am sorry to hear of your struggle to move, but I think we agree that there was really no choice. You did more than anyone could expect. I still marvel at it all.

The accident certainly complicates things, and while any trip to the ER is horrible, yours sounds particularly so. I am thinking that we need to institute an ER protocol for cognitively impaired older adults. I will talk to them about that.

I fear he may not fully recover to his previous baseline, but he should come close to it. We have worked together in the past on the judicious use of Seroquel, and that may be necessary again. Please keep me informed.

Ann to Dr. D.

Thanks for your prompt reply. I'm not sure what to do about his meds. Normally, he takes Namenda and Seroquel at night, Namenda in the morning with 12.5 mg. Seroquel midday. He usually doesn't want the midday Seroquel because it makes him groggy, but I think he needs it. How is the best way to go about this? I don't want to turn him into a zombie. He's so close to that now, without the extra Seroquel.

Dr. D. to Ann

What is the most troublesome behavior problem that we want to control with the Seroquel...or possibly something else?

Ann to Dr. D.

It's really difficult to pinpoint the most troublesome behavior. Every day is different. Now, we can add insomnia to the mix. I was up with him until 3:30 this morning. He's not communicating well at all. Just sits on the side of the bed. He won't talk about the ER experience other than he insists he was attacked in the night, and that it's too horrible to talk about. He's becoming more paranoid, argumentative, demanding, etc. He's lost his ability to do even the simplest of tasks. His hands and forearms shake and twitch when he's getting anxious or frustrated. He's stooped, and shuffles when he walks. He's been unable to get out and really walk here even before the accident, because he's not oriented to the campus. I've had more back problems due to packing, lifting, etc., so I haven't gone out with him.

Socially, it's getting more difficult to take him anywhere. He becomes exhausted if we're in stores, and even the Alzheimer's program at the art gallery seems to have lost its appeal.

Generally, he's become a very unhappy man. I don't know what else to say, except that I'm losing more of the real Ralph every day.

Ann's Note

Months later, I read an article that told of a study by Harvard researchers on the effects of a hospital stay on dementia patients. It noted that the lingering ill effects of being hospitalized seemed to increase the chances of dementia patients moving into a nursing home or even dying within the next year. The stress of new surroundings can send patients with Alzheimer's disease or other dementias into a tail spin. The trauma of being in an unfamiliar place where strangers are performing unfamiliar procedures on them can be devastating to an already damaged brain. The additional effects of administering anti-psychotic drugs (E.g. Haldol) can be irreversible.

Sadly, this knowledge came too late for Ralph and me. I think he suffered untold fears by the well-meaning staff caring for him. I know that many hospitals are taking these new studies very seriously. Meanwhile, here are some ideas.

Regarding Hospitals and Dementia:

- At home, watch for new symptoms, such as irritability or grimacing, which could be a sign of pain. Seek care early to avoid hospitalization.

- Never, ever leave a dementia person alone in a hospital or ER setting. Always have a family member or trusted friend stay with them, especially overnight.

- Bring the patient's glasses and hearing aids to the hospital for optimal orientation.

- Bring the patient's medicines from home in case they are needed.

- Make sure someone (family member or professional caregiver) is always present to advocate for the patient.)

08/09/2011
Vicky to Ann
Funeral Arrangements

You know I have been getting the papers ready for Medicaid filing in case I should need to do that. It's a daunting process getting 5 years of bank statements, etc. together. Well, today I went to the funeral parlor to find out the bottom line for funerals for Jim and me, so that I can prepay them before Medicaid filing. $4,500 for flowers, news article, greeting book, thank you notes, calling hours, funeral in another setting, and cremation. No embalming or casket of any sort. That's the price for each, not for both.

One thing Kip related to me (he has a close friend that just lost his dad to Alzheimer's.) Spend the money on the calling hours and the funeral. His mom didn't, and he feels like he didn't have the chance to say goodbye. He regrets that every day. I know the funeral is for the living, not the dying. It's just that going through all that at such an emotional time is so hard!

08/10/2011
Ann to Dr. D.

I don't know if you had a chance to read my last note, but I think Ralph needs some adjustments to his meds. He's up more in the night with more delusion. I feel some of this is the combination of moving and the accident along with the expected decline. I'd like for him to be able to enjoy the new apartment at least for a little while. I know placing him is probably coming, sooner than any of us expected. We can't really afford this apartment, but my plan was to get him into this system, which in turn would give him a priority for the nursing home. However, if he has another documented episode, the nursing home won't take him. Perhaps I made all the wrong choices. If you think changing or increasing his meds would help, please let me know.

Dr. D. to Ann

Sorry for not getting right back to you. I was wondering how you are using the Seroquel at this point. Doubling the bedtime dose might stabilize his sleep, but he will be less active during the day.

08/11/2011
Ann to Dr. D.

For now, I think I'd like to try 37 mg. Seroquel with Tylenol PM unless you think that's a bad combo for him.

Dr. D. to Ann

It is a reasonable thing to try. Is he out of bed at night to go to the bathroom? How many times? Is he delusional during the day? Is he stable on his feet?

Ann to Dr. D.

He is delusional at night. He is usually oriented in the daytime, but he had me up 'til 3:00 this morning, babbling and blaming me for everything. I finally got him to lie down and sleep, but this morning he is more delusional. I was going to call you, but I'm not sure what you can do. I know he's going to have to be placed and he will not go quietly. It's so ironic. I'm paying this high rent on the hopes he can get into the affiliated nursing home, but if he has another melt down, they won't take him. I'm afraid he's going to end up in a behavioral unit, and spend his last days hating me.

Last night I gave him 37 mg. Seroquel and Tylenol PM. If anything, it made him worse. However, we had dinner at our daughter's home and he was oriented, stable, and seemed to enjoy the evening. He's become a Jekyll and Hyde personality.

I appreciate anything you can do.

08/11/2011
Ann to Dr. D.

Strange disease.

Ralph just woke from a nap and is totally oriented, stable, and compliant. He remembers we had two things to do today, and asked if we were going and what time.

Looking at him now, it seems a shame to place him. He's talking about some day trips he'd like to take when we get a car. Ours was totaled in the accident.

I want to give him time to adjust to the new surroundings before moving him on to a nursing home. We need to do something for the middle of the night episodes so we can both get some sleep. Sorry I'm rambling. Dealing with the mood swings is making me a little off base.

08/12/2011
Vicky to Ann
Dear Friend

I am sorry I had to leave today before giving you a BIG hug! Your sister and Nancy arrived, so I thought I could go as I had to visit Jim. I know by your crying that Dr. D. was telling you that it was time to admit Ralph to a nursing home, and it was just too much for you to bear. I tried to keep Ralph talking so that he wouldn't hear your responses. For a while he wanted to listen, kept telling me to hush, but I think he finally realized he didn't want to listen. I felt so bad for both of you. Very tragic circumstances.

No one could have foretold Ralph's reaction this week. You did what we all thought would work, and perhaps with some additional meds, he could have had a little more time at The Meadows.

Jim was kind of out of it today, but my neighbor, Beth, and I cajoled him into having an OK visit. I just relaxed and thought to myself, the visit is going to be what it will be. As it turned out, Beth rose to the occasion and made it easy for all of us. So, kudos to her!

I am showered and in my night clothes, and feeling so sad for both of us...for the four of us and all our families involved. It really stinks!

I am free this weekend. I just have an appointment at 10 AM on Monday. So, if you need me to sleep over Sunday night, I am only a phone call or e-mail away.

I hope you have a better night's sleep with a quietly sleeping Ralph beside you.

Ann to Vicky

My heart is breaking. Of course, you know Dr. D. told me Ralph has to go into a dementia unit. We must have talked for close to an hour, but the outcome was the same. Ralph has been so sweet to me this afternoon and evening. I think he knows, and that is breaking my heart even more. Dr. D. doesn't think it's safe for me to be alone with him. Nancy will stay tonight, and Brian tomorrow night. May still need you on Sunday. Day at a time. I also met with the elder advocate here for about an hour, and she agrees he must be placed. She feels we should have no problem placing him in the affiliated nursing home because our apartment is already in the system.

Dr. P. called me back and agrees that this is what we must do. I still don't know. Ralph is out in the kitchen cleaning up, and I can't stand it. The tears just keep flowing. He only asked me once why I was crying. I said, "I don't know, just feeling a little sorry for myself," and he said, "I know how you feel."

I'll fill you in Sunday or sooner. I'm having trouble keeping the tears back, and I'm trying so hard to hide it. I can't tell you how much I appreciate you for your help in the midst of all your pain.

Love you,

P.S. I have calls in to a couple of PRI offices. Should have an answer by Monday. Dr. D. said it's important for Ralph to be stable at the time, but not stable enough to screw up the PRI. How do I arrange that?

Vicky to Ann

Love you...and know that I am aching and crying for you too...my arms are around you.

08/13/2011
Vicky's Journal
First Monthly Meeting with Jim's New Doctor

For whatever reason, all the patients were placed here because they acted out or directed their agitation/violence inward. On average, I was told that most residents stay at least 6-9 months. Either they learn better behaviors, or their disease progresses to where they aren't exhibiting the problem behaviors anymore. The staff tries to redirect the residents before behaviors escalate. Medication, I expect, goes hand in hand with behavior modification.

I really like the doctor and the director of the floor for neurobehavioral care. They were compassionate. They answered my questions about why certain medications were no longer prescribed for Jim, and yet they didn't gloss over the reality of the situation. They told me that Jim is in great distress. This was shown by his constant walking and his inability to sleep. They told me that during the previous night, Jim hadn't slept for more than 40 minutes before getting up again. His days and nights weren't switched; he wasn't having any nights. He continues to be intrusive to other residents. He invades their personal space and sometimes gets punched for it. He has been hitting his head against the walls, including the Plexiglas of the nurses' station. He has rubbed his forehead raw doing that. Now, I'm hearing that today he took a run at the window, trying to throw himself out and end his life, but the windows don't break. They are twice as thick as regular windows. He is also expressing suicidal thoughts. He flipped over a table in the dining room, but no one was hurt. No one thought the disease would end like this. It is so tragic, it breaks my heart.

There are two avenues that they could follow:

1)   Slowly increase his medications so that he would be more calm, hoping to quell most but not necessarily all his 'acting out' episodes. This would allow him to be mobile, but he would continue to be a risk to himself and others, so he would have to stay here for a year or more. He could live 6-8 more years, because physically he is in good shape. When he is no longer a risk, then he could be transferred to a regular nursing home.

2)   They will medicate him with one of the valium family of drugs to the point that he would no longer be a risk to himself or others. This would mean that he would no longer be able to walk. At that point, he could be transferred to a regular nursing home. This means he would spend most of his day in a geri-chair, a lounge chair on wheels. He would be moved from chair to bed to chair by the use of a Hoyer Lift. Because he would be too sedated to be active, he would not be able to feed himself. He would also become incontinent fairly rapidly, and would be back in diapers. His physical stamina would decrease because of lack of exercise. At some point he probably wouldn't take nourishment at all. The sedation might also lead to eventual complications with breathing, aspiration of food or saliva causing pneumonia, and death. This scenario might last 1-2 years at most.

I shared with both of them the fact that Jim never wanted to live this long. He had wanted to commit suicide 'when the time was right,' but it seemed he always wanted that 'one more day.' Later he mentioned to me that "I just couldn't do it." I understood his wish to die, and was OK with that, I just didn't want to be aware when he might do it. I didn't want to worry every day at work about what I would find when I came home. I told him no matter what he decided, I would support him and would care for him to the end. We even went so far as to read *Final Exit; The Practicalities of Self-Deliverance and Assisted Suicide for the Dying* by Derek Humphry. Jim was not capable at that time of carrying out the steps.

They gave me all the time I needed to decide. When I came home from that meeting, I went to bed for 4 hours. I just wanted to pull the covers over my head and disappear. How could I choose either choice for my loving and loyal husband of 42 years? I didn't want to see anyone or go anywhere. My heart was crushed and I just couldn't escape the intense and constant hurt. Time to grieve a bit, and then get down to business.

08/13/2011
Vicky to Ann
Sunday

When would you like me to come on Sunday? I could visit Jim in the morning, and then come to your place sometime in the afternoon...whatever time you want after 1:45 PM. I will bring Chinese food for dinner...what kinds do you both like? I will bring my knitted throw so you don't have to worry about any kind of blanket.

I have to leave for my 10 AM appointment at my priority nursing home, but then can come back if you want. It's just a hop, skip, and jump from your place. That way I wouldn't have to visit Jim on Monday at all. I could stay Monday night, too, if you need me. You will probably have to continue the sleepovers 'til Ralph is placed...or sedated more.

Don't know when Kip is coming...we'll have to talk tonight. I didn't call him yesterday. Gave him space and time. I'm thinking that when he comes, he could fly here and then I could drive him back and stay and paint for a few days. We are all like whirling tops on the corner of a table!

Ann to Vicky

Love your analogy.

I'm through telling people they don't have to do anything. I need and want all the help I can get at this point.

I talked to Dr. D. for almost an hour and he says Ralph must be placed for everyone's safety.

He was fine last night with Nancy here. And will be with Brian tonight. Same goes for you tomorrow night. He's wily enough to wait until we're alone to go into his dissertation about 'they' doing us in. Now, he's insisting I finish the plans for some sort of bizarre toilet thingy that is very important for keeping us safe. Stares at me and says I must do it!! It's scary!

Please come tomorrow. I'd like to get Ralph and me out for a ride if possible, but he may be too unpredictable to take in the car.

Re: Chinese food. We eat anything. He's partial to pork or beef and I usually stick with mildly hot sesame chicken.

Gotta run. I'll call you tonight.

Your partner in a criminal disease...

08/14/2011
Ann to Dr. D.
Ralph

You wanted me to be in touch with you today, and I didn't want to call on a Sunday. Ralph is not stabilizing and I'm hoping we don't have any more major episodes before placing him. My goal has always been to get him into the nursing home affiliated with this senior complex, or one of the other top units. We'll have to get him on Medicaid ASAP, but living here will give us an edge on admitting him right away. He's taking Seroquel morning and night. He stays fairly calm after his morning dose, but starts acting belligerent early evening. The evening Seroquel calms him for a couple of hours, but then he's up and acting out. He won't let me near him, orders me out, tells me to shut up, which he's never done. My daughter stayed over Friday night, and my son last night. Brian was able to reason with him more than I could, and got him to the toilet without an incident. I won't stay alone with him at night, so the sooner we get this done, the better. I never thought I would be afraid of him, but I am.

I have calls in to 2 agencies to get a PRI as soon as possible, and I'm working with the elder advocate here; she's been a great help. She has alerted the entire security staff and told them that if they get a call from me, they must be here in 30 seconds or less. This has all taken place since Friday afternoon after your call.

I have had some good cries when he's sleeping, but I know I have to put my emotions aside for the next few days.

One more thing. You said Ralph wouldn't process what's going on, but Friday night he was being especially sweet, and said it looked as if I had been crying and what was going on. I said I was just feeling a little sorry for myself, and he said he could understand that. He was quiet for a while and later he said, "So, are you going to visit me when I'm in the 'bug house'?"

I have gently talked about the fact that we need a little more help, and we both need a chance to rest from all the trauma of the last few weeks. I have no idea what else to say, except he'll know he's not going to a hotel.

Let me know if you want to increase or add any meds. Problem there is, it's getting harder to give him any pills without an argument, much less more of them.

As for the walk, drink, and nap that you suggested; I managed one out of three.

Dr. D. to Ann

I think we should go directly to the Seroquel 25 mg. after breakfast, then mid-afternoon, and then before bed (total of 3x per day.) We might then boost him up to 50 twice a day and a new medicine (Trazodone) at night. I don't recall trying him on Trazodone, and it can help sustain sleep in patients who are activated and confused.

Has he made any threats, been yelling, or wandering?

08/15/2011
Ann to Dr. D.

Last night, he was up a number of times, angry, but not threatening. It takes a lot of coaxing trying to reason to get him to sit on the toilet, so each wake time is at least 30-40 minutes. At 3 AM, he began yelling for help and was becoming more agitated, so in desperation I gave him 25 mg. of Trazodone that our doctor prescribed for me for occasional sleep help. He calmed down and went back to bed after that kicked in. Slept 'til 7 and we went through the whole sad routine again.

I have a little concern about the midday Seroquel. After the AM dose yesterday, he slept 4-5 hours, couldn't seem to wake up even if I spoke loudly to him. When he finally did wake up, he was an angel until about midnight. The night time Seroquel doesn't hold him long enough and the AM dose turns him into a zombie. I'm waiting for a call back from Visiting Nurse Service re: a PRI/screening. I have an application from the nursing home, and will make an appointment as soon as I can. So far, I've had help at night.

In the meantime, I need to finish the house because the closing is next week. Also, trying to find a decent car I can afford. People ask if we're enjoying The Meadows and all that it offers. I just laugh.

Let me know how you feel about the midday Seroquel and how to regulate the Trazodone if we stay with it. Thanks.

Dr. D. to Ann

The low dose of Trazodone might work. Stick with the Seroquel twice a day and use the night time Trazodone as needed. Let's give that a few days and see where we end up.

08/16/2011
Vicky's Journal

Looking back on Jim's wishes, it seemed to me that I should choose the second option. Could I watch the slow withering away of his body, when his mind is tortured every day if I chose Option 1? Could I watch him decline more rapidly and know that I chose that for him? I need to talk with our son, explain the options and get his feedback, even though he is not the one making the decision. Technically, I am the health care proxy, but I don't want to regret what I choose. I will have to live with that choice for the rest of my life.

Kip asked me if there were another option that we had not thought of. What about home care with something like marijuana or some other drug fed to him ... could I manage him...our house is small and isn't equipped with a walk-in shower. We have a tub shower, and the bathroom isn't big enough for a wheel chair or a Hoyer Lift. If two people had to shower him, they couldn't all fit in our bathroom. What doctor would agree to prescribe in such a scenario, and how would I get Jim to be seen? I couldn't transport him by car, and what doctor would make house calls? If he weren't medicated enough, I could be harmed by Jim. If I used nurses or aides from an agency, the agency gets a cut of the person's hourly wage, and it might end up very expensive for 'round the clock coverage...but as expensive as a nursing home? If I didn't use an agency, how would I know they would be reliable, and skilled enough to deal with a dementia patient. What if they didn't show up? In this small house, having two other people around would be stressful, besides having to orchestrate the schedules. It is fraught with all sorts of logistical nightmares. I would have a hospital bed in the living room, and alarms on all the doors. And can you picture me going downtown to score some drugs? We would be putting the aides in legal trouble. It is just too impossible to think about.

I talked with Jim's sister, and she wanted me to know that whatever I choose would be alright with her. Kip and I talked every few days, and I would waver back and forth from one option to another. I talked with Jim's old neurologist. He helped to calm me down and look at the Seroquel/Depakote/Citalopram option (Option 1). He also assured me that if we choose Option 2, that Jim would not be trapped inside his body trying to let someone know he is in there! I also wanted Dr. D.'s opinion. The following is what he told me.

08/16/2011
Dr. D. to Vicky
Update on James Ruppert

I am sorry to learn of your husband's continued trouble. I think that it is very hard to predict how he would respond to a new medicine. I think the most conservative, comfort oriented approach would be to increase the Seroquel to 100 mg. every four hours (ideally q8AM, 12N, 4PM, and 8PM; each dose given if awake.) Still, a very occasional outburst, as you described, should be handled with greater behavioral supervision including re-direction and removal from the precipitating environment. Trying those two things would be a reasonable thing to do. What do you think?

I think that preventing the great discomfort of behavioral dyscontrol is the number one priority. If we need to use more sedating medicine he is likely to become immobile, and he would probably then develop a mercifully intervening acute process. In my experience, people in that condition do not live for more than 1-2 years, but everyone is different.

It is entirely appropriate for you to be thinking of your future. It would pain your husband horribly if he ever understood that his illness might undermine your future security; of course, he will never know that.

08/16/2011
Vicky to Ann
Hope All Is OK Tonight

It didn't sound like this morning went so well, but I'm glad you came to group tonight. I hope Ralph was able to stand the time in his group as well. Is anyone staying the night tonight?

I am going to the banks tomorrow to request all the checks I need from them. I bet they will charge an arm and a leg! I thought about you a lot after I left, but I didn't want to make a nuisance of myself, especially to your relatives.

It really is amazing that there are so many of us in the same situation (almost) at the same time, isn't it? I don't think I've seen so many at one time in all the years I've been in group.

Call me if you need me.

Ann to Vicky

I would have called you tonight, but Lou is staying over, and he gets up at 4:30.

I'm glad I went to group, too, but found it difficult to say enough without saying too much. I talked to Barb a little, because she's getting the same news. All I could think was, "I'd better hurry up with that application or Ralph's bed will be taken."

This is so hard, but this morning was horrible. Ralph lay on the floor looking catatonic for hours. I even called Dr. D. He said to cover him and let him be. When he finally came around, I helped him stand, got him washed and dressed. Believe it or not, we walked the perimeter of the campus, almost a mile, and he was fine! I feel it's almost better when he's in the 'zombie' state, because the thought of placing him when he's doing OK is unbearable.

Both guys are sleeping, so I'll take advantage and get some rest. Brian should be here tomorrow, and he stays up all night, so I'll call you or vice versa.

Thanks again for everything. Can't wait 'til we can get out someplace, and talk and talk and talk.

08/18/2011
Ann to Attorney
Ralph

Ralph is being admitted to St. John's today. They moved really fast to make this happen. I'll call you as I need to. Let me know if there is anything I should or should not sign on admission.

I can't believe how much guilt I'm feeling.

Attorney to Ann

I am so very sorry. You are a great wife...your love for your husband comes through to everyone who has met you. I know you will be his biggest advocate and strongest support through this difficult time.

There isn't a problem with signing the admissions' agreement.

08/18/2011
Ann's Note
The Hardest Day

I realize that probably hundreds of folks are placed in nursing homes every day. But, like death, you don't think about it a lot until it happens to you.

Ralph was admitted to the nursing home on August 18th. The previous evening, I talked to him about how he needed more care than I could give him, and how even though he would be staying at St. John's, I would visit every day. I told him that as soon as he felt better, we'd go for rides, have dinners with Nancy and Lou, and on Saturdays, he could go with Brian and the kids to the Public Market and out to breakfast, a favorite pastime. He was quiet, but totally understood what was happening.

The next morning, I failed to hold back tears as I packed his suitcase. It seemed so odd to be packing for just one of us. We always travelled as a pair, but not this time.

He didn't object to walking out to the car with Brian, but as soon as he was settled in his seat, he closed his eyes. He didn't open them again until he had been in his new room for an hour. Then, he asked, "What am I supposed to do now, just sit here until I die?"

I think Nancy, Brian, and I all died a little that day.

08/18/2011
Brian to Mom
Settling In

How do you think it went?

Mom to Brian

Better than I thought it would. I'll talk more tomorrow. I'm so tired. I went back up tonight, and it was harder because he was in the living (?) room in one of the chairs that were all lined up. They said he ate a big supper, but he was looking for a snack. His evening nurse brought him a sandwich and some ice cream. Then, she brought me ice cream, and I took the sandwich home and ate it. That's about it.

Brian to Mom

I think Dad was admirably strong and prescient about the situation. I'm glad we all spent some time with him; it seemed to have a calming effect on him. Let's see how he gets through his first night. I'm thinking about him like I thought about Hassan's first night at 4-H camp.

Get some sleep. 'Nite.

08/18/2011
Mom to Kip
My Thoughts

In visiting Dad today, it just struck me how poorly his brain is working. He can't get a complete thought out of his mouth, he can't decide whether he wants to walk or sleep, and when I lead him to his bed, he doesn't know how to lay down comfortably any more (fetal position.) He lies in bed all akimbo, I put his legs up on the bed, and he leaves them up in the air. He doesn't even sort of 'nuzzle' to get his head in the right position for sleep. It must be terribly uncomfortable. At least he was walking straight up today.

I told him that Ralph was placed in St. John's today, and Jim's face screwed up like a little kid, and he started crying. I hugged him and told him Ralph would be OK and that St. John's was a wonderful place. I told him Ralph needs the extra care because he gets real scared by the thoughts he is thinking, and Ann can't calm him down.

Basically, after being relieved by the decision to go with the regular medication route, I am having second thoughts. Living like he is...pacing all day...is so unfulfilling. He was guilty about something today, but I couldn't get out of him what made him feel that way. It's really weird, but everyone who knows the two choices have told me they would pick the second. Even the really religious ones...and that shocked me. It hurts my heart to see him so lost.

Kip to Mom

I got your message. I would tend to agree, and I will talk to you about it on Sunday, after I get back from work.

I just need time to really pay attention to this, as we have several drills next week and I am straight out...

Is that OK?

Mom to Kip

No problem...take the time you need. I don't want to push you. I seesaw from day to day. It's just so tragic to visit as often as I do, and see the decline. He is more into his hallucinations than in the real world.

Kip to Mom

Thank you, Mom. I feel guilty that I am not devoting my time solely to this, as Dad deserves it, but I am still doing the same thing that you are doing, back and forth.

I am not sure what I feel.

08/20/2011
Vicky's Journal
The Final Decision

After all the soul searching, I thought more concretely. I am Jim's health care proxy, and it is my duty to do what he would have wanted, not what I want. That actually made thinking about it easier. Time and time again Jim stressed to me over the 19 years that he lived with this disease, that he did not want to go to a nursing home; that he did not want to go 'all the way'. I explained that to Kip and he reluctantly agreed.

I notified Newark as well as Nancy that we were going with Option Two. Before that takes place, however, we were all going to get together Labor Day Weekend to say "Goodbye" to the Jim we knew. The doctor will withdraw Jim's sedative drugs for that weekend, so Jim will be as lucid as possible. We aren't going to tell him what is going to happen, we just want to be with him. Both Nancy and Kip will come in for it.

08/21/2011
Wayne to Ann
Weekend

Hope you got through the Saturday and Sunday OK, even though they are each just another day now. How is Ralph doing? I feel so bad that there isn't more that can be done for him. It just saddens me to no end. Dave and I are both around this week if you need anything, or need some time to yourself. Just let me know. We can always just drink wine, even the 'cheap stuff.'

Ann to Wayne

I haven't really talked to anyone except family yet, but Ralph went into St. John's Home Thursday. It was dangerous for both of us for him to stay here. It's late, so I'll talk to you tomorrow or Tuesday. I'm also in the middle of getting a car and closing on the house, all of which will be this coming week.

Will life ever be quiet again?

Wayne to Ann

Thanks for sharing that news, Ann. I'll not pass that along to anyone. I'm sure it has been a very difficult time and a very tough decision for you all to make. We will get in early this week to see Ralph and spend some time with him. I know you made the best decision for both his and your safety. That is the most important thing right now.

Do you think he needs a walker? He seemed very unsure on his feet. I have one that was Dave's Dad's that I brought back with me from visiting Clara this weekend, in case Ralph could use it.

Let me know if you need to be chauffeured around or need any help this week with your appointments. I don't have anything planned at the moment other than probably an interview at Strong to volunteer, but that isn't scheduled yet.

Hope to talk to you tonight.

Ann to Wayne

Thanks for your offer. I'll keep it in mind.

If you and Dave want to visit Ralph, I think he would enjoy it. I was up there this morning and mentioned you. I asked if he would like to see you and he said yes. I haven't really notified folks about the move. I'm waiting 'til he gets used to the place. Besides, I don't really like to talk about it. It's the hardest thing I've ever had to do.

Wayne to Ann

I would love to visit him. I hope that it will be beneficial for him to see a friendly face, and might relax him a bit.

There is no reason for you to talk to anyone about this until you are ready to do so. We won't say a word to anyone until you do so yourself. I can't even imagine how difficult it must be for you. I hope you have Vicky, Nancy, and Brian to talk to so that you are not alone. You have both been on my mind since yesterday, almost every minute. It is just so hard to grasp what is going on for me, so I can't imagine how you must feel. But, I know that you know you are doing the best thing for Ralph and for you. Don't worry about what others think or what they may say. Dave's mom went through that with people who just couldn't believe that it was necessary to put his dad into a nursing home when she did. They had no idea what she had gone through prior to the decision. Same with you. So, when it is time to tell others, you will know.

08/26/2011
Ann to Dr. D.
Ralph Update

Ralph has been in St. John's Home since last Thursday, 8/18. He was very angry and uncooperative at first. He lashed out at his new caregivers, and we're all keeping our fingers crossed that he settles in. He's doing a little better now and beginning to bond with the staff, but he continues to be a mystery. At times he can't walk at all, can barely move his feet, but today he actually ran down the hall because he thought there was something he had forgotten to take care of. I have been asked by his nurses if Lewy-body dementia has ever been mentioned. He is on 75mg. of Seroquel; morning, midday, and night, and is up and down all night and sleeping a lot during the day. Some of the sleeping is probably because he's bored, but I can't take him out yet. When he can leave for short periods, I'll probably need some help.

Will you still be seeing him from time to time? I would like you to be in on his care, if that's possible. You certainly know him better than the doctor that will be seeing him at St. John's.

By the way, I have nothing but good things to say about the staff. I am so glad we were able to place Ralph in such a caring nursing home.

Dr. D. to Ann

I am glad to hear that you husband is adapting to St. John's. I think it was a very good move for him.

I am happy to be involved with his regular care. He should have a follow-up appointment and you can certainly let me know if new issues arise.

08/27/2011
Dave to Ann
Ralph

It was nice to see you and Ralph the other day. St. John's seems like a very nice facility, pleasant atmosphere, clean, and nice staff. Ralph is where he needs to be.

When people first learned that my Dad was in the nursing home, some of them were very surprised and even asked my Mom why he was there. They had no idea he was as bad as he was. I am afraid you might experience some of those same comments. People simply do not know what the real situation is. But you do, and only you know just what Ralph's condition at home was like. So try not to be bothered and upset if and when people make comments about something they really know nothing about. People will always be like this. You are so good to Ralph, and he is lucky to have such a loving and caring wife.

Just wanted to share this with you, since my Mom and our family went through a very similar situation with my Dad.

See you both again soon.

Ann to Dave

Thanks so much for your nice note. I know what you're saying about people not understanding the situation. I really had no choice. It was either place him or have someone stay with us every night, and that certainly wasn't an option. So far, everyone has assured me I did the right thing at the right time. However, being one of those souls who carries guilt like an albatross, I'm having a hard time. As he settles in and can perhaps be taken out without the chance of his running away, I'll feel a little better about his having to stay there. I would love to be able to drive to your place at least once more.

Ralph remembers you and Wayne coming to see him. He told Nancy about your visit later that afternoon. She wasn't sure if he was imagining it, and called me to verify it.

Tell Wayne to forget the walker for now. His nurse told me yesterday that he was running in the hall. He thought he had forgotten to do something and raced back to his room to do the imaginary thing. The brain is such a mystery.

09/01/2011
Ann to Vicky

I was going to call you last night and then remembered Kip and Nancy were there. Hope it's going well. I'll be thinking of you all this weekend. What a terrible decision you have to make, but we all know it's what Jim wants even though he can't express it. My heart aches for all of us.

I met Beth for lunch yesterday. She's me a few weeks ago. Her husband is getting harder to control and I worry for her safety. She is also going to an elder law attorney that she worked for. Her attorney insists she must apply for Medicaid before any nursing home will take her husband. His PRI has expired, so she has to go through all that again and also re-apply to her preferences. The attorney said the Medicaid application will take months, and I told Beth she can't wait months. I shared all that has happened with Ralph, and how lucky we were to get him in before he went ballistic.

Ralph wasn't doing well yesterday. They gave him extra Seroquel because he was hallucinating big time. He insisted there were people lying all over the floors. He didn't even know I was there. This morning I called and they said he was doing better. Ate breakfast and then said he had to get to work. He went back to his room and his nurse had set up the sketch pad and colored pencils I brought, and he's been sketching like mad. Thank God he's doing something at last.

Take care, know I'm thinking of you, and we will meet sometime next week.

09/04/2011
Vicky to Ann
The Weekend Is Over

Nancy spent 5 days visiting Jim, and Kip came for two. We all had good visits. They actually got Jim up for some walking but he shuffles, and lost his balance falling backwards, hitting his head on the hand rail. It was a small scrape, but the feeling of falling backwards scared him so that he rolled into a ball and cried like a child. We soothed him, and the rest of the visit was uneventful.

We gave him a Snickers bar, his all-time favorite, but fed it to him because he couldn't remember how to eat it. We talked about old memories, and told him how much we love him. And after these days, we are all on the same page. Option 2 it is. It was very hard for Kip to come around to that decision, but Nancy spoke to Kip of all the times in clear mind that Jim told her and me that he didn't want to go all the way, to a nursing home. He feared being trapped in his body, not being able to tell people when he was in pain.

Jim was in a great mood yesterday, laughing and making jokes. Today he was also 'Chatty Cathy', but a little less light hearted. It was weird. It was as if he knew Kip and Nancy were saying in essence, 'goodbye', because he told us that he loved us all, and he said it was good that Kip and I had each other. It was like he was saying 'goodbye' to us, too! It was sad. We were all in tears when we left. He gets medicated on Tuesday. The staff has been really great.

I am off with Kip for the week. I'll let you know when I am coming back. I need some time out of this nightmare. You can always reach me by my cell.

09/10/2011
Mom to Brian
Dad

Were you at St. John's today when Dad fell?

Brian to Mom

No. I've been chauffeuring Kenyans around all day. What happened? I was planning on going up tomorrow.

Mom to Brian

When I went there, his nurse said that he had fallen again but was OK. She said some kids were there, and when he tried to get out of his wheel chair, he fell. So, I don't know of any other kids. Maybe she meant that he was 'seeing' kids???

When I put his clothes away, I noticed that his closet door doesn't work because it was caved in at the bottom. I don't know if he kicked it in or if he fell into it. I couldn't find his nurse after that, and since Dad was eating dinner and wouldn't talk or look at me, I just left.

I wasn't planning on going today, but I got a call at 5:30 this morning. He was up all night, even after they gave him Haldol! They called because he had fallen in someone else's room, but he didn't appear to be hurt. I'm not going to go into all the detail. I'll talk about it when I see you. I talked to the nurse for a half hour. My gut feeling is that they're not going to be able to keep him.

Brian to Mom

Maybe Marissa and Brittany were there with Alan. If you get up before me, which you probably will at this point, maybe you can ask if I can take him out, even if it's in his wheelchair. Hassan has a football game today (as well as yesterday,) and I'm hoping to swing over there while he's playing. I'll be glad when he gets interested in chess again.

Mom to Brian

I'm not going up today. I'm taking a day off. I have to start getting the paperwork together, and I'm going to a BD party for Anita this afternoon. As if I didn't have enough to think about, I realized I'm driving with no insurance. The policy for the new car hasn't come yet. I have to go to the main PO tomorrow to get certified mail that's there for Dad. It can't be the policy because the mail is in Dad's name. I keep getting letters from said insurance company saying they can't pay

Dad's hospital bill until they receive some application that they say we have, but we don't.

Brian to Mom

I thought it was supposed to get easier after you moved?

I miss Saturday morning breakfasts with him. Still hoping he might get back towards his old self a bit.

Mom to Brian

Me too.

09/12/2011
Ann to Dr. D.

My children and I will be meeting with the staff at St. John's tomorrow morning. If you have any observations to help them see a clearer picture of Ralph, please let me know. Ralph continues to be a mystery. At times he walks very well, and other times he can't seem to move his feet. He has frequent falls. He is up and about most of the night even though they've tried Trazodone, and when that didn't work, small doses of Haldol. He can't seem to shake the trauma of the ER and trusts no one. We have not been able to take him out since his admission. He's too unpredictable. He will have a psych evaluation by Dr. H. later this week. Any ideas?

Dr. D. to Ann

It has long been evident that your husband has an atypical dementia syndrome. In 2006 I called it primary progressive aphasia. He then went through a period of looking more like multi-system atrophy (MSA) and in May 2011, I called his illness the Parkinsonian variant of MSA, also called diffuse Lewy body disease, a diagnosis also considered in 2008 and 2009.

I am afraid that none of that matters much, it being an issue of molecular pathology and clinical terminology. However, it reinforces (and is reinforced by) the very difficult time we have had keeping him stable on his feet and dealing with daily visual hallucinations.

When a new doctor sees him, this information should be presented, although my notes document it since 2006. I'd suggest trying some less common medicinal approaches, such as Depakote or Carbetrol, but they really don't do much. He needs supervision, a walker, and all of the emotional support that can be provided.

I know this has been very difficult for you, as hard as it has been on him, and I have tried to shield you from some of the more pointless deliberations, but you seem to want to hear these things. You and I have done everything we could do for him every step of the way. Of this I am convinced. This is a horrible disease, and we can't fix it.

09/14/2011
Vicky to Ann

I am back. Couldn't come home sooner because the storms caused lots of flooding, especially around Route 90. On my way back, I could see the high water level so close to the interstate.

Jim is pretty much geri-chair bound (a lounge chair on wheels.) He's on Seroquel 3x daily and Trazodone twice daily. The nurses suggest that sweat pants and tops will be easier now. Tops should be 1-2 sizes larger. He had a number of accidents in his bed/pants so now he is wearing pull-ups. I read him some of the Hardy Boy Mysteries. Don't know if he heard much of it.

So hard to watch.

09/16/2011
Mom to Brian
PS

Did you hear about Pat Robertson's current 'foot in mouth disease' flare-up?

Brian to Mom

Interesting use of phrase – 'foot in mouth disease' - it serves here as an idiom, metaphor, malaprop, portmanteau, and now ironic pun, since he's been in league with former Liberian President Charles Taylor, an alleged cannibal.

But no, I haven't heard. Who's the latest scapegoat: gays, Muslims, or the intelligent minority?

Mom to Brian

The intelligent minority---us! You'll have to 'Google' it to get the full effect, but a born again in his audience asked if it was OK to date and have a relationship with another person if one's spouse has Alzheimer's. Pat (aka God) said it's OK, but one should divorce the ailing spouse first and then move on to a new life. According to Pat, the one with AD is dead already anyway! Just think of the last six years and all the things Dad enjoyed. He's still far from 'dead'.

Brian to Mom

It makes perfect logical sense.

First you're born.

Then you're born again.

Then you're dead.

Then you're dead again.

Funny how he can preach life after death when he doesn't even allow an Alzheimer's patient to complete their first term.

If it's that easy to pronounce death on the living, why all the fuss over an embryo or stem cell?

So much for tending the sick and comforting the dying. Sometimes I wonder if Jesus wasted his time and talents, seeing how these clowns have twisted his message over the centuries. I'm sure his mother thought so.

09/17/2011
Brian to Mom
Dad – who else?

I was thinking of taking the kids up to see him and taking him to the park around 4:30. Any updates, news, or suggestions?

Mom To Brian

Anne G. and I are going up around noon. We probably won't be there too long because we're going out to lunch after that. Nancy was up yesterday, and he was calm and fairly coherent and 'with it' until he had his midday Seroquel. A half hour later, he began to get agitated and his speech was slurred. Nancy said something about his being better before the meds and he said, "That's what I told you a thousand times!" How horrible it must be for him if he knows inside that the drugs are doing more harm than good. Not being able to express that, he must dutifully swallow them or be labeled difficult, belligerent, and non-compliant. I'm still not comfortable with his meds, but I understand the need for them.

To answer your question though, take the kids and see how he is at 4:30. Never know 'til you get there.

Brian to Mom

OK.

09/20/2011
Brian to Mom
Update

Anything new? It's supposed to rain for the next 40 days and nights, but I think another walk would do him wonders. Even Shino felt better afterward. Of course, she's in Detroit today, Baltimore Wednesday, and Boston on Monday, but other than that, she doesn't get out much.

(This refers to a long wheelchair walk in Highland Park the previous Saturday, where Ralph was cheerful and oriented, and enjoyed showing Shino and the kids, and Nancy and Lou all the places where he played as he was growing up in that neighborhood. We didn't know it then, but that was his last outing, and maybe he somehow knew that, because he enjoyed it thoroughly.)

Mom to Brian

I called Dad's floor this morning and Sue said he was smiling and cheerful today. I told her that I haven't seen him smile since he's been there. He ate most of his breakfast, but didn't eat yesterday. I'm going up in a little while and I'm taking buttermilk (he's been asking for it,) apples, (I'll remember to take a knife,) and some of those mini crackers that he and Aisha love. Maybe he just hates their food. You can take him out for a walk whenever you want. If he's not there when I go, I can always get the latest from Joyce, fill in his menus, and sort the laundry that I do.

I got a bill this morning from U/R for $1250.00 and a rebate check from NY State re: the car for $28.00. Wonder why my budget doesn't balance anymore.

Support group tonight. I'll be home about 8:00.

09/21/2011
Vicky's Journal
The Decline Has Begun

Jim's mouth was very dry when I came in today, so I gave him water...a full glass, then he got his medicine, and had another 1½ glasses of ginger ale.

Jim acted as if he wanted to get up, so I asked the nurses if I could walk him. They preferred that they do it, so they put a belt on him and tried to help him walk. He went about 5-10 feet and started to close his eyes, so they got the geri-chair back.

His body positioning has changed as well. He frequently sits cockeyed in the chair, because he does not know where his body is. If you straighten him up, he moves back to the cockeyed position. I also have to be careful when I give him fluid, that I give it slowly so he doesn't choke on the liquid. It's hard to swallow if your head is tilted up. I am sure he is losing weight. And today, he was in the same clothes he wore two days ago. I know they have changed his pull-ups, but the clothes are the same. You have to choose your battles. It's not the staff being negligent; it's that he won't let them.

Today, Jim's nurse called just as I was leaving the house. She said that in the past few days they had to catheterize him 3 times, because he has gone over 12 hours without peeing. They don't want him to get too distended and uncomfortable. It happened again today, and the doctor thought they should put in a Foley catheter. Continuing to straight cath him could eventually lead to a UTI.

His myoclonal jerks (occasional rapid jerking of a muscle ... arm or leg) are happening about every 5 seconds now. He's had them for years, but they were usually few and far between. Some are really strong. One happened at lunch and his knee jerked so hard that it slammed his hand into the underside of the table. It made his hand bleed.

Jim talks so softly now I can't understand him at all. I have asked him to talk louder, but he doesn't. Maybe he doesn't remember how. I should model it for him maybe. Should I tell him he will die in a few months? Would that give him peace or be upsetting? I don't know. This is all new territory, and it's not going to get any easier.

He did reach out to hold hands today. I long for those gestures from the old Jim who loved me. It tears my heart out. He can't really speak, can't walk, can't pee, wears diapers, and is waiting for his body to fail him.

Ann's Note

August and September of 2011 have become somewhat blurred in my mind. Maybe that's a blessing. I was so bombarded with paper work concerning the accident, applying for the nursing home and gathering all our financial data of the past five years for Medicaid planning, not to mention closing on our home of 40 years and trying to find an affordable car, I think I became emotionally numb. Not numb enough, though, to prevent the pain of watching my sweet, gentle husband decline into someone neither of us would recognize.

In spite of all the care and concern of the staff, Ralph continued his downward spiral. He simply could not adjust to his new surroundings. The ravages of his disease would not allow it. There were times when he seemed reasonably content, ate well, and visited with friends and family, but those times became fewer and fewer. More often, he was uncommunicative, belligerent, and displayed violent behavior toward the staff.

One of the saddest moments for me was the day a consulting psychiatrist told me that it would be dangerous to take Ralph off the premises. Ever! I couldn't believe it! I had promised him we would visit the kids and grandkids, take rides, spend time at my apartment, and on and on. The doctor said he understood, but Ralph's brain was so compromised he could no longer control his behavior. This not only was disturbing to those around him, but absolutely terrifying to Ralph.

He didn't want to live like that and was slowly letting go.

And so it began.........

On Sept. 22nd, Ralph's staff doctor called and told me that when the nurse went to get Ralph up, his arms and legs were rigid and his neck was locked and extended. They were testing him for a condition called 'malignant neuroleptic syndrome', a rare and potentially fatal condition sometimes seen in Lewy body patients as a result of anti-psychotic drugs and narcotics. It became a 'Catch 22'...he couldn't be managed without the drugs, and the drugs were making him sicker.

That weekend, he developed pneumonia. He could no longer swallow pills so they attempted to give him a liquid antibiotic. He managed a couple of doses and then lost his ability to swallow. Early on, Ralph and I both signed forms stating we didn't want tube feeding if it only prolonged an irreversible condition. I struggled with the idea of sending him to the hospital for intravenous hydration, but we (the family) all agreed that would be the last thing Ralph would want.

The family (Brian, Shino, and the kids, Alan, Christine, and their girls, and Lou) and close friends came and went all weekend. Nancy was in New York and due back on Sunday. I decided to stay all night Saturday, and Lou (bless him) stayed until late, and we talked for hours. Nancy was back from visiting Amanda Sunday afternoon, and Amanda decided to take a train in from NYC, travelled all night, and arrived at Grandpa's bedside Monday morning.

09/25/2011
Vicky's Journal

I received a call tonight from Jim's nurse. She has noticed a marked acceleration of Jim's decline. She stressed that he is comfortable and not in any pain, but he is not drinking or eating much anymore. His urine is dark brown...don't know whether it is from blood or dehydration. It was bloody yesterday. They called for Imodium because he is still having some diarrhea as well. She said it wasn't necessary for me to come in tonight, but thought I should visit tomorrow. I will call Jim's sister, Nancy, and Kip tomorrow morning. I guess I had better get Jim's photo story completed in case the funeral is soon. Medicaid may not be needed after all. We will see. More tomorrow.

Ralph is declining with pneumonia and possible malignant neuroleptic syndrome. Amazingly, it looks as if our guys are on the same page.

09/26/2011
Ann to Dr. D.
Ralph

Ralph is declining rapidly. His gag reflex is gone so they can't give him the liquid antibiotic which is probably not helping anyway. He's resting comfortably, and the nursing home is going to bring hospice in tomorrow.

I mailed the form for the anatomical donation, but now they're telling me Ralph has to sign the form himself or they can't accept it. It was always Ralph's wish to donate his brain for research, but they said we couldn't designate a certain organ to be used anyway.

These are stressful days for me and my family and I don't know what to do next.

Thanks for any advice you can give me.

09/26/2011-09/28/2011
Ann's Note

Dr. D. sent his wonderful social worker, Susan, to our rescue. She spent hours on the phone with me and in conference with the Memory Clinic director to see how we could fulfill Ralph's last wish. On the day before Ralph died, Susan made contact with the Brain Tissue Resource Center at the Harvard Medical School. She filled out an online application for me, and the plans were in motion. When I spoke with the folks there, they told me their lab would send samples to neuroscience research centers all over the world. They are all working tirelessly to find a cause and/or cure for this devastating disease. I can't say enough good things about Susan. She went way beyond her job to work with, counsel, and comfort me.

I was so busy making all these arrangements; it took time away from being with Ralph. There was always someone there to hold his hand, though, and when he was awake he looked at me with eyes clear and free of dementia. Just a calm, peaceful, gentle look. On the day before he died, I was holding him and telling him how much I loved him, and he tried to put his arm around me but couldn't move it. His nurse gently placed his arm around me and he whispered "I love you, too." I don't remember his speaking after that.

With the help of hospice and their trays of coffee, tea, and cookies, the family sat vigil those last few days. At times, one would think there was a party going on, and at some point Alan, Lou, and Brian left and brought back a pizza and a box of wine. I hope my dear husband realized we weren't celebrating; we were just trying to deal with it all. One image that will stay with me forever was of Hassan (then age nine) sitting by Grandpa, holding his hand, and telling him how he wished he could see the Lego space station he was building.

All that was heard was the sound of hearts breaking.

09/28/2011
Ann's Note

The night before, Ralph's nurse told me to go home and get some sleep because he wasn't ready to go yet, and I needed my strength for the days to come. She promised to call if things changed. Amazingly, I fell asleep as soon as I hit the pillow. How could that be with my husband so close to death? Maybe my soul knew he would soon be free and whole again.

At 5:30 AM, the phone rang and the nurse quietly said, "He's getting close." I called Nancy and Brian and headed out. Thank goodness the nursing home is just 10 minutes from my apartment. Nancy met me there and Brian promised to head out as soon as he got the kids on the school bus. Isn't it funny how all the ordinary mundane busyness of life keeps going on in spite of the heavy drama occurring in our lives.

I held Ralph's hand and told him how pretty the sunrise was. Nancy arrived and we took turns holding his hand and helping him slip away. He was comfortable and just sleeping. He took a last breath at 9:30 AM and it was over.

09/28/2011
Vicky's Journal

This morning I arranged for our funeral trusts...mine is revocable and Jim's is not...that way Medicaid can't touch it. And while I was doing that...RALPH DIED!! I just can't believe it!

Jim is still having blood in his urine and that worries me. They don't seem to be overly concerned. He is on Ditropan for bladder spasms, and they have discontinued his Trazodone, so he is more awake.

09/29/2011
Vicky to Ann
Specifics on Calling Hours, Funeral...

Please give me the specifics of the service, and I will call everyone from group to let them know. Thinking of you...

Ann to Vicky

I'll try to call you later with specifics. Brian and family and Wayne and Dave are still here. W and D brought Chinese and the kids have talked them into a tour with the pool as an extended stop. Tell me how late I can call you. Nancy and I went to the funeral home today, and she just left for home. If I don't get back to you, the details will be in Sunday's newspaper.

10/04/2011
Ann's Note

The service was simple and beautiful. We held it in the Interfaith Chapel of our local university. Ralph and I always believed in a diversity of faiths, so the chapel seemed a perfect fit. My sister's pastor agreed to officiate. Although we didn't belong to his congregation, he visited Ralph in the nursing home, and he was so kind as he helped us prepare the service. It was filled with some of Ralph's favorite music, hymns, and poetry. Some of the participants were: Brian, grandson Hassan, granddaughter Amanda, Nancy's husband Lou, and Vicky.

Will Bellucci, our friend from South Dakota and our late son's best friend, is a master wood turner. He sent a beautiful pair of urns fashioned out of the same tree for Ralph and me. It's hard to explain how lovely and finely crafted they are, but suffice it to say they are too nice to be buried. They are sitting side by side in my apartment. One journey complete.

10/04/2011
Vicky's Journal
Ralph's Funeral

It was a beautiful service filled with love and family. Many family members spoke as did I. It's a Tuesday evening and the skies are bright with stars. People gathered in the foyer of the chapel for the receiving line and to chat with each other as they exited. After that, I went back to Ann's to join the family for the evening. A great tribute to Ralph. I can't believe Ann's journey with dementia is over now.

10/05/2011
Vicky's Journal
My First Choice Nursing Home

The gal from one of my top choice nursing homes called me today and clarified my financial data. She said that if I agreed to private pay for 2 years, I could have a private room for Jim. I said, "No," that I could private pay for 1 year, but I would actually prefer 10 months, if possible. I heard from the head of Jim's behavioral unit today. She wants me to reiterate that I am willing to offer the year of private pay; she thinks that may be holding them up. I called the admissions person and left a message, but it is Columbus Day. I also gave updated admission forms to my two other choices.

I also spoke to the admissions director at another nursing home. She said that Jim had to be cleared by Medicaid before they could admit him. I told her I wanted to do a year of private pay and I would use Jim's IRA money to do that. She said that IRA's aren't touchable by Medicaid, and I said, "Oh yes they are, as long they aren't in pay out mode." I said that I would be willing to sign a promissory note that was legally binding, that I would do a year of private pay, and she said that she had never had anyone bring that up. She thought I would have to pull all the money out of Jim's IRA and put it in a savings account so that it would be liquid. She gave me the card of someone from finance to call. The finance person sang a different tune. She said all I have to do is sign a form saying that I have liquid money up to $138,000, but that I didn't have to disclose account numbers or anything. How can the admissions director not know this? I know of another person who tried to get her husband in the same place, and they told her the same thing. She then placed her husband in another nursing home with a promissory note!

10/14/2011
Vicky's Journal

Jim was started on antibiotics for a UTI today. He will have a seven day course. They also announced that they would like to place Jim on hospice. However, they are reticent to do it if he will be moving to another facility. Moving would mean changing counties and using a different hospice agency. I would still like to move Jim, so I can spend more time with him and less time commuting. So no hospice yet.

I spoke to my three favorite nursing homes again. Two had no openings because they have to honor their affiliations and take those people first. I left a message for the third, St. Johns. At 11 AM, they called me back and said that they had a spot for Jim on a 'comfort care only' floor. I quickly called the other two nursing homes and told them to stop the admissions process, that Jim had a bed. Then I called the director of Jim's floor, so she could start working on the discharge papers and the transport. She said they would take care of everything. I found out that the social worker for Jim's new floor is a friend whom Jim and I have known for a few years. Jim used to give talks to her support groups occasionally. Perhaps Jim would recognize her voice.

It's amazing how things change so quickly when the timing is right. The behavioral nursing home staff has been wonderful. I couldn't have asked for better treatment for Jim by more upbeat people. The director confided in me that she doesn't think Jim will live to see Christmas. I asked her how she can tell, and she said that after being in the business for some time, she just knows.

I am starting a health update site for Jim on Caring Bridge www.caringbridge.org/visit/JimRuppert so that family and friends can follow Jim's course without my calling each person. This site was created for use when folks have a sick relative. You can journal and post pictures. Relatives can log-in any time they want to get updates. It's free, but supported by donations. Sites like this are wonderful.

10/17/2011
Vicky's Journal
Moving Day

Jim will be moved at 10 AM and will hopefully arrive about 11:30 AM to the new nursing home. I have told him he will be moving, but I don't think he can grasp the concept at this point. My neighbor, also a dear friend, came with me today to help pack up Jim's clothes for the move.

It was a beautiful sunny fall day today. While I was filling out paperwork and signing each page at Jim's destination (almost like buying a house,) I received a phone call that the transport was there early to pick Jim up. By the time I was done with the papers and had proceeded to Jim's new room, he had just been rolled in, and was lifted into bed.

He has a beautiful sunny room facing south out onto Highland Park across the street. Lots of green grass and trees here and there. He was very tired all day, and slept most of it. At 3:30 I went home for a nap, and then went on to dinner and support group, then back to see Jim. He was dressed in his pj's and pretty awake. He has been whispering to himself a lot for a long time, but I have not been able to understand him. While I was filling out his menus for the week, I bent low to the bed and whispered to him that he is my best friend. He responded to that and turned his head to look straight at me, something he doesn't do very often. I know he understood me.

Of late, he has been listing to his left and looking right, something they say many people with Alzheimer's do towards the end of the disease. They choose one side or the other, but are usually consistent. Jim has lost the ability to lie on his side like most of us do when we get tired in one position. He lies on his back where you put him.

I met Jim's nurses and spoke with the social worker. They will set up hospice soon. The social worker is trying to prepare me for Jim dying soon, I think. I also met Jim's doctor who will be making the medical decisions for him from now on. Seemed like a very caring man.

They didn't even want the first month's rent. They said they would bill me. Tomorrow I will get him into a geri-chair and take him for a tour of his new surroundings. I left him in good hands for the night, and hopefully will have a good sound sleep.

10/18/2011
Vicky's Journal

All in all, I think this worked out well. Jim has a social worker whom he used to know, the nursing home is top notch, and it is 15-20 minutes from my house rather than 45! I can visit him as many times as I want during the day, and I don't have to worry about the drive home...and if I need to, I can stay at Ann's. She is only 5 minutes away.

Tomorrow, or the day after that, I will visit the chapel at a local cemetery. I have to pick a venue for the funeral. I don't think the funeral home is big enough for the service, with so many people knowing Jim from where he used to work.

10/22/2011
Vicky's Journal
Hospice Is In Place

Two days ago, Jim was so awake it amazed me! I have not seen his brown eyes so clearly in a long time. He was talking too, and using his normal voice, so most of the time I could even understand him. It was as if he had travelled back in time by a month or two. It was so wonderful to spend time with him like that. It nourished my soul for the path ahead. He didn't take a nap or anything, and was wide awake 'til mid-evening. My social worker friend said to treat each day like that as a gift.

Yesterday he was a bit more subdued...I know now that his behavior will fluctuate as the days progress. Today he is more as I have known him lately...awake for a bit after breakfast. He eats lunch, and then off to dreamland. I came back later today and he was pretty tired, somewhat fidgety, and wincing occasionally, so they gave him a pain pill.

The hospice papers have been signed, and that will be started Monday. He is on a comfort care floor, which is sort of like hospice in that they take no extraordinary measures (generally no IV"s, no antibiotics, just pain management.) Hospice provides an aide to sit with Jim so they are more aware of the signs of decline, and just to be there for him. It will allow me to do some other things knowing someone is with him...that he is not alone. Also, hospice provides counseling and guidance for Kip, Nancy, and me if we need it. It has been helpful to ask whether I should talk to Jim about his death, how to let him know that I will be all right, and that it is OK for him to go when he feels he needs to.

Jim and I have had some very frank talks about this in the past, so they advised me to tell Jim that I love him, that I will miss him, but I will be OK. I am lucky to have had him all these years.

To speak of the mundane, I spent the hours between my visits mowing leaves, cleaning the gutters, and trying to fix my #$%X toilet handle. It won't pop back up after it's flushed, so you have to manually pull it back up. I bought a new one and still can't figure the thing out with the package diagram (made in China!) My neighbor is coming over to troubleshoot tomorrow. Such a simple thing...it can't be that hard. Stuff like that brings me back to reality very quickly.

We know that Jim has entered a different stage in his course, because his breathing is more erratic and apnea-like when he's sleeping, and his myoclonal jerks have become stronger. They are especially strong right after a period of no breathing when the CO_2 builds up. Sometimes they are so big that they scare Jim, because they make him feel like he is falling. He also has had spells where he wiggles his arms and legs all at the same time. Strange.

10/25/2011
Vicky's Journal
A Sense of Humor

Jim is settling in now and seems relatively content. He still shows his sense of humor. He was given Milk of Magnesia the other night. He took one swig and shuddered all over with a face that says, "This stuff tastes horrible!" The next swig he politely turned his face to the wall and spit it out. It hit the wall and ran to the floor. The nurse said laughing, "Jim, you really showed me how you like that one." For the last gulp, the nurse explained to him that he really needed to swallow it, so he did...with a big gulp of water afterwards. No one likes to drink CHALK!

Everyone made us feel welcome, and Jim is getting excellent care. The food looks pretty good too. Jim is sporadic in his eating and drinking, but that is normal for him at this point. I am going every day and sometimes twice a day, but only staying for about 2½ hours each time. Sometimes I am there for meals and help get him organized at the table. As I get more comfortable with Jim's condition, I may back off a bit. For now, I need to see him.

They have an ice cream shop on the first floor that we hope to visit next week. I know Jim will like that.

10/26/2011
Vicky's Journal
Signs

Today Jim definitely has congestion in his chest, probably from aspiration pneumonia. He can't cough hard enough to raise it. They will give him something to dry up the fluid, but no antibiotics. The hospice aide has come every day now, and will sit with him from 12-2 PM. They have also requested someone to sit with him at night for a few hours. They want someone with him, they don't want him to be alone should he die without all the usual signs. Apnea is increasing. The nurse said he wouldn't go tonight, so she didn't think it necessary for me to stay over. They have a room down the hall where I can sleep if I need to. So, I went home to bed, knowing they would call me if things changed.

10/27/2011
Ann's Note
Jim

Vicky called me early this morning to tell me that Jim would most likely die today. I asked if she wanted me to come up. She said that would be nice, but was afraid it would be too hard for me. I took that to mean I should come if I could. Of course, I went.

There were 6 of us, 5 friends and Vicky. Kip was on his way from New Hampshire, in a storm to boot. Hospice, again, provided coffee, tea, cookies, and support. We sat for hours, listening to Jim's breathing, willing him to hang on for Kip. We filled the hours with much talk, laughter, reminiscing, munching, and tears. The usual death bed ritual.

At some point that afternoon, I became brave and decided to go up to the 6th floor where Ralph had been a patient. I wanted to thank the staff personally for his care. It was easier than I thought, and gave me a sense of peace. Most of his caregivers were there, especially his main caregiver, Joyce. I don't know if I could have visited the floor at any later date, but at one month out I was still numb.

The day wore on and Vicky spent much of her time talking with Kip and keeping him apprised of his dad's condition. Finally, at 7:00, Kip arrived. It was time for Kip, Vicky, and Jim to say their goodbyes. The rest of us left. They would need us later, but not now.

Jim died at 9:30 PM.

10/28/2011
Vicky's Journal
Jim's Passing

Jim passed away last night at 9:30 PM. I had received a call at 9 AM that Jim was more labored in his breathing, and his condition was changing every half hour. They thought I should come in right away. I called Kip to warn him that this might be it, so he could drive the 7 hours here, and hopefully make it before Jim died.

I got there, and Jim was definitely on his way, working hard at every breath. He was not conscious. They had put a port in his leg to give morphine and anxiety meds, so that they wouldn't have to stick him every half hour. I called my closest friends (5), and they all came and stayed with me throughout the day to give me comfort. After the first hour and a half, Jim's breathing became a little easier due to the morphine finally taking effect. Mottling of Jim's feet began to be noticeable, but nothing else.

I called Kip again about 1½ hours later, and he had not left work yet. People were urging him to go...but there was some avoidance at play. He had already said goodbye to Dad on Labor Day; I don't think he could face that his dad was going to die today. But as time passed, he then thought, what if Dad is waiting for him before he goes?? That made Kip move into fast gear, get into his car, and begin the long arduous drive in snow, sleet, and rain. It normally took 7 hours. Every hour or so I would call him and ask what town he was passing, and would report it in Jim's ear, asking him to hold on until Kip arrived.

We played Jim's favorite music (John Denver), and reminisced about the old days. We told Jim he was loved in innumerable ways, and held his hand as he progressed. I told him I would be all right, that he could let go when he was ready.

Kip arrived at 7 PM. At that point all our friends left so we could have some family time alone. Kip spent two and a half hours with Jim, and we said all we needed. We thanked him for such a wonderful life. His breathing slowed, and he finally took his last breath at 9:30 PM. He was comfortable and relaxed. It was a beautiful death, filled with love. We couldn't ask for anything better.

Vicky's Journal
Harvard Brain Bank and other things

After Jim's death I called the funeral home and alerted them. Jim needed to go directly to the University Medical Center so that his brain could be saved by Harvard's protocol and received within 24 hours of death. The funeral home told me that the hospital's admission department could not accept pathology patients until morning, and that they were no longer participating in this 'study.' So, to make my emotions run even higher, I had to straighten this out. I knew they could do it, because Ralph's brain was sent a month earlier...but Ralph died in the morning.

I got in touch with the brain bank on-call person and they advised the funeral home how to prepare Jim overnight for transport to the hospital in the morning. The next morning, I called Jim's old neurologist before Dr. D., and asked if he could find me the doctor in pathology who could help me arrange this. He called me back and gave me the name and phone number of the head of pathology. He was very apologetic about the mix up. Admissions dept. was giving out the wrong information. In any event, I called the funeral home and told them everything was ready for transport. The head pathologist called me by 11 AM that the brain was on its way. I was so relieved! To get this far, and try to do a wonderful thing by sharing Jim's brain with scientists all over the world, only to stumble at the finish line was unthinkable. I also received word from the brain bank that they received it within the 24 hour time limit. I now could relax somewhat and go about orchestrating the funeral arrangements.

Kip stayed the entire week until the funeral was over. We went everywhere together from arranging the calling hours, choosing a prayer, to reserving the chapel, a guitarist, and the AV gal who would play the video of pictures set to music I had made years earlier. We bought food and coffee for after the service, and arranged for a big dinner the night after the funeral for those close friends and family who would still be around.

We had calling hours on Thursday night, November 3rd, and many people came. It was a lovely, fitting tribute to Jim. The funeral service was on Saturday morning, November 5th. It was held at the University of Rochester Interfaith Chapel, just like Ralph's (thanks, Ann & Ralph.) The sun was out and it was a bright, crisp day. It was very well attended and many people spoke, besides family. My memorial photo presentation went well, and was a great closing to the service. All our friends pitched in to help make everything come together. Jim would have loved it.

The dinner that night at a restaurant close to our home was terrific, and a great end to the weekend. Family left on Sunday, including Kip. There is silence, and I am alone. I go out in the late afternoon to mow leaves, a mindless activity that helps to ground me somehow. What to do now? My journey with Alzheimer's is over...at least for now. Will Kip follow in his dad's footsteps? I hope not.....

12/11/2011
Last E-Mail Entry
My Message From Jim

I have been hoping that I would get some sign from Jim that he was OK somewhere in the continuum. I have heard of people getting messages through mediums from their loved ones. I wanted one, too. I even joked to Jim as the disease progressed, to please send me a sign that there is a heaven, and let me know he's OK.

Well, on December 11, 2011, a Sunday, I had spent a lazy morning in bed, and I don't think I got up until 10 AM. I don't think I turned the computer on all day, as a matter of fact. On Monday morning there was this e-mail from Jim:

From: James A. Ruppert
To: Vicky Ruppert
Sent: Sunday, December 11, 2011 9:26 AM
Subject: msnbc.com video: Living with Alzheimer's

March 6-7, 2006: WEB EXCLUSIVE: Jim and Vicky Ruppert talk to NBC News about Jim's early diagnosis of Alzheimer's disease. Did he make the right decision four years ago when he chose to find out whether he had the incurable memory-ravaging illness?

http://www.nbcnews.com/id/11715274/

In the video at the end, Dr. Bob Bazell asks Jim what happens if he has to go to a nursing home, even though he doesn't want to go. Jim replies, "I hope I go fast."

I sent it to Kip to see if it was real...could someone else have sent it?...It was the old link to an interview we had done with Dr. Bob Bazell in 2006...how would anyone else know the link or know Jim's e-mail. That was not the e-mail I used to send mail; I always used my e-mail address. Jim hadn't used the computer in years.

This is what Kip replied in an e-mail:

No kidding. I checked this out today, and no viruses were found, and the story is linked to the MSN story as appropriate. And if you watch the video, I would say that Dad is telling us he was OK with the decision we made. You should click the link and watch it again...I can't believe it. This is crazy.

He must love you more than you know to be able to break through the other side like that.

I don't know if you remember, but prior to the weekend we discussed how everyone else was seeing signs, and you wished he would give you a sign to let you know he is OK, or at least here.

You got it.   K.

12/14/2011
Second Sign

That Wednesday morning, I went to put my purse in the back seat of the car. I always did that because it was too big to put by my side, and I still had not gotten used to Jim not taking the front passenger seat. I opened the door, and there was 1 lone Hot Tamale candy on the back seat in plain view. Hot Tamales are my favorite candy, and the last time I had eaten them was on the way back from Kip's at Thanksgiving, a few weeks ago...but I had them in the door pocket on the driver's side. It wasn't there yesterday when I got in the car. I said, "Thanks Jim," and ate the Hot Tamale. I can't ask for more than that.

Chapter Four

2012

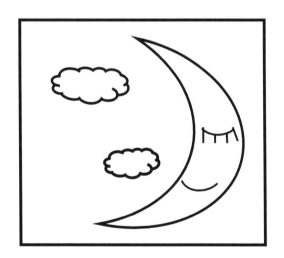

02/14/2012
Neuropathology Report - Harvard Brain Tissue Center
Vicky's Journal

Jim's brain autopsy results came today. Although I felt Jim really had Alzheimer's because of his course and his 2 APOE4 genes, there was some anticipation and fear in receiving the envelope. What if it was something completely different and we didn't know it all this time?

As I read further, though, I read the diagnosis was Alzheimer's disease. Jim's brain was judged to be in the final stage of very advanced disease. Visually, the ventricles of the brain (the pathways that wash the brain in fluid) were quite enlarged, due to the shrinkage of brain tissue caused by the death of neurons. This is a typical finding.

The hippocampus, the entorhimal cortex, and the amygdala all showed moderate to abundant senile plaques and neurofibrillary tangles, classic signs of Alzheimer's. This microscopic pathology mirrors Jim's increasing memory loss and loss of function. These three areas are all involved in the accumulation of memories, and the making of those memories permanent so that they can be recalled time after time. They also deal with emotions. The stronger the emotion, good or bad, the more likely it will be remembered. Because of the plaques and tangles, Jim's neurons couldn't function normally to create and store memories.

There was no evidence of Pick's Disease, Lewy Body Disease, or any other major factor that would cause Jim's course and death.

It is my hope that the donation of Jim's brain will allow more scientists, who are working with the familial form of late onset Alzheimer's (APOE4 gene), to find a way to turn off this gene perhaps by finding other genes that may act as the on/off switches. Our son, by rules of genetics, has inherited one APOE4 gene from his father. I don't expect this defective gene from my side of the family, because none of my relatives died of dementia. I dream that before our son reaches his 60's, the age that the gene will show its effects, that strides will have been made to turn off the expression of this gene. I don't want him to follow in his dad's footsteps or his grandmother &

grandfather, aunts, and uncles. Jim's extended family has been ravaged by this disease emotionally, and financially. This was Jim's last chance to participate in the science of discovery, and I'm sure he would be proud to know that scientists all over the world have access to his brain. He and many others continue to make their final sacrifice for those of us still living by giving their brains to this great cause.

I have learned so much from Jim, and from coping with this disease over the years. The disease has taught me patience and what matters in life; people and the experiences we have with them, those things that Jim lost all along the way... memories. Jim displayed the most wonderful 'can do' attitude, not that he could do anything he attempted, but that he could take on what Alzheimer's threw at him with patience, dignity, and humor. He made jokes about himself quite frequently.

Jim wanted people to know they could enjoy life despite all the concessions that had to be made daily. And to those who weren't familiar with Alzheimer's, he wanted them to learn about the disease so that fear would not stop them from helping others with dementia.

So, yes Jim, you did have Alzheimer's disease. You are the first in your family to actually have the brain autopsy to confirm that, I think. We thank you for that, so that years from now our family will know the truth. Thank you for teaching me patience, and urging me to be present in the moment.

I thank the Harvard Brain Tissue Resource Center for making this donation relatively easy to do, and without cost to the donor and donor family. In some cases a fee may be charged for the removal of the brain, but to date I have not received a bill from our local university medical center. It is wonderful that Harvard shares the autopsy results with the donor's family. I hope this remains a viable way of sharing science around the world so that we can make some well needed strides towards a cure.

03/16/2012
Ann to Dr. D.
Ralph

Last month I received the neuropathology report from the Harvard Brain Bank concerning Ralph's brain autopsy. The letter stated that you had received a copy also. I'm wondering if you would be willing to meet with me (either by phone or in person) at some time to discuss the findings. I know the results (Lewy body dementia) were pretty much in keeping with our thoughts and there were no real surprises.

However, I'd feel more comfortable if I could discuss them with you. (I'm trying not to use the word 'closure' as I dislike that term and feel there's no such thing.) I'm moving on with life and family, but the pain is always there. I know Ralph's final days were probably exacerbated by the use of Haldol, but I believe that was a gift. He no longer wanted to be the person he had become. He had a good death and the look in his eyes told me he was totally at peace.

I never had the chance to thank you for your concern and loving care and I do so now. I couldn't have done it all without you and the Alzheimer's Association.

I think Vicky Ruppert shared with you that we are writing a book from the dozens of e-mails we sent back and forth during the last three years of our husbands' lives. We rarely had the time to phone each other so we would e-mail our dementia stories late at night when our guys were sleeping. If it never gets published, at least it's turning into a fun (???) and interesting project.

Dr. D. to Ann

It is wonderful to hear from you. It is great to know that you have been able to get yourself up from the very difficult experiences related to your husband's passing. The strength you lent to him in his time of need should be what buoys you through your loss.

I read the path report with great interest. As you said, no great surprises there. A lot of brain tissue loss with cellular signs of Lewy body disease. He had a lot of language difficulty as a prominent feature of his disease, but they did not comment on the left hemisphere being more involved than the right; they probably don't do such comparisons.

What they did not say is that he was a great guy who brought a lot of light into the world. Of course, you did not need to hear that from them or from me.

With warmest regards,
Dr. D.

More About Lewy Body Dementia

The FDA recently required a *black box* warning that using anti-psychotic drugs with elderly patients with dementia increased the risk of death. This is especially true for someone with Lewy body disease. A single dose can cause:

- A decrease in cognition, which is often permanent
- Increased and possibly irreversible motor impairment
- Symptoms resembling neuroleptic malignant syndrome (NMS); severe fever, muscle rigidity, and breakdown of the autonomic nervous system that can lead to kidney failure and death

The average life expectancy from diagnosis to death is 2-7 years for a Lewy body patient, as compared with an Alzheimer's patient's expectancy of 3-9 years. This could be a good or bad prognosis depending on cognitive decline, quality of life, general health, and well-being of the individual.

Fluctuating cognition is common with Lewy body disease, but not with Alzheimer's. It's a symptom in which a person shows various levels of awareness over a period of time. There are times when the person shows more confusion, trouble communicating, perception and mobility problems, than other times. Simply put, with Alzheimer's disease, there is a gradual downhill slide, while Lewy body disease is a roller coaster ride.

There is a condition of dementia, more common in Lewy body than in other dementias called *Capgras syndrome*. It causes a person to become convinced that someone close is a look-alike imposter. If the person is married, the imposter is usually a spouse.

Afterword - Vicky and Ann

Dealing with this disease is an act of patience. We developed patience we never thought we had...waiting for the next word to be uttered, helping them find a thought by maintaining silence rather than playing 20 questions...when if 'played,' only made them lose their train of thought altogether. That's not to say that we didn't lose it sometimes. An important part of caregiving was also being able to forgive ourselves for those times when we exploded. There is always tomorrow to 'do it right.' It takes a strong marriage and a relationship of sharing and truthfulness to weather this storm to its conclusion. Not every couple has that. What happens to them is even harder to think about.

Olivia Ames Hoblitzell in *10,000 Joys & 10,000 Sorrows* writes of her husband's Alzheimer's state as being 'serene, deeply peaceful' at times. We could never use those words to describe Jim's state of mind. He had a habit of sitting forward on the couch, holding his head. It ached as if his brain were 'sunburned'. He always wanted relief from that until the day when he felt that he beat the disease. He was always tormented: by trying to make sense of his changing world...the signs that were printed with the letters 'too close together and all jumbled up,' the restaurants that were too loud for him to bear, the menus he couldn't read 'because of the glare,' or the news where people were too cruel to each other. Life was becoming too mean and too threatening. The end of his life was plagued with hallucinations that children were in danger and no one would help him save them. For a family therapist, that is the ultimate pain. Jim's road was anything but serene.

We used to hear that if we developed Alzheimer's or another dementia, not to worry. If we had it we wouldn't realize it. Nothing could be further from the truth. Ralph knew from the very beginning that something was wrong. Neither of us was surprised when he was diagnosed. As time went on and the disease progressed, his efforts and struggles to deal with it all were nothing short of heroic. He spent hours agonizing over and trying to make sense of his world and how he fit into it, and nothing I said or did could distract him. He fully realized that the hallucinations he experienced almost daily for the final three years were his mind playing 'tricks' on him. How horrifying to be trapped in a mind that was constantly betraying him! Was he calm and serene because he didn't 'realize' what was happening? I think not.

This disease is full of surprises. We pictured keeping our husbands at home until the end—hiring health aides to help with their care, and having a hospital bed in the living room with a view of our backyards. Despite our best intentions we were forced to do something so radically different: institutionalizing our husbands because we couldn't keep them safe from themselves.

There was a coming together at the start of our marriages borne by the excitement of discovery of each other and this new life together. We had our children and wove a beautiful and multi-colored fabric of our experiences as 'family'. As our children left, we experienced a life of just the two of us. Then there was the together-ness borne of the discovery and emotional testing we experienced trying to make sense of our husbands' symptoms and what might be the culprit. And finally the slow separation that could not be mended by all the love in the world. There was no solution, no easy fix—not even a hard and painful one—a wall of protein filtering out their ability to make sense of their world and verbalize it. A heavy quiet overtook our lives as our caregiver minds were running 100 miles an hour inside. A tiredness in all of us that no amount of sleep could fix. Nap time was a luxurious escape from all that we feared. But it backfired for them because their waking was filled with the unknown. What day is it, is it morning or night? Do we have anything planned? Will I be able to cope, to make it through? Will I embarrass myself?

And the end filled with the deepest pain, and yet at the same time relief. No matter how awful the decline and the behavioral changes, we wanted our guys back. We caregivers dreamed of a time when we would be free, but not now. We're not ready. We will never be ready. To be alone the rest of our lives. In a sense we were alone for years, but not. Now it will be permanent, so final.

Grief and Recovery - Vicky

It took months of sleeping at all hours of the day and some wakefulness at night to find some rhythm to my life, and recuperative rest for those last three years of Jim's illness. My friends and neighbors gathered around me and kept me attached and engaged.

After slogging through the funeral, I had to have patience and let some meaning creep back into my life. Joining a grief group wasn't necessary for Ann or me. We, instead, kept attending our Alzheimer's support group with the blessing of its facilitators. It is comfortable there for us to talk and share.

Ann and I still relied on each other as a thermometer for how well we were dealing with our grief. I went for the longest time before allowing myself to break down. I did have moments when a song or a TV show would elicit tears, but the sobbing didn't come until springtime. I don't even remember what brought it on the 1st time. I was watching TV and I just let myself go. It felt good. It also happened once at group when Ann was talking and I just couldn't keep the grief to myself. I just silently shook with tears.

Ann and I had always wanted to rock babies in the nursery, and so we signed up as 'cuddlers' at the hospital where I once worked. For me it was a chance to hold a baby. I didn't know if I would ever be a grandmother, so it was a way to give my love. It was also a chance to give back to society in a very undemanding way. No stress in this job – just pure giving and joy.

I knew I needed more love in my life. I missed having someone in the house, someone to talk to. In February, I decided I wanted a dog, so I looked at all types and reached out to a breeder of Pocket Beagles. I went to visit her and her present litter, and fell in love! By chance, one became available because of severe allergies in a family who had adopted her. Although I didn't want one 'til summer, because of a trip to Europe I had planned, I couldn't say "No." I figured that the time commitment I would have to devote would not be a problem. I'd just finished 19 years with a man with Alzheimer's and 42 years of marriage. I could handle it.

Lily, as I called her, has been a joy no matter how much frustration or what I have had to sacrifice with friends to train her. She is spoiled rotten, but has given me so much love, and I have given her so much in return.

After all is said and done, monetarily Jim left me in a place where I don't have to work if I am careful, and vet bills don't impact my life in any major way. It also has opened up a world of friendships with other pet owners on my street, and through puppy classes. I take Lily to puppy day care twice a week so I can devote 2 full days to home care, gardening, and appointments while Lily plays with other dogs. The sacrifice of making spur of the moment decisions to go somewhere or attend unplanned activities has been worth it for me. I am also glad I adopted a puppy rather than a rescue dog. I wanted to experience the world of puppyhood from the beginning.

The holidays have not been so bad for me. Last year, I spent Thanksgiving with Kip and his girlfriend's family. Christmas was spent with Jim's sister, Nancy, and her family in Florida. This year I spent

Thanksgiving with 2 close friends, and Christmas was spent at Kip's home in New Hampshire. New Year's Eve was harder for me than all the rest. I miss Jim so, but I have to look toward this next year on my own. I've been dreaming about him a lot lately, always when we were in our 20's.

Moving On - Ann

After the fast decline, after the last breath, after the service, the flowers, the outpouring of love and support from family and friends, after the piles of paper work were dealt with; one glaring truth remained; Ralph was gone and I wasn't.

Grief is described as: a multi-faceted reaction to a major loss, a painful, unhappy response to the death of a loved one. I wouldn't presume to give advice on how to deal with it all. I just know what seems to be working for me.

First of all, I miss him terribly. Not a day goes by that I don't wish he were here beside me. We were together almost sixty years and I don't like living as half of what should be a whole. But, I'm learning how to be just me and there's a lot to learn.

Grief, for most dementia caregivers, begins with the dreaded diagnosis. Many illnesses end with the loss of a loved one, but there's always the hope of a cure. With most dementias, the medical world isn't even close to a cure, or at least, a drug that might turn a death sentence into a controlled, chronic illness. We caregivers experience an ongoing grief as we watch our spouse (partner, parent, child) disappear little by little and bit by bit. It's not surprising that when the end comes, there is a mixture of anguish and relief. Fortunately, as time goes on, one (at least me) remembers more and more the person that was, not the tortured soul they had become. Remembering the sweet, gentle, creative and loving Ralph is incredibly bittersweet.

I figured out early on that a drawn out mourning wasn't for me. I decided to use the philosophy both Ralph and I aspired to during his illness. 'One day at a time.' We have to get through each day one way or another so we might as well get on with it. I try to concentrate on the blessings and joys of 'now.'

As our friendship grew, Vicky and I found we had more in common than just our husbands' disease. We both always wanted to volunteer in the newborn nursery where we could help the staff by rocking babies. In January '12 we interviewed at a local hospital. What we thought was an original idea by us turned out to be a volunteer idea with a waiting list. In the meantime, I took a job in the Patient Discharge Department, and Vicky in one of the other areas. Two weeks after I began, I was asked to fill a space in the NICU (neonatal intensive care unit.) I said yes to both jobs and I enjoy them both. People tell me, "It's wonderful that you're giving back." No, not really. I get as much out of it as I contribute. It's a win-win situation.

The support I've received from family and friends has been invaluable. Nancy, Brian, and Alan and their families include me in most of their plans and I'm ready to go at a moment's notice. My youngest grandchildren and my great granddaughter are still enjoying overnights and weekends with Grandma. It took a while, because they all missed our house. Now, I guess my apartment 'feels like Grandma, and besides, she has a swimming pool right in her building!' My sister has an apartment near mine and while we've always been close in spirit, we raised our families miles apart. Now, we can be special friends as well as siblings.

All in all, it's been a rough road, but Ralph and I had more years together than many folks, and I feel truly blessed, loved, and very, very grateful.

When All Is Said and Done

If Vicky and I had set out to write a novel about dementia, it wouldn't have seemed plausible because there would be too many coincidences. Imagine. Two couples meet in a support group for dementia. They are separated by a generation, length of their illnesses (19 years vs. 7,) and lifestyles. However, in the space of three years, they all become close, share their stories, hopes, and fears. Then, suddenly, both men's illnesses accelerate at about the same time, and their final hours take place in the same facility. They die just one day short of one month apart. Their brains are sent to Harvard Medical School for research, and their memorial services are held in the same place. All neat and tidy, like a 'made for TV' movie. . . . . . . Ann

Chapter Five

Caregivers 101

Things We Have Learned

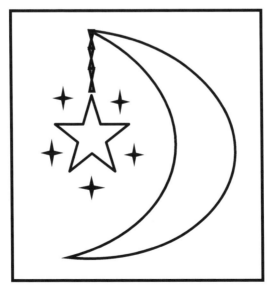

Picking a Doctor to Follow Your Loved One

1. This doctor should be a neurologist. Of course, your primary care physician will also follow your loved one, and advise you if they think you should plan a visit with your neurologist before your regularly scheduled visit. (We have found that a general practitioner or family doctor may not always have the expertise in recognizing all the nuances of the disease as it progresses, and may not know what drugs to try when problem symptoms are interfering with life.) You should feel comfortable speaking your mind with the neurologist you choose. Your neurologist should be your partner in this journey and should be willing to 'play the bad guy' when restrictions of activities are necessary (giving up driving for example.)

2. At the time of diagnosis the person thought to be suffering from dementia should be given extensive psychological and functional testing to help pinpoint what areas of thinking are affected, as well as some blood tests. Other diseases can look like Alzheimer's, but are curable. You don't want to miss a window of opportunity if it is curable! A geriatric neurology clinic or memory clinic is your best bet for this testing and future follow-up. If not found through your local hospital, you can find them through the nearest university medical school.

3. Generally the dementia patient is seen about every six months until closer management is necessary. It is helpful to either write a note to the doctor that he/she can read prior to meeting with you, or at least jot down notes of changed behaviors or important things you want to address while in the meeting. That makes the most of your time with the doctor. A written note is especially helpful when you want to convey things to the doctor that you may not want to say in front of the person with dementia.

4. If you can locate a clinic that also has a social worker on staff to help with the support of the patient and the caregiver, that is a great combination. They are more aware of local community resources and can help steer you towards a solution to a particular problem.

Not every physician will be as committed to providing such open communication as ours was. He was instrumental in solving small problems with a phone call, when a full appointment may not be needed, or for severe problems when you can't wait for an appointment. It is a truly dedicated person who makes themselves available to their patients, because it adds many, many hours to their day.

What to Do After the Diagnosis

1. **Have family meetings** to discuss a workable plan to handle the dementia as it progresses. If you can be open enough, try to have the person with the dementia there so they can tell you their wishes for the future. This is a tall order, but if the person with dementia and their spouse know everyone in the family will work together to give them the best care, then it may give them some peace of mind.

2. **Get your legal house in order.** Health care proxies, living wills, powers of attorney should all be decided upon. At this time, it is a good idea to have a family member sit in on the discussion with you and your Elder Law attorney, so that they understand your position. Discuss the holdings of the care-partner and whether you have enough money to afford nursing home care for your care-partner or whether you will likely need to apply for Medicaid when the time comes. Familiarize yourself with Medicaid rules (as of 2013 a 5-year look back period) so that you don't unknowingly gift money away, and keep all financial records for future filing purposes. This includes complete monthly bank statements, etc. If a house is in the care-partner's name they might want to make other arrangements that your elder lawyer advises. Check the beneficiaries on all the holdings the care-partner has for optimal Medicaid/estate consequences.

3. **Organize your important papers** and make your legal/financial status known to an appointed person in your family.

4. **A life insurance policy** owned by the care-partner may need to be transferred so that it is owned by the beneficiary or caregiver. Again, ask your lawyer.

5. **Get a Safe Return bracelet** for the care-partner (it's very difficult to take off once put on) and either a bracelet or necklace for the caregiver. The back of the jewelry lists a

phone number and Safe Return identification number. The Safe Return agency will reveal the wearer's name and address and whether they are a caregiver or a care-partner to whomever calls.

6.   **Try to be open about disclosing the diagnosis.** It will make it easier for both of you if you don't have to try to hide the truth. Our Alzheimer's Association has a 7-week course for both the caregiver and care-partner to address all sorts of topics, including divulging the diagnosis. Because the care-partners talk openly in the course it makes it easier for them to talk to friends and family.

7.   **Participation in Alzheimer's studies can be very rewarding for both caregiver and care-partner.** Not only will you both feel that you are doing something for society and research, but patients are also followed very closely during the study period. Possible studies can be located through your Alzheimer's Association web-site or your local research hospital/university.

8.   **Join a support group in your area.** The Alzheimer's Association has support groups in many locations. They actually cover dementia no matter what disease process the dementia is from. Much of the advice is the same. Referring to www.alz.org will help you find your local association website.

9.   **Volunteer for the Alzheimer's Association.** You can be part of a panel to educate the general public about what AD is like, or help the association to advocate for funding. You could volunteer to be filmed for a local or national TV station doing a story about dementia, or just help the association run their office by doing things to help. All these activities bolster self-esteem!

10.   **Volunteer** somewhere else if the care-partner has special skills they have not yet lost.

11.   **Become physically active** doing activities you like.

12. **Take vacations while your care-partner can still adjust to change**.

13. **Make humor a part of every day**.

14. **Either have the person with dementia stop driving**, or if they continue to drive, make sure they have passed a driving test.

15. **Begin to appreciate each day** as it comes rather than constantly looking toward the future. This does not mean don't do future preparation, but don't dwell on the future. Prepare, then let it go!

16. **Be cognizant of signs of depression** in you or your care-partner. Dealing with dementia can be stressful for the caregiver as well as the care-partner. Discuss these symptoms with your doctor. It is not a sign of weakness that you or your loved one might need an antidepressant at some time during this illness.

Shelter from the Storm-Ideas That Get You Through

1. If you have met one dementia patient, <u>you have met one dementia patient</u>. No one is exactly like another in symptoms, steps of progression, length of life, etc. It all depends on what areas of the brain are destroyed. There are also many subsets or types of dementia, Alzheimer's disease being predominant. The one thing you can depend on is that <u>some part of the person's memory is affected</u>.

2. <u>Never make a promise to your loved one that you cannot keep</u>. "I'll take care of you at home for as long as I can" is the most you should promise. Things can escalate quickly into a situation where it may no longer be safe to care for your loved one at home.

3. Working with people who have dementia brings to mind the Alcoholics Anonymous slogan, 'One day at a time,' only in this case it is 'One step at a time.' If you get too far ahead, you lose them.

4. Somewhere around <u>50-70% of patients become agitated /belligerent in their end stages</u> which makes the placing/continued care in a regular nursing home dicey. If the personnel can redirect the patient, medicate, or distract the person so that violence does not occur, then they are better off. That is why it is very important that the staff know how to interact with the dementia person, and be trained in doing so. Acting out behavior towards staff sometimes can be overlooked. However, when it is directed at other residents, it may be necessary to refer them to a behavioral nursing home. Behavioral facilities are structurally designed and decorated differently with safety as the highest priority. This means a higher staff to patient ratio, better trained staff for dealing with intense behavioral issues, more intensive monitoring of each patient, and big bucks in monthly fees. This can sometimes be a temporary assignment until the behaviors are remolded, or until that 'rough spot' in their disease

has passed. Generally, this means at least a 6 to 9 month stay.

A very good summary of agitation and dementia can be found on the website for Progressive Supranuclear Palsy. Although it was printed in 1998, it is a great overview of the subject. The drug section may need to be updated with more recent methods, but I find it still to be very informative.

http://www.pspinformation.com/disease/dementia/guides.html.

5.   Depending on where the person is in the disease when diagnosed, it is always better if the person can be given the chance to understand the disease and what is happening to their brain. Knowing, in a way, seems less scary than having relatives constantly 'placating' them. If they can learn to be open with their family and friends, there is less time spent using valuable energy to hide the condition. It also gives the person a chance to 'give something back' by helping explain to others what it is like to have dementia. Being open also gives friends and family in daily contact with the person the chance to ask about what is going on and how they can help. People tend to shy away from things they don't understand or are fearful about.

6.   Although getting a dog or cat is the last thing a caregiver would want to do at this stage, if you have an animal already, think seriously about keeping the pet. A dog or cat gives unconditional love. They don't judge, but accept you the way you are! If you don't have an animal, volunteering at a local animal shelter may be just the thing in the early stages. Dogs always need a walk or a brushing. You can define the hours that work best for you and your loved one. In our community, we have a program through the Alzheimer's Association where a handler can bring a dog to your home for an hour

a week. That program has been very successful, and the people they see always look forward to it.

7.   At some point during the disease, a technique called <u>therapeutic fibbing</u> will come in handy. The primary caregiver has to determine at what point this is appropriate vs. responding to the dementia patient by telling them the truth. Here is an example: Marion asks her daughter where her husband is, because she hasn't seen him in a long time. Instead of responding to Marion that her husband died a few years ago (which will cause her to grieve all over again every time she hears it) the daughter tells Marion that he is on an important business trip and will be gone for a while. This response saves Marion and the daughter many tear-filled moments.

8.   Another completely different scenario describes <u>going where the patient is.</u> In other words, going to the patient's 'reality' rather than giving further explanations. Example: Marion says to her daughter that she wants to go home (she is in her home of 30 years with all her possessions around her.) Her daughter responds by saying, "Yes, Mom, let's go home." They put their coats on and drive around the block. They pull into the driveway. The daughter remarks about a number of 'familiar' things as they enter the home, such as the flowering bushes by the door and how lovely they look. Marion now accepts that she is home. This very scenario happened to Ralph. Ann called her son, Brian, to come over. Brian took his dad to the end of the driveway and brought him back, this time pointing out things that reminded Ralph that he was home. It worked!

9.   <u>Distraction</u> is also a wonderful tool. In keeping with the prior example, the daughter might have responded the first time with, "Yes, that old home brings back a lot of good memories doesn't it? Remember when I told you I was going to run away from home when I was five, and I got three houses away and then came back?"

10. <u>Have your doctor be the 'bad guy.'</u> When your loved one wants to continue driving and you don't think they should, ask the doctor to inform the patient that he should not drive any longer. They will take the news a lot better than from a spouse, or the family, because the doctor is an authority figure. This approach can be used for a number of instances.

Driving, of course, can be a very 'sticky' subject. Once the Alzheimer's diagnosis is given, I think by law they have to give up driving. In Jim's case, because he lived with the disease for so long, he drove while having the diagnosis of minimal cognitive impairment, but when it became probable Alzheimer's, Jim took a driving test and failed it, so he stopped driving. The neurologist should be able to give you an idea of whether or not he/she is safe to drive. If the doctor says he/she can drive, then if the patient has an accident, the neurologist's opinion should be given in court. The best solution is a driving test. If they pass then you have proof of their legal status, and you can bring that to court if something happens. In our city there is a rehabilitation center that offers the driver's test. It is not cheap, but worth it in the long run. That is another example of having someone else acts as the 'bad guy.'

11. <u>Be mindful of crowds.</u> Crowds can be very confusing for a person with dementia because they don't necessarily remember what kind of clothing the caregiver is wearing. If the caregiver is moving in front of them and the person with dementia can't recall what they look like from behind, how are they ever going to keep up? It can be a very scary scenario. If the caregiver holds onto their hand, then they feel they are being treated as a child. I would try to hold Jim's arm or hand as if we were strolling along, conveying some warmth and love, rather than grabbing him by the arm and 'dragging' him through the crowd.

Although, I do admit doing that when I lost sight of Jim, and then found him again in a crush of people.

12. <u>Try to keep the dementia person involved and engaged in life.</u> Sometimes this is easier said than done, especially in the later stages. Have them do what they still can, like drying the dishes, setting the table, folding laundry, sweeping the driveway, vacuuming, sorting screws, etc. Make sure to compliment or praise them for their actions. Early in the disease, if they can volunteer using skills they still have, that's a great idea. Because Jim was a family therapist for many years, the Alzheimer's Association used him as a facilitator for their dementia patient support group. Being a facilitator was so natural for Jim, he could do it appropriately without thinking.

Asking the dementia person's opinion makes them feel involved. Even if they can't dress themselves, if you give them a choice of what to wear, they have a say in the process. That does not mean asking "What would you like to wear today," (too broad), it means "Would you like to wear the red shirt or the blue one?"

13. <u>Let trusted neighbors know</u> the code for your key pad garage door opener, if you have one. That way if your loved one can't work the key pad, neighbors can help him get in. Also let your loved one know they can go to the neighbors for help. Our neighbors were always very helpful and sometimes if they saw Jim way down the street, they would go fetch him and bring him home. They always kept an eye out for him. Sometimes Jim got away while I was in the side garden, but I didn't see him leave!

14. When placing your loved one, <u>choose a facility that is easy to visit</u>. Even in excellent facilities, the residents with the most frequent visitors are the ones who receive the best care.

15. Once your loved one needs assisted living or nursing home care, <u>get to know the aides and nurses giving care on the floor</u>, especially the aides and nurses ministering to your loved one. Ask about their families and engage them whenever you see them. The better you treat the

personnel taking care of your loved one, the better care your loved one will receive, and the more receptive the staff will be to your needs. Yummy food is always appreciated!

16. Bring your loved one 'to life' by <u>showing the caregivers who they were</u> and what they did in their profession, childhood stories, hobbies they loved, etc. The caregivers may understand the person better by knowing some of their history, and it allows more 'food' for discussion and humorous exchanges.

17. Rochester is on the forefront of two new ways of thinking about what nursing homes should be: The <u>Eden Alternative</u>, and the <u>Greenhouse Project</u>. The Eden Alternative is an organization that promotes the continuation of learning and discovery as aging continues rather than just a period of decline. They promote designing nursing homes more like homes than institutions where there is increased interaction with others, including children and animals. The Greenhouse Project is a new type of nursing home on a smaller scale, in a regular neighborhood. It is a building designed for 10 residents with a main living room, kitchen, and 10 bedrooms with baths adjoining the common areas. This is more like living in a home-like atmosphere with a smaller staff who become more like family.

<u>Aids to Help Make the Journey Easier</u>

After diagnosis, as things begin to get harder for your loved one, it is important to work as a partnership. If you try to discuss openly what will happen in general terms, and that the both of you will make a valiant effort to keep life 'normal' and fulfilling as the disease progresses, that will be a very good thing. If you can impart that the aids you use now or in the future are to make life easier and less frustrating, then maybe they will be more easily accepted. Everything is purely by trial and error. Not everything works for everybody, so be creative and try not to put a lot of emotional weight on these cues that you do try. Just be cool and accepting and see if they help.

Different things can be tried at different stages of the disease. You don't want to insult your loved one by using certain cues too early when they don't need them, or too late when they obviously won't work. Start out printing reminders, but eventually reading may become very difficult. At that time you can try shifting to pictures that tell a story to convey what you mean.

The very first thing to do post-diagnosis is to make a card to be carried in the wallet that gives the carrier's name, address, and phone number. Write I HAVE ALZHEIMER'S. Also list the phone number of the spouse or other person to be contacted, and other names and phone numbers of contacts in case the family member cannot be reached. Make it the size that will fit comfortably in the wallet, and either put clear tape over it to preserve it or have it laminated. Jim carried his for years until he stopped carrying a wallet. I also always made sure Jim had $10 to $20 in his wallet so he could buy things. I took the credit card out of his wallet fairly early on to prevent it from getting lost. Even if you are worried that they may lose the money, give them some so they feel they have autonomy, just not a lot at any one time.

The second thing is to apply for a **Safe Return Bracelet** for your loved one (as mentioned before) and get either a bracelet or necklace tag for yourself. Safe Return assigns a number to your loved one and registers where they live and who their caregiver is. If they get lost, there is a phone number on the bracelet, and if called, will identify the person and where they live with important contacts. If anything happens to you, authorities will know you are a caregiver for someone with dementia, and will take action to make sure that person is being properly cared for.

Here are some other things that may be helpful:

1.   Phone List – Create a phone list in a fairly large size and simple font so that your care-partner can easily read it. Put the phone numbers they would use first for best access. As time progresses you may need to increase the size. Make sure there is enough space between listings such that each listing is clear. Display it next to the phone(s). Another handy list to make on the computer is a list of people's names on the left and the word "called" on the right. All your loved one has to do is circle the correct name. Then you know whom to call back. When the memory is really compromised, try to let the phone ring so it will go to voicemail. Then they don't have to remember anything.

2.   A Day and Date Pad – I took a 5 x 8 inch pad, one with a thick top cover. I folded the cover back on itself so that it formed a stand up part at the top of the pad, and then folded it under the pad, stapling it in place.

On the stand up part I printed in Sharpie pen, 'TODAY IS' in large letters. I used the pad paper itself to write the day of the week, then the month and date with any major things that were happening that day that he would need to remember.

Tear off each day when it is over. You can fill out a week in advance, or more if you like. Keep it wherever they will see it every day. I put ours right above Jim's placemat. For example, TODAY IS …. Wednesday May 5th… Jim has dentist apt. 3pm. I printed rather than using script because Jim could read it better. I also kept my printing fairly large so that it took up most of the page. This way Jim didn't have to make sense of a big calendar and what day it was among crossed off squares, etc.

3. Tasks To Do List - Early on I made Jim a "Tasks to Do" List that I printed on the computer as a long strip of paper. I only included items that Jim could do by himself. I could fit 3 lists on a sheet, printed them up on card stock so they would be sturdier than paper. I would usually circle things that needed to be done and would leave them on Jim's placemat when I went off to work in the morning. Some examples of things Jim could do early on were: pick-up sticks in the yard, mow the lawn, water the lawn with a sprinkler, fill the bird feeder, blow the deck and driveway, do hot tub chemistry, clean the dish drainer, clean the tub and shower, vacuum living room, get the mail, take out garbage, wash windows outside, wash windows inside. As the disease progressed, I dropped some items off the list. This made him feel that he was needed, and that he had accomplished something good during his day.

4. I AM AT WORK...I will be home at 5:45 p.m. This I made out of a manila file folder. I folded the flat closed folder in half horizontally and then formed the folder into a triangle with the base being double and the bottom of the folder sticking up. Staples kept it together. I wrote across in large letters I AM AT WORK, then down below the time I would be home. Below that line I wrote the work phone number so that he could carry it to the phone and call the number if he needed to talk to me. I put it away when I wasn't working. Jim would know if he didn't see the sign, then I wasn't at work. I worked part time, and it was difficult for him to keep my schedule straight.

5. Colored Paper Cups Marked with a Mailing Label 'Breakfast', 'Lunch', and 'Dinner Pills' - Fairly early on I took over filling Jim's weekly pill box with pills. It was just too hard for him to remember when and how many of each he was supposed to take. Every morning I would put each meal's pills into the cups and set the appropriate one by his plate. As he became more confused I would only put the cup he was supposed to take in front of him. Evening pills I put by his tooth brush at bedtime. If I did that earlier, he might take them earlier!

6. <u>Key Lock For Bicycle</u> – Jim used to cycle on the Erie Canal path to our town recreation center, work out, and then cycle home. The key was on a plastic expandable key ring he could wear on his arm. He had a bike bag that always held the lock and key when he wasn't using it. No combination to remember. Remember to label the bike helmet and bike as well! As the disease progresses they may not remember what color the bike or helmet are, and the name will help them identify their own possessions. Regular address labels are good for this purpose. I gave him a key to the house on a key ring that had a big animal figure at the other end so he could find it. This was in case he could no longer remember the code to our garage door opener. Eventually, I just had to leave the back door to the garage open all the time so I knew he could get in if I was not at home. Although this may cause security worries, its better knowing your spouse can get in. Sometimes we have to let things go by the wayside in order to make life for our loved one better, and give them some autonomy.

7. <u>Name Labels On Jackets, Hats, etc. As Needed</u> - You can have labels printed that also have your phone number on them, then just sew or iron them into the clothing. I also made a tag saying JIM that he could take to the rec. center and put over the hanger so he would recognize his coat. Without it, Jim came home a couple of times with someone else's coat... once with their car keys inside! Oops! When situations like this arise, if you explain the reason to people they are usually very accommodating. We have never had a problem with someone's reaction. A bottle of wine as a gift helps!

8. <u>Signs Showing Where You Have Gone</u> – I used a number of these. They were downloaded pictures from the internet placed in sheet protectors. I showed them to Jim beforehand to make sure he would understand what I was trying to convey.

    a. 2 women walking briskly in athletic clothes – my sign for <u>"I went for a walk."</u> If Jim was asleep when I left I would place it on the floor in the hallway so he would have to walk over it to go anywhere.

b. A hairdresser working on a blonde woman (can't see the face) – I'm at the hairdresser.

c. A woman kneeling in a garden – I'm gardening.

d. A pill bottle with a big Rx and pills spilling out – I went to the pharmacy.

9. Introduction Cards - Cards that say "The person I am with has Alzheimer's disease. Thank you in advance for your understanding and patience." You can make them on the computer. These are helpful in a restaurant or in a clothing store if the person who has dementia is being waited on. Give them to the waiter, waitress, or salesperson as discretely as possible. If you call a local small store, and explain that you want to bring the person with dementia in and need special assistance (you can't always go into the dressing room with them), they can tell you a time when the store is not very busy and they can give you 1:1 help. This makes it a better experience.

10. Shuttle To Rec. Center Schedule – After Jim gave up driving and the weather wasn't conducive to bike riding, I made time schedule cards for various days of the week and the phone number to call so that Jim could ride to and from the rec. center at minimal cost on our town elder bus. That way he knew he was going to the rec. center, it was a reminder to call for pick-up, and what time to be ready.

11. Very early on in the disease I moved all my clothes out of our bedroom closet and into a guest bedroom nearby. Then I arranged Jim's closet with all pants on one side, and all shirts on the other. He also had a chest of drawers that was filled with only his clothing. That way I didn't wake Jim up getting ready for work in the morning, and

he knew all the clothes were his because it was his closet. There is a point in the disease where they don't recognize their clothes from anyone else's. Before I moved my clothes, there were many times Jim would try to put on my jeans and then get frustrated because they wouldn't fit.

12. Time & Date Cube – This is a 4 x 4 inch cube that is black. It has two buttons. When pressed, one button says the time with a.m. or p.m. The second button says the day, date, and year "Wednesday, May 25th, 2013." The bottom of the cube has the setting buttons. I covered that with cardboard so the settings could not be changed by accident. This was available through a visually impaired website, and was called Reizen™ 3 in 1 Talking Super Cube Clock for the visually impaired ($24.95.) This was especially helpful when Jim was looking for TV shows and had no clue of the day or date.

13. Favorite TV Shows List – printed on cardstock for durability, I listed them by days of the week with the time, channel, and name of the show. Jim used this until he could no longer change the channels.

14. Picture Phone – These are available on the internet by searching for Picture Button Phones. They may have 8 or 10 square buttons that you can insert photos and program with speed dial numbers, so your loved one can push the photo of the person he/she wants to call. It also works normally too. This is a great idea when the phone numbers either can't be read anymore, or the number can't be held in the brain long enough to press it. Don't wait too long to switch to this type of phone, however. I did and by the time I got one and programmed it, Jim couldn't recognize any of the pictures, even though one of the pictures was me!

15. Pictures on cabinets - Pictures of a glass, a plate, a bowl, or a fork etc. can be printed from pictures on the internet, and taped to the cabinet in the kitchen where they are

stored. I found that pictures work better than the printed word. You need to choose a picture of the item that is well defined and simple so it is not a confusing image. The background should be white. This can also work in the dresser drawer. Jim had V-neck and U-neck undershirts. I didn't use pictures, I just wrote V-neck and U-neck on index cards and put them on the top of the pile of the appropriate shirts.

16. <u>Change The Background And Simplify The Table</u>-I realized by watching Jim eat, that he was having trouble distinguishing his plate from the place mat and all the things on the table. I did away with a lot of the extraneous items on the table, and changed the placemats for a dark green piece of vinyl that I cut to the exact size of the table top. That way our plates 'popped out' so he could see the plate much easier. Simplifying or clearing surfaces that your loved one uses like the coffee table also helps. A table with 5-6 things on it makes it more visually confusing for the dementia person's brain to pick out what he wants-the TV remote. I noticed that with Jim. If a lot of different items were on the table, he couldn't separate his wallet from the other things even though they were different shapes and colors.

17. <u>Cut The Meat Before It Is Served</u> - I cut both our meats before bringing the plates out so that Jim wouldn't be 'singled out'. I started this when I noticed Jim couldn't distinguish one food from another. Other meal changes may need to be made eventually. Jim had a habit for years of chewing ice. So much so, that he wore down all his teeth. I didn't realize it at the time that his teeth weren't working for him, and he started complaining that his meat was full of gristle, but my piece never was. Or his meat was too tough. Finally I realized what the real problem was, and tried to serve softer foods. This is the time to avoid steaks, etc. in restaurants or you might have some embarrassing moments. No explanation that the problem was his teeth was acceptable to Jim. Another suggestion when things get harder for your loved one is to secretly

ask the waitress to have the meat for both of you cut before it is presented.

18. Change The Style Of Clothing - Change the clothing style that your loved one wears as dressing becomes more difficult. The pants went from jeans to jeans that I put heavy duty Velcro in place of the button. Shortly after I switched to a waist that was elasticized. Shirts went from button down to T shirts or sweatshirts. When Jim was geri-chair bound, the clothes were about 1-2 sizes larger so they were easier to get on and off.

19. Changing The TV Viewing Habits – As the disease progressed, Jim favored short TV programs, ones without complex plots that he could follow more easily. He became more upset by shows or news where people were harmed, even if it was not real. He could no longer watch war stories because he would begin crying about all the horror that his dad witnessed in WWII. Even if we were in the movie theatre and it was a short clip, he would cry and become all upset. I had to look for happy, funny, or scientific shows that interested him. Everyone is different. You just have to pay attention to how they react to various programs and avoid the ones that may be problematic.

20. Cover The Mirror - In assisted living, Jim complained about all the people in the bathroom. I realized he was seeing but not recognizing himself in the mirror. He didn't want to go with people watching him, so I covered the mirror with a Hawaiian scene. If you are at home and your loved one becomes upset when viewing himself in the mirror, take the mirror down, or cover it if you can. Some people will begin to talk to their reflection in the mirror, thinking it is someone else. Sometimes this is O.K., but occasionally they are hurt because the person they see doesn't answer them. In that case, covering the mirror may be helpful.

Also watch out for large expanses of reflective glass, say, in restaurants. Make sure to sit away from glass reflections.

21.   Changing Door Knobs - Once Jim's confusion reached a stage such that I began to worry about him locking himself in our bedrooms or the bathroom, I changed the door knobs to the press down kind with no lock rather than the knob type. I used the excuse that the knobs were worn and I had noticed they were sticking at times (a fib.) Jim helped me change them.

22.   Anti-Theft Precautions- I replaced the knob on the den where all our finances were kept when I was getting close to hiring part-time companions for Jim. I bought one with a lock, and took the key with me, hiding another key in the house. I moved my jewelry box in the den as well, just to be on the safe side.

23.   Creative Ways To Dispel Agitation – Jim's cousin used some great aids to help soothe her mom when she was in a nursing home:

   a.   The first was a book in which a loving message is recorded as well as her voice reading the story. The story subject was "Counting the ways I love you." The aides where Jim's aunt lives found the book very helpful in calming her when her daughter couldn't be there.

   b.   The second was a reproduced photo of mother and daughter on one side, and basic information about where the aunt lives, a description of her family, etc. on the other side. It was laminated to keep it clean, and a few copies were made.

   c.   The third idea was a clear plastic tub filled with reproduced family photos and mementos that her mom can look through, kept in the activity room where her mom spends most of her time.

d. <u>Russ Carlton DVD's</u> are wonderful for Alzheimer's patients. He sings a lot of familiar songs, but at a slower pace and with words displayed on the screen. It is amazing how even the 'non-talkers' and 'nappers' will awaken and sing along when they hear the old songs they knew way back when. Jim's cousin bought all his DVD's for her mom's nursing home. They kept the residents engaged.

http://russcarlton.com/singalongs.htm.

Having a Safety Evaluation of Your Home

We had a safety evaluation through a grant that the Alzheimer's Association received. I am reasonably sure that Lifespan or ElderSource may offer them also. Even if you don't implement everything that they suggest, it is an eye opening experience and makes one more sensitive to your surroundings. Sometimes just another point of view is what is needed to highlight those things that could become problems in the future.

Here is what they suggested for our 1029 square foot ranch house:

Garage:

- Put poisons out of sight.
- Install a gate on cellar stairs.

Kitchen:

- Put a grab bar on the wall next to the step-down area by the door.
- Place yellow tape at the edge of the step so it is always visible.
- Remove stove handles when not in use.
- Install an alarm on the door or an alarm mat by the door so you know when the door has been opened.
- Removal of throw rugs.

Living/Dining Room:

- Replace stationary dining room chairs with swivel chairs. (I agree that swivel type chairs make it easier to get in and out of near a table, but I also see problems with swivel chairs that could cause falls.)
- Remove coffee table and foot stool and add a small side table instead.
- Remove coat rack on wall in front hallway in favor of a railing.

- Remove bookcase in hallway to bedrooms for wheelchair access if needed.
- Angle the sofa if a wheelchair is needed and build ramp off back deck for wheelchair accessibility.

Bathroom:

- Take door off bathroom (If someone falls against the door on the inside, no one will be able to get in. Use pocket door between living room and bedrooms for privacy.)
- Get a toilet seat with arms for stability.
- Put swivel chair in shower/tub.
- At night close guest bedroom and den doors, leaving bathroom open with night light. This will lead him to the toilet.

Bedroom:

- Raise bed up on cups to make it easier to get in and out.
- Put a railing on the bed.
- Close the pocket door between the living room and bedrooms/bathroom and put an alarm on it that can be set at bedtime so you know if he's up.

This is meant as a springboard to look at your own surroundings with fresh eyes. Not all suggestions will apply to everyone. Simplify things visually so there are less distractions and pay attention to footing issues. Grab bars in the tub/shower area are not mentioned because we already had them installed when we remodeled. Also railings in pertinent places next to stairs sturdy enough for the person to pull themselves up are a good idea. Because of 'the lay of the land' our home didn't require them.

The Best Defense Is a Good Offense

'The best defense is a good offense' occurred to me suddenly one day when I was tired of dealing with the spoils of situations, always reacting to some consequence of Jim's increasing memory loss. Sometimes it meant dealing with Jim's frustration over my doing tasks Jim had already done, because they were blatantly inadequate, things I just couldn't let go. Sometimes it was spending time looking for misplaced items during a chore Jim had accomplished. Other times, it was trying to muster the energy to 'go along with' Jim's choices rather than 'bucking him every step of the way,'(or at least that is what it felt like to him.) Acting offensively eliminated the problem before it happened, and made life much smoother in the long run. Here are a few examples:

1. **Mowing the lawn:**

    Jim had been chomping at the bit one spring day to get out and mow the lawn. After sitting idle most of the winter with only a few tasks to keep himself occupied like snow blowing the driveway and washing the dishes, he was anxious to exert himself doing a worthwhile activity that he thought was in his realm of possibilities. I had reservations about his mowing the lawn, and didn't know if when finished, he would feel that sense of pride of doing a job 'well done.' So one day before Jim began his season of mowing, I got the lawn mower out while he wasn't there and checked the oil, filled it with gas, and adjusted the wheels so that they were all even and a bit lower than he had them the previous season. I would 'maintain' the mower each week throughout the mowing season. That way he would have to refill the tank less often, thereby hopefully avoiding the situation of a missing gas cap on the gas can or mower due to his forgetting to replace them when he was refilling the tank. Many times the previous season I had spent time walking patterns on the lawn looking for those missing gas caps!

Lowering the wheels a bit made it easier with Jim's decreasing perception, for him to see the difference between the mowed and unmowed areas. The previous season Jim had the wheels on the left lower than the wheels on the right, which made every pass that he did look funny, but Jim never recognized the problem.

I also made a deal with Jim, that after he finished, if there were any big patches left unmowed, that I could 'finish up' those areas without his getting all bent out of shape. I explained to him that he was doing me a big favor by mowing the lawn and he saved me oodles of time if he mowed while I gardened, then I would just neaten it up at the end. It was too hard and maddening for him if I directed him to the patches left undone. I looked like an airport traffic control person with the signal lights out there on the tarmac directing plane traffic. I also found out years later that our neighbor would sometimes sneak out while Jim was showering after mowing the lawn, and he would cut the missed areas.

The last thing I did in regard to mowing was to buy replacement gas caps for the mower and gas cans so if Jim lost one, no big deal was made, I just gave him a new one. Hopefully one of us would discover the misplaced one as time went by.

2. **Shearing the hedge and weed whacking the edge of the gardens:**

The privet hedge that followed the contours of our back property line only needs trimming approximately 4 times a year, thank heaven, so this wasn't too much of a problem. If I saw it needed trimming, I would do it when Jim was away, then he would just see that it didn't need trimming, but he wouldn't register that I had just done it, because he wouldn't remember what it looked like before. Again, due to his perception problems, he could whack the hell out of it and butcher it, but not see that he was doing a bad job. Other times I would let him do it, but would neaten it up days later when he was out. Because I was out doing the gardening, I could also weed whack the edge of the gardens when he was gone, and he would just see that they didn't need doing, but would not remember when he did it last. This saved face for Jim, even though he didn't know it, because when he did do it, it was really awful. Yes, it made me more work, but it kept our relationship in harmony.

3.   **Dressing:**

Weed out the closet or dresser so that it only contains clothes that the person with dementia will wear. That will help lessen the confusion of making choices. If the person wants to choose what they wear, have them choose between two things, rather than the entire closet of clothes.

Getting clothes out while the person is showering is also helpful. I would discard the dirty clothes and put clean ones in proper order on the bed so that underwear is on top and pants and shirt are on the bottom. Later as Jim lost my identity, I would sneak in while Jim was in the shower and put the dirty clothes in the wash, leaving clean underwear on the sink for him to put on so it preserved his dignity (he didn't want me to see him naked.) Then he would come out to put his shirt and pants on.

Give him choices. "Jim, do you want to wear a belt today? How about a handkerchief for your pocket? Do you want two?" That helps him feel more in control of the situation. Helping a person with dementia dress is so heart wrenching, because sooner or later they lose the orientation of clothing...don't know front from back, and see sleeves as pant legs, etc. Despite the fact that your heart is breaking, be as patient and nonjudgmental as possible in re-orienting the clothing to where it must go. Before frustration becomes a daily part of the dressing procedure, change the style of clothing so that getting dressed is made easier…from button shirts to over-the-head or zip front style, from zip front waists to gathered waistbands.

4. **Trimming, cutting the meat before it is served:**

    This again deals with the perceptual problems that may occur as the dementia becomes more advanced. They eventually don't recognize what they are eating, so announcing what is on the table can be helpful. Not only won't they recognize what is on the plate, but they eventually won't remember that meat may need to have fat cut off the side before eating, or how to cut it into bite sized pieces. It is belittling to them to have you reach over to cut their meat while they are seated; so if you are out, quietly ask the waitress to discard all fat and cut the meat before serving it if you can. Do the same at home with both you and your loved ones plate before they are brought to the table.

5. **Buy a grabber if you don't already have one:**

    It's a tool that allows you to squeeze the handle and pick-up sticks or other things on the ground. Jim loved to use his…he found it fun, and it gave him hours of pleasure picking up sticks (even if he didn't get them all because he didn't see all of them.) Our neighborhood is mostly locust trees and they are messy, always dropping sticks on the lawn. It gave him something worthwhile to accomplish.

6. **A trip in the car:**

    Before leaving the house in the car with a dementia or health compromised individual, think of all the things they might need during the trip that they may not have. I don't know how many times we had left the house and I didn't bother to even notice that Jim didn't have his glasses on! You are in the mindset so many times that they will have what they need like any other person that gets into your car, but they won't! It may be eye drops, medication, glasses, a cap to keep the sun out of their eyes, a jacket, or gloves. Sometimes it's good to keep extras in the car, but then you have to remember to replace them if they are used.

If you have some reservation about what your loved one might do during a car ride (open the door and try to get out) get in the habit of locking the doors if your car doesn't have the automatic locking capability. If this behavior does become a problem you can encourage your loved one to ride in the back seat where the child safety locks are employable.

These are just a few examples where you and your loved one's life can be made easier. In general, think of ways to circumvent problems that may arise before they happen, and take steps to make sure they don't. The fewer problems that arise when a person is trying to be successful, the better they feel, and the better the caregiver will feel. A nice quiet meal is so much better than a scene in a restaurant about the supposed poor quality of the dinner!

You are their memory, their eyes, and their ears. You have to be that for the both of you, but it is well worth it.

Have a Little Compassion

There have been many beautiful vignettes written by caregivers about those with Alzheimer's: the love they have for the person; the yearning for just a little bit of the person they once knew to surface and show some real recognition of us; or to hear them say 'I love you' one more time.

I think most caregivers can't help but feel shock and fear, deep hurt, and regret for the embarrassments, the frustrations, the humiliations, and the losses that those with AD endure in their downhill slide into the disease. We experience these things profoundly, but that doesn't mean that we can always show compassion. Most of us aren't saints, and eventually our aggravation may surface when we deal with the day to day care of a person with dementia. No matter how hard I tried, there were times when my frustration got the better of me, and I would 'fly off the handle' and express anger as a raised voice or a demeaning tone. For the longest time I didn't register that my tone of voice was anything but patient. Being a family therapist, there were a few times when Jim sat me down and said he didn't like my expressed anger, and that he was doing the best he could. The weird thing was, I hadn't interpreted what I did as anger...or shouting. When trying to coach him toward a specific task, I would raise my voice. Maybe I thought if he heard me better, he would respond more favorably, but I would also speak a bit slower with a lilt in my voice. When discussing these incidents with my son, he said, "Oh, Mom! I remember that voice because you used to use it with me when I was growing up, and it would drive me crazy. It was condescending!" That really had me wondering about it. How could I see it one way, and the two of them see it so differently?

As time went on, I started to pay attention when Jim would aggravate me, and all of a sudden 2-3 days later, BINGO! It registered as I was using that same voice. Now I knew what Kip and Jim meant. I really hadn't intended to sound condescending, but I could certainly see how it could be interpreted that way. My voice response was so a part of me as the 'patient caregiver', and now I had to try to change it. Every time Jim wanted to help, I had to be very careful about how I said what I said. Hopefully, I am changing my behavior. I grew up in a relatively poor family. It was not uncommon to hear my dad yelling about the money they owed, and how he was going to pay the bills with the money they had. To me, yelling was anger. In Jim's family, however, he rarely heard his mother and father raise their voices. A raised voice, even not at the decibel I would consider as anger, was definitely so to Jim!

As caregivers, our days are so filled with being patient as we lay out the morning clothes, hang up the ones that have been discarded, or put them in the wash, make sure they take their pills, turn the TV on after their 4th or 5th try, try to keep them occupied while trying to do the household chores, make sure they wash, shave, brush their teeth with tooth paste and not suntan lotion, eat their breakfast, lunch, and dinner that we prepared, and take them places to exercise so they are not so sedentary. Sound harried? Is it any wonder that occasionally we lose our composure and begin to steam or completely explode? That is when we should remove ourselves from the situation until we have cooled off. There is nothing the person with dementia can do about it but try to forgive us for the outburst, and for us to forgive ourselves. We should apologize for the incident, and just move on.

Part of the problem that contributes to our outbursts is that we tend to look at our loved one and compare them to a person without dementia...how they once were. We let the behavior anger us when there is no possibility that they can do what we want them to. "Why can't he hang up his clothes like a normal person!" Even though realistically we know that the person with dementia can't do the things that would make our lives so much easier, we need to sit ourselves down and think over the things that have us upset. We need to put ourselves in their shoes and realize what a day is like for our loved one. They feel lost trying to navigate their day to day world with the millions of things that are a puzzle to them. How scary would it be if we were them? How nervous would we be if we couldn't find our caregiver, would they leave us? Who would help us?

The losses they have suffered are devastating. Not to be able to do their job anymore, possibly being fired because of some behaviors elicited before the disease was diagnosed. They can't work on their hobbies because their thinking skills are too fuzzy, and they feel they can't contribute to the household. They can't button their shirt or zip their coat, things that they considered so simple only a few years previous. Not being able to read, or watch television or a movie and come away with the meaning of it all. Their world is a frightening place. When we think of their world in these terms, hopefully it will help us to have a bit more compassion when dealing with them.

Fear of the unknown adds to our stress level too, and brings us closer to 'shorting out' periodically. It seems that no matter where Jim is in the disease, I get used to where he is and how he acts and I make a 'new normal' in my head. Despite what is staring me in the face, I can somehow convince myself that things won't get any worse, and I say "I can deal with this." I go through my days not really thinking about the future and what will be until one day when Jim does something that screams at me, "I AM GETTING WORSE!" Then the dread hits me and I grieve all over again for where we've been and where we are heading, and the person I am losing. It causes anxiety, depression, sleepless nights, and just general dread. It takes a lot of energy just to pick myself up and go on. After all...what choice do I have anyway! And staying in a funk only makes my life less rewarding. So I try to stay positive, and live from day to day, moment to moment.

So try to remember – besides showing compassion and understanding for your loved one, have compassion for yourself. Be forgiving, cut yourself some slack, and know that you are doing the best that you can at that moment! **There is always tomorrow to do it better** (phrase by Angela Dentz).

When Looking For Resources In Your Community, Know the Partnerships That Exist Between Institutions

When looking for an alternate living arrangement for a dementia person, there are many things to consider that are not obvious when making your choice. In the Rochester, New York area, some nursing homes are abandoning the locked units for dementia care in favor of placing the patient among other nursing home residents. Their thought process in this decision may seem crazy at first, but this is their reasoning.

Nursing homes are expensive – at the time of publication (2013) approximately $12,000 per month. Many families are trying to avoid the high cost of nursing home care for those with Alzheimer's by placing their loved ones in locked assisted living facilities. For many, this eases their pocketbook. Assisted living facilities are about half the price of a nursing home per month. Then, when the patients can no longer feed themselves (the definition of assisted living is that residents must be able to feed themselves,) they are moved to a nursing home. By this point, many of the loved ones are past the wandering stage, and so can be reasonably placed in a facility that does not have a locked unit.

For those patients who are still wandering, however, if they are placed in a facility that has no locks, a great disservice is done to the patient and their fellow residents. The wandering in and out of rooms, and the 'pilfering' that is a normal part of Alzheimer's /dementia could be a real source of friction. Therefore, it is important to find out the specific nursing home's orientation in regard to locked units. Most admission forms ask if the patient is wandering, and if so, you would be wasting your time trying to get them in a facility that does not have locked units.

While the choice of an assisted living facility saves you money in the short run, you will have to balance it against the need to offer 1-2 years of private pay when you are ready to admit your loved one to a nursing home. By offering 1-2 years of private pay, the nursing home is enticed to accept you over a Medicaid-eligible patient, because they receive more money from you than Medicaid. This is your bargaining chip to get your loved one in the nursing home of your choice. Medicaid-eligible patients are sent to nursing homes with a vacancy in a Medicaid bed, not necessarily one of your choosing. {If your loved one was lucky enough to have long term care insurance, then they will be looked upon favorably by the nursing home and you won't have a problem gaining entrance to a nursing home.}

So, ultimately, you have to weigh cheaper assisted living sites against nursing homes and hope that if you choose the assisted living track, that you have enough money when they need nursing home care, if they do, to get them in a good one. This decision should be made along with your Elder Law attorney and financial advisor so they can guide you.

When choosing an assisted living facility or a nursing home, it is important to know the partnerships that exist in your community. There are many senior living places springing up all over the country that have everything from independent living to assisted living to nursing home care available to their residents, all within a short distance. They may have to move apartments from one classification to another, but residents are automatically eligible for the next step in the continuum. They are called continuum of care senior living centers. Although these places are pricier than going the independent route, they provide a great level of confidence and peace of mind knowing where one will go if increased care is needed. They may have to wait for a bed to open up, but when one does, they are automatically eligible. This is what saved Ann and Ralph when Ralph needed immediate admission to a nursing home. They had just moved into a continuum of care independent apartment a few weeks previously. Within days of determining that Ralph needed more care, he was admitted to their affiliated nursing home.

If one chooses an assisted living facility that does not have any partnership with a nursing home, then one has to wait while people are admitted from the assisted living facilities that do have a partnership with that particular nursing home. Only when the partnerships are fulfilled, are open beds offered to the general public or nonaffiliated facilities.

It is also important to research what doctors will be assigned to your loved one upon entering a facility (some insist on your loved one using only their assigned physicians.) That physician group may be easier to use because the group actually comes to the facility for regular patient visits, rather than having to transport the person to a doctor's office. That particular physician group may have an alliance with a certain hospital in your area. This means that if your loved one needs to be admitted or have emergent care, that they will usually go to the hospital where the doctors covering the patient have an alliance. This sounds good on face value, but if that particular hospital emergency room does not offer a psychiatric ER, and your loved one happens to be sent to the ER for agitation and violent behaviors, the staff may not be appropriately trained to handle the situation. This can drastically exacerbate the behavior of the patient. What happens if this hospital does not have a partnership with a behavioral nursing home and your loved one acts out while in the ER or on a floor of that hospital? It goes in their record, and those notes of violent behavior may prevent them from being taken back to the facility they came from. In that case, the hospital social worker may have to look for a placement for your loved one in one of the state's behavioral nursing homes.

New York State has three behavioral nursing homes. Some hospitals have affiliations with them, so if you are in one of those hospitals that does have an affiliation with a behavioral facility, and you are in need of that care, then all you have to do is wait for a bed opening. As with the scenario described above, if you are in a hospital with no affiliation, then you have to wait until other affiliations are satisfied if patients are waiting for admission, before you are even considered. Some patients have had to wait in the hospital for as long as a year awaiting behavioral placement and some have had to be placed out of state. Can you imagine not being able to visit your loved one because they are too far away? Talk about 'abandonment issues'.

That could have been us. Jim was sent to a non-affiliated hospital ER for his violent behavior because that was where the assisted living doctors practiced. They needed to find out if there was a physical reason for his violence (UTI, lung infection, etc.) He was denied re-entry to the assisted living and was in need of a behavioral placement, once they determined that there was no underlying physical cause for Jim's behavior. At first there were no beds available in any of the three. The one I visited that week happened to have a death a day later, and I had money I could spend (rather than Medicaid) for Jim's care, so I think they chose Jim over 7 other patients. We were lucky. They do look at the needs of each possible admission, but the fact that they had a face to go along with Jim's paperwork didn't hurt. The social worker at the hospital stressed that point...even if there are no openings, make a visit anyway, it might work in your favor! If Jim had not gotten that placement, we could have been waiting for months! If you have to wait in the hospital for a behavioral placement, the hospital &/or your health care plan can try to make you pay for your hospital stay from that point on, rather than your health care paying for it.

A Word about Behavioral Nursing Homes:

Their purpose is to retrain, divert, or distract patients displaying violent behaviors so as to keep themselves and other residents safe before the violent behaviors are elicited. Patients are placed there because of various diseases or trauma to the brain causing the behaviors. Although many people with Alzheimer's display agitated and violent behaviors in their latter stages (50-70%), they are not the sole population in behavioral facilities. The average stay is about 6-9 months, during which time they are either retrained to elicit more acceptable behaviors, or medicated to prevent or reduce them, or they have transitioned out of that behavior to a more restrictive physical state.

The Need for Separate Emergency Room Dementia Areas

Easter 2011, I had to initiate a mental health arrest for my husband, Jim. (A mental health arrest is a nice way of saying a trip to the Emergency Room.) He was in his 19th year of Alzheimer's, and wanted to leave home (Rochester, NY) and walk to New Jersey, his childhood home. While in the Emergency Room (ER) he became very agitated, screaming and pounding on the glass door of his room to go home. Later that summer he was also sent to the Emergency Room twice for agitation and violence issues. These two other 'admissions' provoked further violence because he was disoriented and frightened. That caused a mental decline that was unrecoupable.

Agitation and violence happen frequently in the later stages of Alzheimer's disease (50-70% of the time). The agitation begins when the person with dementia cannot express something that is bothering them. Perhaps it is something they want to do or are afraid of, something surprises them, or it may be that they have pain or feel ill but can't express this to those around them because of their dementia. When their needs in response to this agitation aren't met, it can escalate to violence. At this point, whether they are at home or in assisted living, or even a nursing home, they may be sent to the Emergency Room for a workup. They want to determine if there is something physically wrong that is causing the patient to act this way.

Once the tests are complete, if there is no indication of disease, then social work must decide whether they can return home, or whether they should be placed in a nursing home or a locked assisted living facility for safety reasons. This was the case for Jim. He was threatening to leave home on foot, and because of his dementia history, could not be permitted to do as he wanted. The violence that he displayed while he was in the hospital put him on a path of no return.

People with dementia have very special needs that are not usually met in today's Emergency Rooms. Because of memory problems, they may not remember from one second to the next what brought them there or when they will be able to leave. They are usually confined to a relatively small space, sometimes with other patients. Unless someone they know is with them all the time, it may be very hard to keep them oriented, and they can become very frightened. This exacerbates the behavior that brought them there in the first place. The longer they have to stay in this confusing place that is not soothing to them, the more severe the sundowning effect. (Sundowning is an increased confusion and agitation occurring at the end of the day perhaps because of tiredness, overstimulation, decreased lighting which causes problems in interpreting their environment, hallucinations, etc.)

Alzheimer's disease and other forms of dementia are on the rise because people are living longer and the wave of baby boomers reaching retirement age is just beginning. At age 65 approximately 10% will develop Alzheimer's. By age 85, 50% will develop Alzheimer's. That is a large number that will keep on getting larger. It will be increasingly common for that population to have ER admissions because more and more families will try to take care of their loved ones at home to avoid nursing home fees, until some uncontrollable event happens. Violence may not even be an issue in the admission. Implementing the following suggestions will not only help the dementia patient have a better stay that impacts them negatively less often, but it will also make the nurse and doctor in charge of this patient have a smoother and shorter interaction time with the patient.

Here are our suggestions:

1) The rooms should be private and should provide more space so the dementia patient doesn't feel closed in. Small spaces feel claustrophobic and increase sundowning.

2) The rooms should provide enough space so that a lounge chair can be included for the family member to stay with the patient. This will help to ease the fear the dementia person feels, because they don't know where they are or why they are there. Soft music should be available for playing.

3) If a family member cannot stay overnight, a 1:1 aide should be provided to serve the same function as a family member, to keep the dementia person relaxed and oriented. Presently instead of this, they may simply medicate the

patient for the overnight, sometimes with something like Haldol, a psychotropic drug, if their behavior warrants it.

4) Provide space for the dementia person to walk accompanied by family to get rid of the tension without interfering with the ER staff. They were apprehensive about Jim walking freely because of the violence he previously displayed. If it were a separate area or hallway, no one else would be in harm's way.

5) Have access to a larger bathroom so the caregiver or aide can more easily go in as well.

6) Better access to their meals and medications so their schedule is not thrown all out of whack. At one hospital, Jim waited eight hours for a meal and meds. I finally asked why neither had been given in that length of time, and then finally they brought him something to eat and some of the meds he should have been getting all along. I didn't ask sooner because I thought they were waiting for test results, which they weren't. I would advise bringing any meds along with you, if you can, when going to the ER.

7) Provide a clearer explanation to the dementia patient and caregiver what the ER staff is doing and how long it will take. Frequently the dementia patient is ignored in favor of talking to the caregiver, if they even do that.

8) Some sort of scrubs should be provided or permission for the patient to wear their own pajamas so they feel comfortable, rather than having to wear the cold hospital gowns. Many dementia patients feel cold either due to the destruction of the temperature sensing areas of the brain, or due to a side effect of their

medications. This will help with toileting issues too, if they are in their own pajamas.

9) Very strict use or prevention of the use of Haldol, because of the possibility of diagnosed/undiagnosed Lewy body disease. Haldol given to Lewy body patients can cause Neuroleptic Malignant Syndrome.

10) Faster turnaround time to get the dementia patient in and out helps the patient, family, and the ER. Many times, hours are spent waiting for a simple physician's release signature.

11) Extensive training in dealing with dementia patients is needed so that their stay causes the least amount of trauma to everyone involved. There are very specific skills used with a dementia patient that aren't used with the 'normal' individual. If their stay in ER causes agitation in the patient, violent behaviors can be the result. This can be very costly to the patient if it is documented in their record. The behavior doesn't need to happen if they are dealt with properly, and feel comfortable in their surroundings. It may cause the refusal of admission to a nursing home, and may require them to be admitted to a behavioral nursing home. Empty beds in those nursing homes are rare and extremely expensive ($21,500/mo. in 2011.) Every admission to the hospital or ER sends a dementia patient to a lower functioning level, which in most cases is not recoupable.

We have sent these ideas to all our local hospitals in hopes that they would consider implementation.

What Is a PRI and How Do I Get One

PRI stands for patient review instrument. It is an 8 page form that evaluates a person both physically and emotionally to see what level of care they need, and if nursing home placement is fitting. It must be done before a person is admitted to any nursing facility.

In New York State, there is also a preadmission screen that is done at the same time as the PRI to comply with law DOH695i (Omnibus Budget Reconciliation Act.) The screening focuses on protecting the mentally ill. In the 60's and 70's there was a big shift from mental institutions to nursing homes. When this happened, the mentally ill were found not to need skilled nursing, but there was no appropriate housing option for them. This screen was created to catch those mentally ill whose mental health needs were not being met, so that they could be addressed. Those patients who have dementia as their primary diagnosis do not have to undergo this screening according to this law.

The PRI addresses the evaluation of the activities of daily living: does he need assistance with personal hygiene (bathing), does he need assistance dressing and undressing, can he feed himself, can he make his own transfers from bed to chair etc., can he walk without assistance, does he have bowel and bladder control (presence of an ostomy or catheter.) This also includes whether the person has trouble hearing and seeing, and whether he displays disruptive behavior and psychopathology.

The PRI and screen are performed by specially trained technicians, usually nurses or social workers. If the person is coming from a hospital to a nursing home or assisted living, the hospital staff will do the evaluation without added cost. If the person is coming from home, there are trained personnel from home health care agencies who will do it. You can look them up under home health services in the Yellow Pages or the internet. There is a fee for service that must be paid, and prices vary. Ann's PRI cost $200 in fall 2011. The PRI and screen and usually a medical summary from the person's doctor as well as the admission documents are submitted before entrance to a nursing facility is permitted. If the PRI and screen are done in your home, you will receive a copy of the review, and copies will be sent to all nursing homes or other institutions being considered for placement by the PRI provider.

The PRI is good for a maximum of 90 days, or expires sooner if the status of the patient has changed.

The Nursing Home Interview

1. How does the facility smell?

2. Does it look clean?

3. Is it pleasantly decorated, easy to clean, relatively up to date?

4. Does the person giving you the tour interact with the residents? Call them by name?

5. What types of things are included in the basic monthly rate? Laundry? Do you label the clothes of each resident or does a family member? Are there types of clothing that I should avoid bringing? What clothing is best for my loved one and easy for the staff to help with dressing?

6. Are haircuts extra? Do they appear on my monthly bill or do I have to have a separate account for haircuts (petty cash account?)

7. Can the resident retain his private doctor, or does he/she have to switch to a doctor on staff?

8. Do you have dentists and podiatrists who regularly visit or do I have to take my loved one out of the facility to see these types of professionals?

9. If the resident needs emergency or hospital care, are your doctors affiliated with a specific hospital? If they become violent, are they sent to the hospital? Is that hospital affiliated with a specific Behavioral Nursing Home?

10. If a resident is hospitalized, how long will you keep their bed available for them?

11. How are medications handled? Does the floor nurse order them when they are needed? Is there a pharmacy in-house? Do I have

to pick up prescriptions, or are they delivered to the nursing home?

12. What is the resident's diet like? How far ahead are choices made and who makes them? If they don't like what is sent to them, can they get an alternative? Is there a place where snacks can be held for them?

13. Do you have a resident animal on the floor? Cat, bird, etc. What about residents who are asthmatic?

14. Semiprivate or private rooms – What furniture is included? Is television and cable included? Phone? Dresser? Chair? Is the bathroom shared? Pictures? Who hangs them? (Depending on the resident, a phone may or may not be a good idea.)

15. How long is your waiting list for private pay? How long do you have to guarantee private pay before going on Medicaid? Do you have an affiliation with a continuum of care senior living center, so that they are accepted before private patients?

16. Can I make an application and turn it down if we are not ready to make the move yet? If I turn it down will I remain at the top of the list or go to the bottom? (Remember that a PRI is needed with the application and that is only good for 90 days.)

17. Are there visiting hours or can family visit at any time?

18. What kind of programs do you offer to engage the dementia residents? Do you seek them out to join in the activities?

19. Does this include physical activities?

20. Are there supplies available for programs?

21. If a resident wants to go back to bed after breakfast, do you allow them to? What if they are up walking the floor in the middle of the night? Do you give them sleeping pills? Do you let them establish their own schedule of waking and sleeping?

22. How many nurses and aides are present weekdays, nights, weekends, holidays?

23. Will my loved one always have the same staff taking care of them all the time or do they rotate? This is an important question. It is much better when the staff don't rotate so that they truly know the resident in time. They can more easily respond to a resident if a problem arises because they are more familiar with them.

24. How many times a week are they bathed? Are men bathed by men?

25. If they are incontinent are they bathed more often?

26. Is there significant staff turn-over?

27. Is this nursing home part of an Eden Alternative, or do they have a Greenhouse Project setting in the community? If so, how are residents chosen for these areas?

28. Do you have a resident council?

29. Do you have a family council to provide feedback to the staff?

30. What signals you that a resident is getting in the elevator or leaving the floor?

31. Am I notified with each change in medicine or a change in the care plan?

32. Am I notified when there is a change in my loved one's behavior?

33. Can I bring my loved one outside for a walk, for lunch? How do I notify staff and how far ahead? (This will depend on the status of the patient and whether they can transition to a car, etc. safely.)

34. Monthly fee (remember there is a state tax of 6% for New York State – check your state for tax consequences.)

35. Ask for an application and an admissions contact person including their phone number.

Medicaid Overview for Those Needing Nursing Home Care

Medicaid is a national health care program designed to help low income families and individuals as well as the disabled for such things as health care, home care, and nursing home care. It is administered by each individual state and the rules differ significantly from state to state, but it is funded by both the federal and state governments. Because nursing home costs are so expensive, and many caregivers are extended family of the person with dementia, an increasing number are looking to Medicaid to foot the bill for their loved one's final years in a nursing home. Seniors are worried because the high cost of nursing homes can put an enormous drain on the spouse's nest egg, making what once might have been a secure retirement into a very precarious or desperate situation.

Many nursing homes require applicants to know their Medicaid eligibility prior to the admissions process, in particular when placement is being made from the community. This means that they must have already submitted the appropriate forms and paper substantiation, and have received their results as to whether they are eligible for Medicaid. Most caregivers seeking nursing home care for their loved one, especially in the case of Alzheimer's, aren't prepared for this requirement up front. They have been too busy caregiving, and all of a sudden things change and they are forced to take the nursing home step way before they anticipated.

That happened to us. Applying for Medicaid before making a nursing home application wasn't necessary when we first looked at nursing homes just a year ago (We were trying to be proactive.) How quickly the field can change. It generally takes 2 months once the paperwork is submitted to receive an answer, and most of us can't wait two months when circumstances sour, and we need placement right away. We were lucky that we could maneuver around that requirement by signing an agreement that I would pay for one year privately, and that I had enough money available to do so. This is called private pay. Some nursing homes are even asking for two years of private pay before going on Medicaid. At this time in Rochester N.Y., that comes to about $140,000 (1yr) to $276,000 (2 yrs.)

The Medicaid application for New York State can be found online, called Access NY Health Care Application, or by going to your nearest social services department. There is also a Supplement A that must also be filled out for those who are blind, disabled, chronically ill, or need nursing home care. This is also available online. The plethora of paper documents that must accompany your application will take quite a while to accumulate, so don't wait until the last minute to gather them.

The law that guides Medicaid eligibility as of 2013 is the Deficit Reduction Act of 2005, enacted in 2/8/2006. It states that there is a look-back period now of 5 years (60 months) for resources/assets that may have been transferred to someone else without reimbursement dollar for dollar in order to fit into the eligibility window. If there was disposal of resources in that five year period, it calculates a penalty or waiting period for eligibility for the institutionalized spouse. It also poses limits on home equity and a requirement for the state to be the beneficiary on annuities.

In this discussion the institutionalized spouse is the person needing nursing home care and the community spouse is the person living at home in the year 2013 in New York State.

The institutionalized spouse can have:

$50 in income per month (amt. over this goes to nh)
< $14,400 in savings & other liquid assets
$ cost of health care premiums per month
Irrevocable burial trust/plot
Personal property (no collections)

The community spouse can have:
Auto, home (may be limited in equity value)
Property, Prepaid burial account
$74,820 - $115,920 assets (see attorney)
$2,898 monthly income (25% excess goes to nh)
$ cost of health care premiums per month, including
      Long-term care policy, if any

Any assets over the stated amounts that are considered to be liquid are to be used for the institutionalized spouse (spending down). Because Roth IRA's are tax free, they are considered more favorable for liquidation by Medicaid regulations. Regular IRAs and other retirement accounts are considered available also, unless they are in pay-out status (you are receiving regular distributions.) The pay-out sum must be added to monthly income. Unfortunately, the cash value of your life insurance also counts as an asset, and they may force you to take a loan out of the policy(s) in order to meet the asset limit.

The income figure includes social security and any pensions you are getting. For the community spouse any thing over the $2,898 and the health care premiums would be multiplied by 25% and that amount would be paid to the nursing home for the institutionalized spouse's care. For the institutionalized spouse, any amount over $50 + monthly health care premiums, 100% would go to the institutionalized spouse's care unless the community spouse does not have enough income to bring him/her up to the $2,898 plus health insurance premiums.

When Jim was in assisted living, I used money from a non-IRA fund of mine to get that down to my accepted asset level for the community spouse. I also purchased an irrevocable burial fund for Jim and a revocable one for myself. Medicaid would not touch those. When Jim went to the behavioral nursing home, I liquidated some of our small IRA funds and cashed in my life insurance policies (because Jim wouldn't need them as beneficiary,) and then began withdrawing from Jim's IRAs so I would have enough money to pay for a few months out. I was working on getting all the Medicaid substantiation papers together for the 5 year look-back, and would apply for Medicaid for Jim as soon as the paperwork was complete. Just before the time of making the application to Medicaid (which in our case was the 1 year private pay), our financial advisor would put the rest of our IRAs in pay-out mode so they would not be touchable. The payments I would receive from my IRAs, however, would have to be added to my income figure. For anything over the $2,898, I would have to pay 25% to the nursing home. The payments from Jim's IRAs would automatically go to pay for his nursing home care (as well as his social security and his pension.) That is better than having the entire IRA wiped out by the nursing home costs.

As you can see, spending down to the allowable levels for Medicaid does gain the institutionalized spouse some time to private pay, and a year or two of private pay will allow you to place your loved one in the nursing home of your choice. Otherwise, you are at the mercy of the nursing home that happens to have an open Medicaid bed when your loved one needs it. It may be a good nursing home, or it may be a place that would be at the bottom of your list if you had a choice.

On the other hand, for a relatively young spouse, how can they be expected to live on the $74,820-$115,920 asset level and have it last to the end of their life? All the time spent accumulating a retirement nest egg, and it can be exhausted in the matter of a few years! Somehow it doesn't seem fair. You are robbed of a spouse, and also robbed of your security as well. It's a very stressful scenario.

I guess you could say I was lucky that Jim died with only a few months of nursing home care 'under his belt.' He died before I could apply to Medicaid for him, and before our IRAs were put into pay-out mode. He died before I had to borrow on one of Jim's life insurance policies that would help me in my retirement (I was beneficiary). And after nineteen years of the disease, it was a blessing that he did not have to spend years in a nursing home. He already had no quality of life. His nursing home stint didn't put my retirement money at great risk. Not everyone is so lucky, if you want to call it that.

Medicaid Application Checklist - Copies of the following:

Social Security Card
Birth Certificate with state seal
Marriage Certificate
Military Discharge Paper if in the military
Alien Registration
Health Insurance Card
Health Insurance Bill (proof of payment by employer & if employer
    pays)
Divorce Papers where applicable
Spouse's Death Certificate if applicable
Power of Attorney
Proof of Citizenship (Passport-expired acceptable) – in lieu of Birth
    Certificate
Proof of Residence prior to admission

Resources (provide 60 months of statements for the following - open and closed accounts, for both spouses, verify source/purpose of deposits/withdrawals greater than $500)

Bank Accounts
IRA/Annuities
Trust Funds & Agreements

Mortgage and Notes
Life Insurance (copy of policy and face values required; also
    beneficiary designation)
Stocks/Bonds (if sold, redemption paperwork) Personal
Collections
Inheritances
Real Estate
Motor Vehicles (copy of title/registration, payment book
    and contract)
Safe Deposit Box (inventory required)
Pending law suits or legal cases
Child support income
Tally of gifting amounts with cancelled checks over last 5
years
Burial Items:
Burial Space Items
Burial Trust Funds (Keep revocable until time of Medicaid
    application)
Burial Plots (Deed)

Income(Gross Monthly amt. for applicant and spouse, if applicable):

Social Security (current benefit statement)
Railroad Retirement
Union Benefits
Retirement/Pension (current statements or letter from company)
Veterans Benefits
Rental Income
Disability
Workers Compensation
Wages
Dividends
Trust Payments
Alimony
Mortgages/Note Payments
Annuity Income
Gifts
Payments from Insurance
Copies of income tax information for last five years (including tax
    returns and/or 1099's)

It can't be stressed enough how important it is to have an elder law attorney guide you through the process of understanding Medicaid eligibility. They can also provide help for Medicaid filing and the nursing home application. It is also important to have a trusted financial advisor to help you decide what should be done with your assets during this time so that you preserve as much of your wealth as possible. [During the entire time Jim was going from home to hospital to assisted living and nursing home, I was in constant contact with both my lawyer and my financial advisor so they could assist me in each step.....what move to make and what funds to withdraw money from for payment.]

The above explanations are merely a tool to help you understand the rules put forth by Medicaid and how it affects your money. They are not meant to provide legal advice. Please do not act or rely on this material without seeking your own legal counsel. The Medicaid rules change year by year and from state to state. Therefore, the advice of an attorney is crucial.

Spousal Refusal Document

A spousal refusal document is a paper in which the community spouse signs a denial of payment for the institutionalized spouse's long term care bills. It is usually signed to protect the money that the community spouse has in his/her name from being used for the spouse. If a copy of this document is filed with the Medicaid application, then if the institutionalized spouse meets the requirements for Medicaid, and forms with all necessary documents are submitted and approved, supposedly Medicaid would pay for the institutionalized spouse. This does not mean that by signing this document that the community spouse pays nothing, however. Presently these refusals can be challenged. For example, New York has a spousal support requirement. Medicaid may later send you a letter requiring you to pay the amount that they have paid for the spouse to date, as if the refusal had not been in effect. That amount, however, would likely be much less than what you would have paid outright in the beginning because Medicaid payment rates are much less than regular room rates paid by a private pay customer.

Also, sometimes the case may be deemed valid. With the escalating costs of nursing homes, one year of a nursing home fee in Rochester at the time that Jim was institutionalized was $11,500/month x 12 or $138,000 per year not including pharmacy bills. For Jim's behavioral placement, the fee was $21,500/month x 12 or $258,000 for one year. That doesn't leave much left for the community spouse, in case they need nursing home care down the line. What if the person is fairly young like Jim at 64? I am presently retired so I could be home to take care of Jim, but if they use all of Jim's money and start siphoning mine, how will I live from 64 to the age I die? I would definitely have to go back to work! And it leaves a very uncertain future for those of us who did save for our retirement but had to spend it all on our spouse's nursing home care.

I chose not to use spousal refusal even though it was signed years ago in order to obtain placement for Jim, guaranteeing 1 year of private pay. That doesn't lock me in to Jim staying there if the situation changes. All nursing homes would rather have a private pay patient than a Medicaid patient because they are reimbursed more. Eventually the promise will be going up to two years of private pay before claiming Medicaid eligibility. As the baby boomers are reaching their 70's and 80's, more people will need nursing home beds and the fewer open beds there will be, so having some leverage to place your loved one in a good facility will be paramount. So it is good to plan on using a fair chunk of money to get them in, pay the year, and then try to protect the remaining assets. The spousal refusal document creates much less 'flutter' with the institution if the dementia patient has been already living there for a number of years. At that point, they are less likely to go after the spouse for Medicaid reimbursement.

The future of spousal refusal is uncertain. There have periodically been proposals to do away with it, so make sure you are aware of the current laws in effect in your particular state and get the advice of a good Elder Law attorney!

Seeing an Elder Law attorney and a good financial advisor is money well spent, especially with a disease like Alzheimer's. There are all sorts of 'refinements' that should be made as soon after diagnosis of a debilitating disease in order to protect as much of the assets as possible. Again, this explanation of spousal refusal is not meant to provide legal advice. You should rely on your attorney and financial advisor to guide you because they know your particular situation.

24127283R00202

Made in the USA
Charleston, SC
16 November 2013